# Practice Knowledge and Expertise in the Health Professions

Edited by

**Joy Higgs** BSc, GradDipPhty, MPHE
Director, Centre for Professional Education A
The University of Sydney, New South Wales,

and

**Angie Titchen** DPhil, MSc, MCSP
Senior Research and Practice Development Fe
Honorary Research Associate, Faculty of Hea
New South Wales, Australia

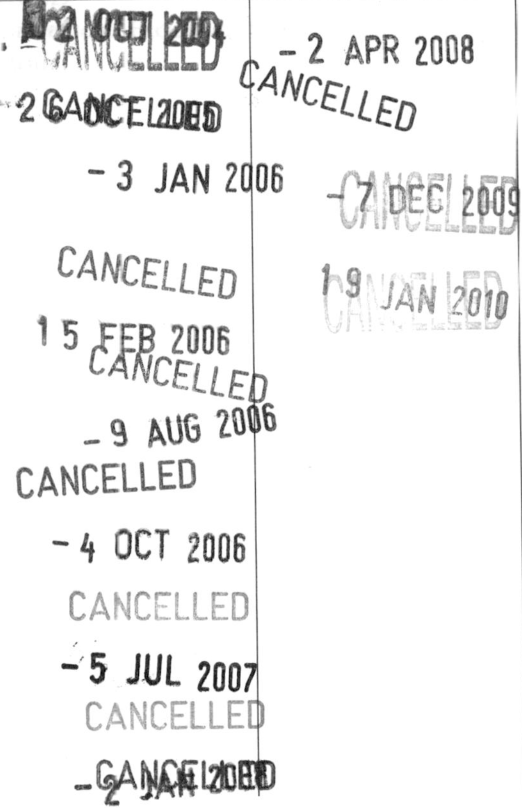


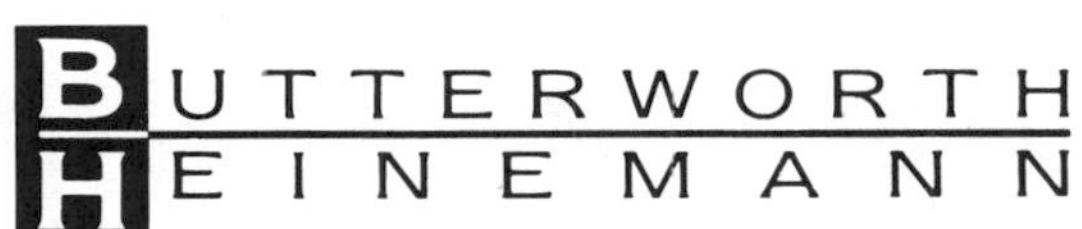

OXFORD AUCKLAND BOSTON JOHANNESBURG MELBOURNE NEW DELHI

Butterworth-Heinemann
Linacre House, Jordan Hill, Oxford OX2 8DP
225 Wildwood Avenue, Woburn, MA 01801–2041
A division of Reed Educational and Professional Publishing Ltd

A member of the Reed Elsevier plc group

First published 2001



**British Library Cataloguing in Publication Data**
A catalogue record for this book is available from the British Library

**Library of Congress Cataloguing in Publication Data**
Practice knowledge and expertise in the health professions/
edited by Joy Higgs and Angie Titchen
p.cm
Includes bibliographical references and index
ISBN 0 7506 4688 8
1. Medicine–Philosophy. 2. Medicine–Practice
3. Expertise I. Higgs, Joy II. Titchen, Angie

R723.P734 2001
610–dc21 2001018075

ISBN 0 7506 4688 8

Composition by Genesis Typesetting, Rochester, Kent
Printed and bound by MPG Books Ltd, Bodmin, Cornwall

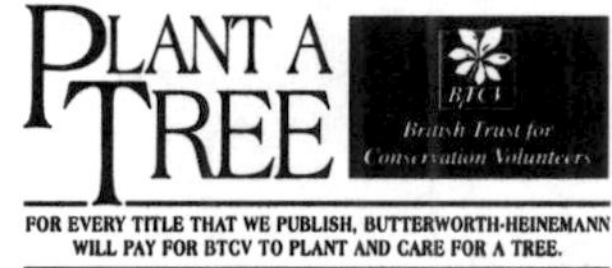

# Contents

# Contributors

**Clare Amies** BA, BSW
Western Region Health Centre Limited, Melbourne, Australia

**Lee Andresen** BSc, DipEd, PhD (*)
Consultant in Higher Education and Academic Development, Ballina, New South Wales, Australia

**Sarah Beeston** MA, FCSP, DipTP
Department of Health Sciences, Faculty of Science and Health, University of East London, London, UK

**Dawn Best** DipPhysio, MEd (*)
School of Physiotherapy, La Trobe University, Melbourne, Victoria, Australia

**Christine Bithell** MA, DipEd (*)
Head, School of Physiotherapy, Faculty of Health and Social Care Sciences, Kingston University and St George's Hospital Medical School, London, UK

**Philip Chan** MAppSc, DipOT, TDipCOT, RN
School of Occupation and Leisure Sciences, Faculty of Health Sciences, University of Sydney, Sydney, New South Wales, Australia

**Sherrill A. Conroy** N, BN, MEd (*)
Collège de la Région l'Amiante, Thetford Mines, Quebec, Canada

**Anne Cusick** BAppSc (OT), MA (Psych), MA (Interdisc Stud), PhD (*)
Faculty of Health, University of Western Sydney, Sydney, New South Wales, Australia

**Hal Davey** BA, BEd, MA (Educ)
School of Occupation and Leisure Sciences, Faculty of Health Sciences, University of Sydney, Sydney, New South Wales, Australia

**Jan Dewing** RGN, MN, BSc, DipNursEd, RNT, Dip Nurs (*)
Senior Fellow for Dementia Care, Gerontological Nursing Programme, Royal College of Nursing, Radcliffe Infirmary, Oxford, UK

**Helen Edwards** MA, PhD (*)
Centre for Higher Education Development, Monash University, Clayton, Victoria, Australia

**Steven J. Ersser** PhD, BSc (Hons), RGN, CertTHEd
Head of Nursing Development, School of Nursing & Midwifery, Faculty of Medicine, Health & Biological Sciences, University of Southampton, Southampton, UK

**Robyn Ewing** BEd (Hons), PhD
School of Social Policy and Curriculum Studies, Faculty of Education, The University of Sydney, Sydney, New South Wales, Australia

**Maureen H. Fitzgerald** RN, BIS, MA, PhD
School of Occupation and Leisure Sciences, Faculty of Health Sciences, The University of Sydney, Sydney, New South Wales, Australia

**Jane Gamble** BAppSc (OT), MHPEd
School of Occupation and Leisure Sciences, Faculty of Health Sciences, The University of Sydney, Sydney, New South Wales, Australia

**Elizabeth C. Henley** BSc, BPT, MClSc
School of Physiotherapy, Faculty of Health Sciences, The University of Sydney, Sydney, New South Wales, Australia

**Joy Higgs** BSc, GradDipPhty, MPHEd, PhD
Faculty of Health Sciences, The University of Sydney, Sydney, New South Wales, Australia

**Ian Maxwell** BA (Hons), PhD, DipArts (Dram Arts)
Department of Performance Studies, School of Society, Culture and Performance, The University of Sydney, Sydney, New South Wales, Australia

**Brendan McCormack** DPhil (Oxon), BSc (Hons) Nurs, PGCEA, RGN, RMN
Director of Nursing Research, The Royal Hospitals, Belfast, Northern Ireland

**Victoria Neville** BSc, GradDipPhty, MPHEd, MA (Interdisc Stud)
School of Behavioural and Community Health Sciences, Faculty of Health Sciences, The University of Sydney, Sydney, New South Wales, Australia

**Anne Parry** PhD, MCSP, DipTP (*)
School of Health and Social Care, Sheffield Hallam University, Sheffield, UK

**Margot Pearson** BA, MA (Hons), EdS
Director, Centre for Educational Development and Academic Methods, The Australian National University, Canberra, Australian Capital Territory, Australia

**Barbara Richardson** PhD, MSc, FCSP (*)
School of Occupational Therapy and Physiotherapy, School of Health, The University of East Anglia, Norwich, UK

**Ann Jervie Sefton** AO, MB, BS, BSc (Med), PhD, DSc
Department of Medical Education, Faculty of Medicine, The University of Sydney, Sydney, New South Wales, Australia

**Jennifer Simons** MA (USyd), MA (UNSW)
Faculty of Education, The University of Sydney, Sydney, New South Wales, Australia

**David L. Smith** BA (Hons), PhD
School of Social Policy and Curriculum Studies, Faculty of Education, The University of Sydney, Sydney, New South Wales, Australia

**Annette Street** BEd (Hons), PhD (*)
School of Nursing, Faculty of Health Sciences, La Trobe University, Bundoora, Victoria, Australia

**Angie Titchen** DPhil, MSc, MCSP (*)
Senior R&D Fellow, Royal College of Nursing Institute, Radcliffe Infirmary, Oxford, UK

**Robyn L. Twible** MA, DipOT
School of Occupation and Leisure Sciences, The University of Sydney, Sydney, New South Wales, Australia

**Richard Walker** BA, DipEd, MEd, PhD
School of Educational Psychology, Literacies and Learning, Faculty of Education, The University of Sydney, Sydney, New South Wales, Australia

**Shane Weir** BA, BSW
Narrative Solutions, Melbourne, Victoria, Australia

**Karolyn White** RN, Oper.ThMCert, BA, MA (Hons)
Department of Nursing Practice, Faculty of Nursing, The University of Sydney, Sydney, Australia

(*) Honorary Research Associate, Faculty of Health Sciences, The University of Sydney, Australia

# Foreword

I accepted the invitation to write this foreword to get an early sight of this promising book; and my patience was richly rewarded. While centrally situated in nursing, physiotherapy and occupational therapy, individual chapters range much wider to include medicine, midwifery, education and even drama. More important, however, is the cross-professional relevance and focus of the problems and issues discussed. One never feels that an author's first profession dominates their writing. Another important feature is that the majority of authors have a common second profession, that of being a teacher in a university-based professional school. Thus their daily work involves trying to bridge two very different professional cultures with a constant risk of being marginalized by both.

Most authors come from Australia or the United Kingdom, where the initial training of nearly all health professionals has moved into universities since 1950, mostly during the last 20 years. Only medicine trained all its new entrants in universities before that date. This coincided not only with a period of determined expansion in university intakes, the demise of elitism, but also with an increasing emphasis on the importance of scientific research. It is interesting to speculate whether this latter trend has peaked. We may certainly expect to find a growing tension between research as an increasingly specialized, globalized and competitive activity employing large funded groups of researchers who have almost ceased to engage in teaching, and research as a more local activity performed by university–practitioner partnerships seeking to improve local practice. In general, this book treats these different organizational approaches to research as complementary: the former may be important for the discovery of new possibilities in the scientific domain, but the latter is essential for learning to incorporate new thinking from a range of sources into the holistic care of clients.

A central assumption of this book, is that the gap between universities and health care organizations is best perceived not as a gap between theory and practice or between 'idealized' practice and 'real' practice but as a gap between two different cultures of practice. Yet both university workers and health practitioners use a similar range of practical knowledges; knowledge which is personal, tacit and multi-faceted rather than exclusively scientific. Hence the debate which this book seeks to inform is both cultural and epistemological and the mode of engagement with the reader reflects this dual concern. The epistemological debate is about the relative priority accorded to different types of knowledge. While a range of typologies are usefully explored and the diversity of perspective encouraged, some coherence is introduced by the frequent use of a tripartite typology – propositional knowledge, professional craft knowledge and personal knowledge – which reflects the authors' two professions as well as their personal life experience in non-professional contexts. There are many excellent characterizations of the nature and role of various forms of non-propositional or pre-propositional knowledge in health care settings. Given that the general ethos is that of challenging the perceived hegemony of propositional knowledge, the book could well have been subtitled 'Practice fights back'.

Several chapters discuss these issues in the particular context of moving towards more client-centred forms of professional practice. This is a key part of the argument because it provides the moral justification for the development of a broader and more integrated range of professional knowledge in both initial and continuing education. Moreover, this argument can be taken much further outside the world of the professions. Do not clients also need to develop a wider range of knowledge and a more confident, reflective use of that knowledge if they are to participate more fully in discussions of their own health needs? Cannot a similar range of knowledge types be found in other areas of human activity? Can we not argue, therefore, that a wider range of knowledge should be developed in schools and universities as part of our general, rather than vocational, education?

This line of thought leads directly to the need to reconceptualize the role of universities in our society. As I first wrote in 1985:

> The barriers to practice-centred knowledge creation and development are most likely to be overcome if higher education is prepared to extend its role from that of creator and transmitter of generalisable knowledge to that of *enhancing the knowledge creation capabilities* of individuals and professional communities. (Eraut, 1994, p.57)

*Professor Michael Eraut*
*University of Sussex*
*Institute of Education*

# Preface

Practice knowledge in the health professions is a fundamental tool of clinicians, educators and researchers. This book explores this fascinating topic through the eyes of a community of scholars from each of these three categories. It is the product of research and scholarship. The authors have utilized a range of knowledge generation and investigation strategies to explore the breadth and depth of practice knowledge. We invite readers to join this journey of exploration and contribute to the ongoing challenge of testing, extension and informed use of practice knowledge.


## Acknowledgements

We would like to thank our team of authors and peer reviewers for their scholarly, creative and critical input. Their contributions have expanded our understanding of practice knowledge.

We also wish to pay special tribute to Joan Rosenthal for her invaluable role in facilitating the process of collaboration and review of this book.

*Joy Higgs and Angie Titchen*

# Section One

## Knowledge and practice

# 1

# Professional practice and knowledge

**Joy Higgs, Angie Titchen and Victoria Neville**

***Reflections on our cover artwork***

As with all artwork the viewer cannot fully know what lies in the mind, heart and imagination of the artist. Our cover illustration was painted by a member of our community of authors, Cathy Charles. We invite you to consider four interpretations or images created by this painting. The first is a sea anemone, a living creature flourishing in the rich, warm waters of a reef; growing, changing over time, giving birth in its time to many new and varied offspring to continue the living history. The second image is a frozen kaleidoscope image, showing the momentary alignment of countless pieces of coloured glass, creating an image which can be variously meaningful to the creator and other viewers of this unique picture. The third image is a view from above, a helicopter view if you like, of a child's play-time construction of coloured rods and wheels. The shape, intricacies and purposes of this imaginary structure, labyrinth or puzzle were born of the complex imagination and aspirations of the builder. The final image focuses on the background, seeing a living, changing river carrying along a water flower released from its quiet pool to travel a journey of knowing.

In this deliberate use of a creative artwork to illustrate professional practice knowledge and in the above interpretations of the painting we are seeking to open our imaginations (as well as those of our readers) to the fascinations, intricacies, growth, complexities and limitless potentials we see in practice knowledge.

From interpretations such as those considered above, we can derive a composite picture of professional practice knowledge as:

- A living thing, a dynamic phenomenon (whether we are speaking of the practice knowledge base of an individual or the profession).
- A generative, creative, reproducing collective of past, present and future knowledge generations and variations.
- A constructed, rapidly changing nexus and entity, pausing for no more than a brief instant in its creation of multiple perspectives, deriving an endless array of ideas, images and realities from changing patterns and formed and barely formed ways of knowing, even when using the same colours – glass fragments of events and ideas.
- A mysterious dynamic construction of countless paths and possibilities, with today's marvellous creation gaining from, but not limited by, yesterday's learning.
- A result of learning, creativity, experience and personal knowing, with some known or unknown knowledges of things like gravity, survival, refraction and improvization hovering in the background.
- A river, its flow constantly changing with the topology of the landscape, sometimes rushing and rapid, sometimes falling, and sometimes resting still in a pool. The qualities of the river, its fluidity, mystery, transformative capacity and uniqueness are those of professional practice knowledge.

This book enters the discourse on practice knowledge in a turbulent and challenging time in the evolution of knowledge, society and health care. We live in a postmodern era, one that rejects grand theory and certainty, when rules and absolutes are replaced by radical relativity. We live and work in a society that is dominated by globalization and concomitant demands for high levels of demonstrable accountability, cost-efficiency and measurable quality. We live and learn in a world where knowledge is socially constructed. We practise in contexts where evidence-based practice is an expectation and fashion, often emphasizing the grounding of practice in research knowledge that provides measurable evidence for best practice. We belong to professions that have strengths and limitations in dealing with the competing demands of these three contexts (accountability, evidence-based practice and socially constructed knowledge). We are people with our own values, goals and personal frames of reference, which will continue to influence our intentions, actions and performance as professionals.

In this chapter we present five key arguments in the exploration of professional practice knowledge:

1. The divide often made between theory and practice needs to be removed to understand better the nature of practice and knowledge. Practice and knowledge in the professional context are deeply embedded in each other and operate interdependently.
2. There is a need to ground and illuminate practice in an applied understanding of practice epistemology.
3. Professional practice requires three forms of knowledge (knowledge derived from research and theory, from professional experience and from personal experience).
4. Blurring the boundaries between different knowledges and their generation is an important part of understanding the strength and scope of practice knowledge.
5. Professional expertise in the human service professions such as the health professions resides in practice wisdom and practice artistry, both of which require the integration of the three forms of knowledge.

## The theory and practice divide

A 'profession' is an occupational group that is able to claim a body of knowledge distinctive to itself, whose members are able to practise competently, autonomously and with accountability, and whose members contribute to the development of the profession's knowledge base (Higgs, 1993). In the emergence of the health occupations as professions, propositional knowledge, derived from research and scholarship, was sought to provide the foundation of the professions' knowledge base and their theory for practice, and to establish the professions' status and credibility.

Professional practice is concerned with the manner in which practitioners perform the roles and tasks of their profession in conjunction with individuals who are their clients or patients. It includes, but is not limited to, the application of theory and practice principles to real world problems. The difficulty for practitioners lies with the 'messy' nature of these problems, unlike their 'sanitized' textbook counterparts upon which much professional preparation is focused.

Schön (1987) called the field of professional practice a 'swampy' area, because many of the decisions made in managing problems are based on data that are often uncertain, ambiguous or hidden. Situations to which professionals apply their practice are often complex because they involve people. People bring to the situation their own perceptions, needs and experience. These features influence the nature of the problem. Problem clarification and management decisions, then, cannot be made without reference to the person concerned. The nature of professional practice requires health professionals to develop knowledge from their practice about the variety of contexts in which they practise.

Developments in theory may influence professionals' actions in practice. Practice experience may influence professionals' interpretation of theory and its use in practice, and also contribute to the elaboration of existing theory and the generation of new theory (Eraut, 1994; Titchen, 2000). Effective professional practice relies on both theoretical knowledge and knowledge from professional practice experience. Both are embedded in the context of professional practice, yet are interdependent. This interdependency is largely ignored in the contemporary evidence-based health care focus.

Theory for practice and the reality of practice context complexity necessitate the development of practice knowledge. Professional practice without underpinning theory is guesswork. Applying theory without considering the practice context may result in ineffective treatment and management decisions, or decisions considered irrelevant by the patient. In addition, mere application of theory may be more indicative of inexperience than expertise. Eraut (1994) and Titchen (2000) suggest that expert practitioners transform theory in a variety of ways in order to make it useful to particular patients in their particular situations. (This point is elaborated in Chapters 7 and 10.) In addition, Titchen claims that experts generate new knowledge, for instance in the form of practical principles.

The divide between theory and practice is explored further in Chapter 4.

## Practice epistemology

Epistemology is the study of knowledge and knowledge generation. It is concerned with the relationship between the knower and the known. Effective practice utilizes different forms of knowledge. Understanding professional practice requires an awareness of the ways in which knowledge informs practice and is developed from practice. There is a need, therefore, to ground and illuminate practice in an applied understanding of practice epistemology. This understanding will help expert practitioners and educators to guide less experienced and beginning practitioners in acquiring and integrating these different kinds of knowledge and pointing out their source.

In Chapter 5, Titchen and Ersser examine contemporary thinking in this area, and in Chapter 7 they develop an analytical framework to advance understanding of practice epistemology in the context of the health professions. In Chapter 6 Richardson examines the evolution of practice knowledge and the role of practice epistemology within the process of professionalization. White, in Chapter 18, explores practice epistemology in the context of ethical decision-making.

## Forms of knowledge for practice

Professional practice requires thoughtful action. Health care professionals are faced with situations in which patients require their help. Patients expect that health professionals will take some action to relieve or improve their health problems. Taking effective action, however, depends on the health professional's ability to identify and analyse the problem and its related factors. Health professionals then try to make sense of patients' problems by drawing on their knowledge. The knowledge that clinicians bring to the clinical encounter is a primary feature of the therapeutic intervention (Jensen et al., 1992). Higgs and Titchen (1995) suggest that this knowledge takes three forms:

1 propositional, theoretical or scientific knowledge – e.g. knowledge of pathology;
2 professional craft knowledge or knowing how to do something;
2 personal knowledge about oneself as a person and in relationship with others.

Each form of knowledge has a distinct nature. This is summarized here, and discussed more fully in Chapter 6. In short, propositional knowledge is formal and explicit, and is expressed in propositional statements. Relationships between concepts or cause and effect, for example, are set out. This form of knowledge is derived through research and/or scholarship. Claims about the generalizability or transferability of research knowledge to settings other than that in which the investigation was carried out are made. Scholars who develop 'armchair' theories may draw on the empirical work of others, or use other devices to make claims for generalizability or transferability.

On the other hand, professional craft knowledge and personal knowledge may be tacit and embedded either in the practice itself or in who the person is. Cervero (1992, p. 98) describes professional craft knowledge as a 'repertoire of examples, images, practical principles, scenarios or rules of thumb that have been developed through prior experience'. Professional craft knowledge comprises both general knowledge gained from health professionals' practice experience (e.g. knowledge about how a population of patients responds to disease or disability) and also specific knowledge about this particular patient, in this particular situation and context at this particular time. Professional craft knowledge can be expressed in propositional statements, but here no attempt is made to generalize beyond the individual's or a group of colleagues' own practice.

Personal knowledge is accrued from life experience; for example, knowledge about an individual's need for dignity, independence and meaning. This kind of personal knowledge might be general in nature, uniquely conceptualized from the collective knowledge held by the community and culture in which the individual has been brought up. It could also be particular in nature; for instance, knowledge about self as a person, in different roles and relationships. In its general form, it may be accrued more or less unconsciously through socialization. In its particular form, personal knowledge is perhaps acquired more consciously by reflecting upon one's knowing, being, doing and feeling in each unique situation. Chapter 11 pursues further the topic of personal knowledge.

All three forms of knowledge are important. Propositional knowledge provides the basis for analysing patients' physical and psychosocial problems. Practitioners must be able to recognize the meaning of the results of their assessments in terms of underlying pathology or illness. Knowledge errors at this stage ultimately may lead to errors in treatment management decisions that may not help, and may hinder, recovery.

Professional craft knowledge enables professionals to place the physical and psychosocial analyses within the context of particular patients' needs and to integrate different forms of data (Rew and Barrow, 1987). Such knowledge enables clinicians to determine the timing and selection of important data collection to consolidate their understanding of the particular clinical problem (Jensen et al., 1992). Indeed, research has demonstrated that it is the ability of experienced professionals to integrate propositional knowledge with professional craft knowledge that enables them to know what information is important and to distinguish and comprehend the significance of crucial cues (Larkin et al., 1980; Payton, 1985; Dreyfus and Dreyfus, 1986; Elstein et al., 1990). The integration of both forms of knowledge into 'well-developed and easily accessible schemata . . . [enables practitioners] to evaluate and treat different patients efficiently and with confidence' (Jensen et al., 1992, p. 718).

Working with people lies at the core of health professional practice. In order to make treatment more effective, health professionals must be able to communicate with patients and listen to their interpretations of their problems. In seeking to understand patients' problems, concerns and lived experiences of health and illness, health professionals must enter the life-world of their patients. Health professionals draw on their personal knowledge from their life experience to help them recognize the meaning behind patients' hopes, fears, dreams and current experience. In personal knowledge lies our recognition of individuals and of those aspects of ourselves that are common to all individuals. Carper's view is that personal knowledge 'promotes wholeness and integrity in the personal encounter, the achievement of engagement rather than detachment' (Carper, 1978, p. 20). Thus health professionals are able to tailor treatments to meet patients' specific needs. The ability to place the clinical problem within the patient's world and to design personalized care and interventions that take the patient's experience into account is recognized across the health sciences as a key element of expertise that develops from clinical practice experience (Benner, 1984; Burke and DePoy, 1991; Crepeau, 1991; Jensen et al., 1992).

The health professional's use of professional practice knowledge ensures that clinical assessment includes the whole person and that clinical management is meaningful for the patient. Clinical practice that includes propositional, practice and personal knowledge provides a sound foundation for practice, reflects the humanity and caring and ethical aspects of the health professions, ensures a holistic approach to therapeutic care, and is more likely to result in assessment and management decisions that meet the patient's needs.

## Blurring the boundaries of knowledge

The credibility of the health professions in the eyes of the public and the body politic may depend on their propositional knowledge. This form of knowledge is tested and verified in the public domain. In contrast, as already indicated, professional craft knowledge is often tacit in nature. Practitioners simply 'know' what decisions or actions to take in a particular situation but often are unable to make explicit their 'knowledge' that underpins those actions (Schön, 1983; Eraut, 1985).

When a health professional encounters a situation that 'feels' familiar, 'unconscious processes trigger expectations that structure explicit mental activity' (Boreham, 1992, p. 73). This mental activity takes the form of challenging, refining or confirming those expectations (Benner, 1984; Jarvis, 1987). An important goal for professional groups and individuals is to reflect on these mental challenges and to seek to make explicit and test the underlying knowledge which enabled the seemingly 'invisible' decision-making.

The process of acquiring the tacit or implicit knowledge of practice involves two steps, according to Jarvis (1992). The first step occurs when professionals 'forget' the original rules from propositional knowledge learned in their professional preparation education. This knowledge transforms into a type of knowledge that is internal, expressed in habit and difficult to articulate. The knowledge becomes 'embodied' in the individual practitioner (Mattingly, 1991) and embedded in professional practice that is directed towards action (Cervero, 1992).

In the second step, professionals monitor their own performance with varying levels of conscious awareness. The degree of conscious awareness, however, influences the extent of the learning (Watkins and Marsick, 1992). Professionals then adjust their understanding and practice rules/principles based on their own performance evaluation in the new context. These adjustments to their knowledge become internalized, so that professionals are often unaware that their professional craft knowledge has developed through the experience (Jarvis, 1992).

Titchen's research (Titchen, 2000) reveals more about this process of acquisition. She identified three ways in which professional craft knowledge is accrued. First, theoretical principles are used in practice, enabling the practitioner to understand them more fully. Over time, the principles become internalized, fine-tuned and elaborated as they are transformed into practical principles. Second, professional craft knowledge is gained merely by being there, immersed in the situation, encountering a puzzling or confusing situation, or feeling irritated by something, and then working things out for oneself. The third way combines the first two. A problem is encountered in the use of theoretical principles and a problem solution is generated through a process of trial and error as the 'nitty-gritty' practicalities are worked out. Learning comes about not only through close involvement of heart and head in the situation, but also through being able to stand back and reflect upon the experience.

Eraut (1994) argues that it is not possible to separate the acquisition or learning of professional craft knowledge from its creation and use. This is supported by Titchen's (2000) research. She found that professional craft knowledge can be acquired through the experiential facilitation strategy of 'critical companionship' as well as through experience. (See Chapter 10.)

Implicit knowledge, especially from incidental learning, is inherently context-bound (Berry and Deines, 1993; Johns, 1993). This is where evaluation and testing of the knowledge is essential to enable the learning to be used in future practice (Jarvis, 1987; Malkin, 1994). This testing of knowledge in a variety of contexts clarifies the situations in which particular actions are appropriate or inappropriate. Without this critical analysis there is a danger of actions becoming routine and applied in an unthinking way (Baskett et al., 1992). Actions without thoughtful consideration of the context in which they are applied are merely habits and do not demonstrate the use of professional craft knowledge.

Professional craft knowledge, then, is developed from each individual's practice experience, and is tested and modified in daily practice. Yet the knowledge of individual practitioners may also be shared with others in their profession, thus contributing to the professional craft knowledge of others. This sharing of knowledge may occur at an informal level, when practitioners talk to each other about their practice, or more formally in conference presentations or in professional journals with sections devoted to practical reports or clinical notes. The professional craft knowledge shared in this way does not become part of the individual's knowledge until it is tried and tested in the individual's own practice and becomes part of the process of adjustment of the individual's practice principles.

The nature of professional craft knowledge is inherently focused on the individual practitioner. Yet it also has the potential to contribute to the knowledge base of the profession. The initial part of this process requires research that identifies the professional craft knowledge of experienced practitioners with regard to particular problems and/or contexts. Then, when the related variables have been clarified, empirical research may test the efficacy of that knowledge more broadly across a range of practitioners and settings. Confirmation of the efficacy of this knowledge then transforms the professional craft knowledge of individuals into propositional knowledge of the profession as a whole. In this way, the knowledge developed from each practitioner's professional experience may contribute to enhancing the knowledge base of the profession. This point is elaborated more fully in Chapter 7.

Thus, while different types of knowledge may appear distinct in their characteristics, the nature of professional practice serves to blur the boundaries. Herein lies the strength of practice knowledge. Not only does professional practice comprise the three forms of knowledge, but also these knowledges can transform or inform each other. Propositional knowledge can be transformed by professional craft knowledge and professional craft knowledge has the potential to elaborate and inform propositional knowledge. Personal knowledge can also be transformed into professional craft knowledge if practitioners use themselves as a person therapeutically. This interdependency is furthered by the fine interplay between the three forms of practice knowledge.

## Professional expertise

In order to practise as health professionals we need a solid foundation of theoretical knowledge and a thorough understanding of the nature of our professional practice, understanding of the forms of knowledge that we use in our practice, and an understanding of the ways in which we develop our knowledge about our practice from our practice. The different knowledges upon which we draw in our practice constitute only one aspect of the development of professional expertise. It is the ways in which we use our knowledge and understanding that contribute to our development of expertise. We need to use our creativity, imagination and sensitivity to patients' needs in order to use our knowledge in appropriate ways. Our professional expertise resides in our practice wisdom and professional artistry (see Table 1.1).

This argument is supported by Benner et al. (1996), who recognize the place of Aristotelian practical reasoning in expert clinical judgment.

Other chapters in this book specifically address the nature of expertise (e.g. Chapters 8, 12 and 14), whilst further chapters address aspects that are relevant to the development of professional artistry and expertise: the nature of knowledge derived from practice experience (e.g. Chapters 5 and 7); the variety of ways in which practice knowledge can be understood and generated (e.g. Chapters 2, 3, 13 and 27); and strategies for enhancing individuals' practice knowledge (e.g. Chapters 10, 15–17, 19 and 20).

Implications and strategies for teaching practice knowledge are examined in Chapters 21–24. Chapters 25 and 26 explore research issues associated with directions in practice knowledge.

## Conclusion

In these opening pages, we have attempted to provide a taste of professional practice knowledge from a postmodern perspective. Our cover has suggested to us four images of professional practice knowledge: a sea anemone, a frozen kaleidoscope pattern, a child's play-time construction and a river. Ancient wisdom tells us that 'we can never step into the same river twice'; so it is

**Table 1.1 Practice wisdom and professional artistry**

**Professional artistry** is the meaningful expression of a uniquely individual view within a shared tradition (see Chapter 5, 9 and 14). It involves a blend of:

- **practitioner qualities** (e.g. connoisseurship, emotional, physical, existential and spiritual synchronicity and attunement to self, others and what is going on);
- **practice skills** (e.g. expert critical appreciation, ability to disclose or express what has been observed, perceived and done, and metacognitive skills used to balance different domains of professional craft knowledge in the unique care of each patient, and to manage the fine interplay between intuition, practical reasoning and rational reasoning and between different kinds of practice knowledge);
- **creative imagination processes** (imagining the outcomes of personalized, unique care interventions and creative strategies to achieve them).

By using cognitive, intuitive and sense modes of perception, professional artistry enables the practitioner to:

- mediate propositional, professional craft and personal knowledge in the use of applied science and technique in the messy world of practice through professional judgment;
- realize practical principles;
- use the whole self therapeutically.

These qualities, skills and processes and their blending are built up through extensive introspective and critical reflection upon, and review of, practice.

**Practice wisdom** is the possession of practice experience and knowledge together with the ability to use them critically, intuitively and practically. Practice wisdom is a component of professional artistry.

with professional practice knowledge. With each patient, situation and context, the practitioner transforms his or her knowledge to provide unique, personalized, effective care. Like the river which contributes its flow to the sea, this unique knowledge contributes eventually to the restless knowledge base of the profession. Other chapters in this book examine many different aspects of practice knowledge and will contribute to a greater understanding of professional practice.

## References


Baskett, H. K. M., Marsick, V. J. and Cervero, R. M. (1992) Putting theory to practice and practice to theory. In *Professions' Ways of Knowing: New Findings on How to Improve Professional Education* (H. K. M. Baskett and V. J. Marsick, eds), pp. 109–118. San Francisco: Jossey-Bass.

Benner, P. (1984) *From Novice to Expert: Excellence and Power in Clinical Nursing Practice*. London: Addison-Wesley.

Benner, P., Tanner, C. and Chesla, C. (1996) *Expertise in Nursing Practice: Caring, Clinical Judgement and Ethics*. New York: Springer Publishing.

Berry, D. C. and Deines, Z. (1993) *Implicit Learning*. Hove: Lawrence Erlbaum.

Boreham, N. C. (1992) Harnessing implicit knowing to improve medical practice. In *Professions' Ways of Knowing: New Findings on How to Improve Professional Education* (H. K. M. Baskett and V. J. Marsick, eds), pp. 71–78. San Francisco: Jossey-Bass.

Burke, J. P. and DePoy, E. (1991) An emerging view of mastery, excellence, and leadership in occupational therapy practice. *American Journal of Occupational Therapy*, **45**(11), 1027–1032.

Carper, B. A. (1978) Fundamental patterns of knowing. *Advances in Nursing Science*, **1**, 13–23.

Cervero, R. M. (1992) Professional practice, learning, and continuing education: An integrated perspective. *International Journal of Lifelong Education*, **10**, 91–101.

Crepeau, E. B. (1991) Achieving intersubjective understanding: Examples from an occupational therapy treatment session. *American Journal of Occupational Therapy*, **45**(11), 1016–1025.

Dreyfus, H. L. and Dreyfus, S. E. (1986) *Mind Over Machine*. New York: The Free Press.

Elstein, A. S., Shulman, L. and Sprafka, S. (1990) Medical problem-solving: A ten year retrospective. *Evaluation and the Health Professions*, **13**(1), 5–36.

Eraut, M. (1985) Knowledge creation and knowledge use in professional contexts. *Studies in Higher Education*, **10**(2), 117–133.

Eraut, M. (1994) *Developing Professional Knowledge and Competence*. London: Falmer.

Higgs, J. (1993) Physiotherapy, professionalism and self-directed learning. *Journal of Singapore Physiotherapy Association*, **14**(1), 8–11.

Higgs, J. and Titchen, A. (1995) Propositional, professional and personal knowledge in clinical reasoning. In *Clinical Reasoning in the Health Professions* (J. Higgs and M. Jones, eds), pp. 129–146. Oxford: Butterworth-Heinemann.

Jarvis, P. (1987) *Adult Learning in a Social Context*. Kent: Croom Helm.

Jarvis, P. (1992) Learning practical knowledge. In *Professions' Ways of Knowing: New Findings on How to Improve Professional Education* (H. K. M. Baskett and V. J. Marsick, eds), pp. 89–94. San Francisco: Jossey-Bass.

Jensen, G. M., Shepard, K. F., Gwyer, J. and Hack, L. M. (1992) Attribute dimensions that distinguish master and novice physical therapy clinicians in orthopedic settings. *Physical Therapy*, **72**(10), 711–722.

Johns, C. (1993) Professional supervision. *Journal of Nursing Management*, **1**, 9–18.

Larkin, J., McDermot, J., Simon, D. P. and Simon, H. (1980) Expert and novice performance in solving physics problems. *Science*, **208**, 1135–1142.

Malkin, K. F. (1994) A standard for professional development: the use of self and peer review, learning contracts and reflection in clinical practice. *Journal of Nursing Management*, **2**, 143–148.

Mattingly, C. (1991) The narrative nature of clinical reasoning. *American Journal of Occupational Therapy*, **45**(11), 998–1005.

Payton, O. D. (1985) Clinical reasoning process in physical therapy. *Physical Therapy*, **65**, 924–928.

Rew, L. and Barrow, E. (1987) Intuition: A neglected hallmark of nursing knowledge. *Advances in Nursing Science*, **10**(1), 49–62.

Schön, D. A. (1983) *The Reflective Practitioner: How Professionals Think in Action*. London: Temple Smith.

Schön, D. A. (1987) *Educating the Reflective Practitioner*. San Francisco: Jossey-Bass.

Titchen, A. (2000) *Professional Craft Knowledge in Patient-Centred Nursing and the Facilitation of its Development*. University of Oxford DPhil Thesis. Oxford: Ashdale Press. [Published version of original 1998 DPhil thesis of the same title]

Watkins, K. E. and Marsick, V. J. (1992) Towards a theory of informal and incidental learning in organisations. *International Journal of Lifelong Education*, **11**(4), 287–300.

# 2

# The knower, the knowing and the known: threads in the woven tapestry of knowledge

**Joy Higgs and Lee Andresen**

The texts that speak most directly to . . . our question, that is, in terms of life, are the texts where it is most difficult to discern the answers we need. The answers are in the stories; indeed, the answers are the stories.
(Clandinin and Connelly, 1995, p. 79)

*Imagine, if you will, a great hall in an ancient Tudor mansion. Near lofty ceilings, great coloured windows allow the traveller to look out beyond the here and now to view forever. Around each wall hang endless tapestries, a record of history and knowledge through the ages. Yet these are living tapestries, forever growing on limitless ('Tardis')*[1] *walls as new knowledge is continually added to the great history of ideas. The coloured lights streaming through rose-coloured windows pick out patterns made real through the imagination of the watchers, each person viewing the knowledge vista through the frames of their own knowing and experiences.*[2]

*One traveller, a carpet-weaver by trade, places his creation on the flagstones. The carpet grows under his busy fingers as he draws on the knowledge of the ages in the tapestry designs. His imagination is fired by the patterns of other people's knowing and by his own carpet dancing. (See Plate 1, at the front of Section 3, p.119]*

In this chapter we explore ways of knowing on several levels.[3] We model different kinds of knowledge and ways of knowing by exploring our topic through theoretical perspectives; and by illuminating and interpreting knowledge through our own and others' experience. We hope to empower our readers to take risks and be adventurous in their own projects of seeking to know.[4] This chapter is the outcome of our own adventure into exploring knowledge. We chose to work in a jazz mode of exploring the nature and nuances of knowledge, and of our own understanding of knowledge. We planned together, wrote individually and responsively, improvising, mirroring and countering each other's ideas and expressions.

As a result we created a metaphor for knowing and knowledge. It is the picture of threads of understanding being woven into tapestries and carpets to illustrate, respectively, the collective and individual bases of knowledge.[5] This imagery arose from Lee's personal journey in which he came to see the historical evolution of knowledge as resembling a never-ending tapestry coming down to us through history as an unbroken artefact, a product of centuries of human thought. It comprises not only what we know, but what we know about what we know. Professional practice knowledge is presented as a family of coloured threads being woven in new shapes, patterns and textures within and across the ancient tapestry of knowledge.

Joy uses an image with research students that 'picks up this thread'. She encourages her group to construct the theoretical framework for their research in the form of a virtual carpet. Building on the image of research as a process of seeing more clearly (since we can stand on the shoulders of the giants who have gone before), she describes the individuals' knowledge base, as the foundation for their new knowing, as a carpet woven from the tapestries of the knowledge of time, capturing and transforming their patterns and designs. The students are encouraged to view their own knowledge generation[6] as not just 'standing' on the carpet, but rather as 'dancing' on it.

This tapestry/carpet metaphor also has a time–space dimension, in the form of a continuum. This emerges from time to time via references to past and future images, and to the frame of reference historicism provides for knowledge generation and interpretation.

## Exploring knowledge concepts through the metaphor

Exploration of our metaphor allows us to identify concretely different conceptual threads in the ground of the tapestry of knowledge. The threads connect with and emerge from questions such as 'What are the different matters (the objects of knowledge) about which people believe they know something?' 'What kinds or ways of knowing are they engaged in?' 'In what manner do they appropriate and communicate their knowledge?' A comprehensive interrogation through questions of this kind would lead us to uncover virtually all of epistemology,[7] which is the study of knowledge.[8]

### What did the weaver know about his visit to work in the great hall?

*The weaver knew that he had come to weave a carpet, that the owners of the manor wanted the carpet to reflect the tapestries, and that the knowledge of the ages represented in the tapestries had been created by generations of skilled craftspeople before his visit.*

There are two ways of 'knowing that' something happened: either you are there yourself or (if you weren't) you believe reliable evidence, sometimes from witnesses who were there. 'Knowing that' commonly produces propositional **knowledge**. It can only be known 'after the event' (a posteriori) on the basis of (generally observational) **evidence** together with **induction** based upon that evidence. The weaver's knowledge of the tapestries was knowledge about things and events. It was public, collective or shared knowledge. Such knowledge is **objectively** held, available for being discovered by others. It is **communicable** and explicit knowledge and (potentially at least) practical in the sense of useful knowledge (Connelly and Clandinin, 1985; Sternberg and Caruso, 1985; Rorty, in Eisner, 1993). This knowledge contributes directly to explaining things (e.g. the history of the manor), and it is entirely particular (e.g. to the history of the family). Knowledge of the tapestries was a highly **verifiable** matter; the weaver could accept this knowledge without doubt as a form of true knowledge. If he wanted to prove the truth of this knowledge the weaver could question whether it corresponded with his other knowledge (of the manor/of the history of tapestries), whether this knowledge was justified by relevant historical events or objects and whether from his experience he felt able to commit himself to the truth of this knowledge. The things about which we believe in this propositional sense comprise a large part of the inner 'furniture of our existence'.

It would be a mistake to think that such concrete things as these are what scientific knowledge is composed of. Scientific knowledge, despite the myths that surround it, bears only an indirect and uncertain relationship to observation and evidence. It is comprised not of 'facts' (e.g. Eisner, 1993) but of highly elaborated and abstract explanatory theories, high-level propositions that form webs or networks of interconnected meanings. The philosophy of science would suggest that these theoretical edifices are neither susceptible to 'proof' (**verification**) nor even to 'disproof' (**falsification**) – at least not in any simple, direct or obvious manner. The reasons that particular theoretical **constructs** in science become and remain dominant have mostly to do with their explanatory power as sets of ideas rather than with their precise 'fit' with 'reality' (see e.g. Bruner, 1985; Phillips, 1985). There probably exists a particularly close affinity between rational science and intuitive artistry. They appear to be parallel or complementary ways by which the human imagination operates in its highest-flying and most transcendent modes.

We can at this point in the search declare with some confidence that we have now encountered most of the elementary technical terminology of epistemology (see Audi, 1995). Table 2.1 provides a list of these and other epistemological terms.

### What frame(s) of reference guided the weaver's knowing and action?

*The weaver brought to the act of weaving the carpet a variety of knowledges encapsulated in the art and craft of his occupation including educational (e.g. history, mythology), religious, personal, aesthetic (see Eisner, 1985), intuitive (see Dewey, 1960) and technical knowledge received from long tradition and training.*

The weaving task required the practitioner to take **abstract** ideas from the tapestries and make them

**Table 2.1 A list of epistemological terms, arranged in pairs**
These pairs and triads of terms as set out appear to be presented as oppositionals. However, that is not literally the case, and each pair of terms is not necessarily antonymic. We place them against one another because epistemology customarily uses them as binaries to convey either opposing, competing, contrasting or sometimes merely alternative positions about knowledge.

| | | |
|---|---|---|
| A posteriori (after the event, on evidence) | | A priori (before the event, on premises) |
| Abstract | | Concrete |
| Academic | | Everyday |
| Aesthetic | | Intellectual (Dewey, 1934, in Eisner, 1993, p. 11) |
| Belief, commitment | | Disbelief, detachment |
| Communicable (explicit) | | Tacit (implicit) |
| Congruent | | Adversative |
| Correspondence | | Non-correspondence |
| Discovered (emergent) | | Received (handed down) |
| Explain | | Understand |
| Falsified | | Non-falsified |
| Hypothetical | | Literal, actual |
| Illegitimate (unauthorized) | | Legitimate (authorized) |
| Induction | | Deduction |
| Justified | | Unjustified |
| *Knowledge THAT | Knowledge HOW | Knowledge OF |
| Narrative | | Paradigmatic (e.g. Bruner, 1985) |
| Particular (*ideographic*) | | Universal (*nomothetic*) (Eisner, 1993, p. 10) |
| Personal | | Collective (shared, social) |
| Practical (useful) | | Impractical (useless) |
| *Propositional (THAT) | Procedural (HOW) | Experiential (OF) |
| Public | | Private |
| Rational | | Intuitive (Pre-rational or non-rational) |
| Scientific | | Traditional |
| Subjective | | Objective |
| *Technical | Practical (moral) | Emancipatory |
| Things (concrete objects and events, *phenomena*) | | Truths (abstract propositions, *noumena*) |
| True (believable) | | False (non-believable) |
| Verbal (linguistic) | | Non-verbal (pre-linguistic) |
| Verifiable | | Non-verifiable |
| Holistic | | Atomistic |

* Denotes ternaries or triads, which can be thought of as forming a triangle of forces pulling in three directions rather than a simple linear pair pulling in two.

**concrete** and specific in his carpet. Religious and mythological concepts in the tapestries needed to be understood. This illustrates one of the challenges practitioners need to face in their roles. Some hypothetical claims may be difficult to verify. In some knowledge areas such as religion and mathematics, most people who believe this knowledge do so on the basis of either faith or pure reasoning (*a priori*) rather than on the basis of evidence (*a posteriori*). Often it is a deduction (something that logically follows) from other things they believe (such as the existence of God), beliefs which are handed down (they are traditional, or received) as distinct from knowledge which people discover or create for themselves (see, e.g., Huebner, 1985).

We can talk about the frameworks through which people view the generation and use of knowledge by using the concept of **paradigms**. Imagine the great hall (like a futuristic holosuite[9]) sequentially framed in different paradigmatic contexts of rules, **ontologies** (world views) and **epistemologies** (approaches to the study of knowledge).[10]

'Enlightenment thought' in the seventeenth and eighteenth centuries operated squarely within the **scientific paradigm** (as understood at the time). It was held as an article of faith that through the method underlying the Science of 'nature' (namely study involving observation, experimentation, rational induction and universalizable theory generation), humans had the power to answer all conceivable questions of existence. Scientists today, even those of the 'hardest' variety, no longer (with any unanimity) hold such dated utopian views. The enlightenment project failed, and it left a mixed legacy, part of which is our loss of the possibility of belief in progress, via Science, towards a perfect world. We must approach questions about the application of contemporary science to human problems with extreme caution because of this legacy. We witness these days a passion to apply 'scientific rationalism' to human problems (education, management, health), but this has little or nothing in common with either the values held or the methods used by scientists. It represents a prescientific value-position more correctly termed 'technical rationality' (Schön, 1983), and it makes unjustified and illegitimate usage of science's status to forward its own particular moral position in human affairs. That position is the belief that for every conceivable human problem there exists a technical-rational fix. (See, e.g., Fish and Coles, 1998.) Science, as such, supports no such premise.

But there exist research paradigms other than that of Science. Among others, the **interpretive paradigm** celebrates subjective knowing and multiple perspectives, and the **critical paradigm** seeks to empower through emancipatory knowledge (Higgs and Titchen, 1995). Whichever frame of reference the seeker for knowledge brings to the task, we can imagine a community of like-minded researchers/practitioners working together on an inquiry challenge or setting the guidelines for the individual researcher. This family and tradition of scholarship determine which hypotheses are regarded as legitimate and authorized.

Other ways of knowing, beyond research, can also be labelled paradigms. Within theology, for instance, a religious community shares collective knowledge which may be proclaimed publicly as universalizable truths.

It is characteristic of most religious or metaphysical world views that (at least in the best cases) they are **holistic**. That means that the knowledge constituting true belief is held in a web or interconnecting network in such a way that each separate item of knowledge is understood in relationship to the whole. Such fully developed interpretations of life or existence tend also to be held and sustained **dialogically** (also called **hermeneutically**[11]). Religious/metaphysical world views are, however, only one instance of hermeneutic systems, but a useful one for studying.[12]

If we turn to the **personal** knowledge of the individual, we find that it includes intuitive (Dewey, 1960), moral, aesthetic and artistic (Eisner, 1985) knowledge. Its content is not in the first instance intellectual or rational (although it can become intellectualized and rationalized after the event) (Arnheim, 1985). It could be called prerational or pre-linguistic, consisting of impressions, images, movements, shapes, smells or colours, rather than words as such. Personal knowledge can also arise from experience. Experience can bring a sense of verisimilitude or believability to ideas previously known in an abstract sense (Bruner, 1985). This process is not truth but is analogous to truth in that it provides grounds for some form of grounded commitment to the proposition. Believability is also one of the tests for good practice in narrative writing, as well as being a test for good theory in one (interpretive) paradigm of the social and human sciences. Through engagement in events the individual gains **experiential** or **phenomenological** knowing and self-knowledge. This kind of direct involvement in events (as distinct from merely hearing or reading about them) supplies a ground of knowledge categorized as **non-propositional**.

## Professional practice knowledge

This chapter asks the question 'What do we know about professional practice knowledge, and how should we respond to what we know?' What does professional practice knowledge mean to professionals working in clinical practice, in research and in education? In answering it, we continue to weave, adding threads of our own to the knowledge of the field (the tapestry) and to our own knowledge base (our carpet) as we make sense of what it means both to know something confidently and to act wisely upon that knowledge.

Patterns are recognized against a ground, becoming distinguishable only against some stable background, which has its own textures, hues and patterns because it also has been woven to create meaningful images of generations of ideas. We can approach that ground, the ancient story of knowledge, in part through the history of ideas which reveals some of the 'givens', out of, against and through which new designs daily emerge. New threads, freshly visible from today's vantage point, become traced upon the same ancient tapestry, by the deft hands of today's weavers, as they draw upon and add to the ongoing fabric of knowledge.[13]

Within the context of professional knowledge (e.g. the health sciences professions) the wall tapestries can be viewed as the broad spectrum of existing knowledge, which includes the knowledge of the field of the profession(s) in question.

Such knowledge includes the propositional knowledge and the professional craft knowledge that are together owned collectively by the profession. The weaver's carpet, by comparison, represents the knowledge base that the individual professional brings to his or her professional practice, including propositional and professional craft knowledge learned from the knowledge of the professional field and from the wider breadth of propositional knowledge across the knowledge tapestry, together with additional knowledge deriving from the individual's own research, theorizations and experience. The latter can include professional craft knowledge (gained from professional experience) and personal experiential knowledge. This experiential knowledge can take the form of procedural knowledge and highly tuned **intuitive/aesthetic** knowledge (gained and cultivated through extensive experience, plus natural grace and giftedness). As with all expert practice it probably also involves **tacit** knowledge (know-how which is revealed only in and by our actions and within events, but which we can find neither words to describe nor formulae to account for). The sometimes elusive intersection of all these knowledges may be what Donald Schön (1983) tried to capture with his term 'thinking in action', and what Connelley and Clandinin (1985) described as 'minded practice' and 'personal practical knowledge', and what Grimmett and Mackinnon (1992) called 'craft know-how'.

## Knowledge and history: another way of appreciating the ground of the tapestry

Understanding professions as human practices involves perceiving the intertwining of knowledge and history. Far from being a mere academic (in the pejorative sense of impractical, irrelevant) pursuit (see Sternberg and Caruso, 1985), history is a repository of knowledge about what it means to be human, and what humans are capable of thinking, doing and being.[14] Thus the history of each profession is an integral part of the history of human practices in general.[15] On entering a professional calling we each inherit a history and take our turn at becoming an author of its ongoing story – weavers of the tapestry.

The role of history in knowledge generation involves two key concepts. The first is the 'history of ideas' (see, e.g., Berlin, 1979), which refers to the birth, impact, decline (and re-emergence) of ideas on the human scene. The history of ideas within a field is larger than the history of any particular practice, characters or events. At its centre is the history of knowledge itself. That is, how people at different historical times (including the present) understand what it means to 'know' or to 'have knowledge' about things.

The second concept is 'historicism'. This concept refers to 'the recognition that all social and cultural phenomena are historically determined, and therefore have to be understood in terms of their own age ... each (phenomenon) has its location in space and time; such phenomena therefore cannot be subsumed under laws or generalisations that transcend the limits of their age or their society' (Stanford, 1998, p. 155).

In bringing these two concepts together we see that the evolution of professional knowledge involves both individual and collective reflection on what the profession knows and what it does, in the context of the particular times in which this evolution occurred. From today's vantage point we locate that historical professional knowledge within the wider history of ideas, and we interpret (and re-interpret) it by drawing upon a broader knowledge of society and its historical transformations.

A new way of understanding history and engaging in historical research, and historicism itself, evolved in opposition/resistance to the Enlightenment of the seventeenth and eighteenth centuries. These trends were a response to the utopian belief in the possibility of a perfectible world. That world, it was hoped, would be brought about by accumulating knowledge of timeless truths regarding everything in human affairs, using the methods of the natural sciences.

Historians and philosophers, including Vico and Herder in earlier times (Audi, 1995) and later Berlin in the twentieth century, felt obliged to counter this Enlightenment revolution in thought (Berlin, 1979, 1990; Stanford, 1998). Vico, for instance, introduced the idea that every culture was explicable only in its own terms; Herder emphasized the uniqueness of each human being which could not be brought under general principles; and Berlin attacked the 'monism' of science and rationalism with the contrary notion of 'pluralism', the possibility of more than one true answer to any genuine question (Berlin, 1990).

'Much of our knowledge and understanding is relative to where we happen to be living in history' (Stanford, 1998, p. 159). Stanford interprets historicism in a way that distances it from naive relativism (i.e. the view that there are no 'truths' and that everything is relative to the observer, the writer or the speaker). He adopts the stance of partial or epistemological relativism rather than full or metaphysical relativism. The latter 'denies that there is a reality independent of our understanding or interpretation' (Stanford, 1998, p.160). He concludes that historicism requires a position between the extremes of full relativism and the Enlightenment's ideal of applying science to all possible human affairs.

Giambattisto Vico of Bologna (1668–1744), an Italian lawyer who taught at the University of Bologna, argued that a true understanding of any knowledge is historical, and that 'every society in all its aspects is characterised by its own particular pattern or style; and each successive stage of a society grows from its predecessors by human effort not natural causation. This involves both the concept of a culture and that of historical change' (Stanford, 1998, p.156). Vico warned of the risks inherent in new directions the world was wanting to take. Though this notion was taken up by a few others at the time, it was not until the twentieth century, largely through Isaiah Berlin's work (e.g. Berlin, 1979, 1990), that it re-emerged as an idea to be reckoned with for many reasons, one of which is that the notion of pluralism (many correct answers to one question) depends largely upon it; this idea will be returned to later in our discussion. We need to understand and generate knowledge today within the context of the past history of knowledge evolution in our profession.

## Professional practice in the tapestry: new figures or old?

We might now ask whether, and in what way, professional practice knowledge creates fresh designs or new figures on the ancient ground of the history of knowledge and human ideas. Are its figures unique, novel, self-standing, or are they composed of threads, lines and patterns that can be traced back to other forms of knowledge?

Our answer was anticipated in Chapter 1, where it was claimed that professional practice is built up from various forms of knowledge. Figure 2.1 is based on Vico's categorization of knowledge.

His view was based primarily on the distinction between those things which 'Man' has created or is responsible for (which humans are capable of understanding fully) and those matters which 'Man' did not create (particularly the world, which natural science studies) and which humans are never capable of fully understanding. Science, being uncertain and imperfect knowledge, is represented by the circle to the left; other

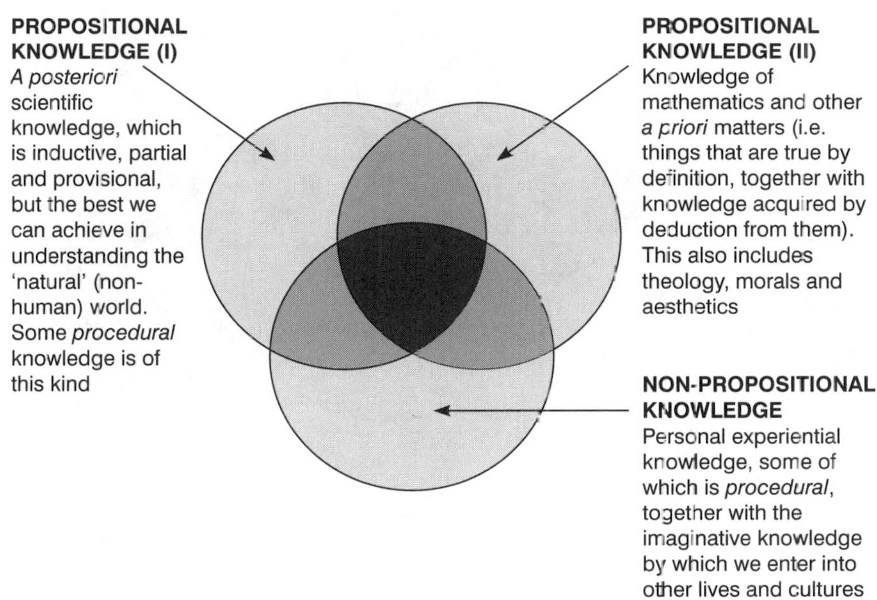


**Figure 2.1** Overlapping knowledge types (after Vico)

more certain, reliable, trustworthy forms (including mathematics) are encompassed in the circle to the right. All this knowledge (in the two upper circles) is propositional in nature.

Berlin (1979) argues that inherent in Vico's historical theories is an additional, third category, which he calls **personal experiential knowledge**. Inherently fragile and in need of verification from other knowledges, this is nevertheless the knowledge that alone enables us to imaginatively understand history, other lives and other cultures. It is represented by the lower circle, and is **non-propositional (phenomenological**). From a Vician perspective, the professional practice knowledge of any particular professional community could be interpreted as involving elements of all three knowledge categories. Similarly, individuals can draw on knowledge they possess (or can acquire or generate) from each category. In any specific situation (e.g. the management of an actual clinical problem) we can imagine the interaction or overlap between the three knowledge circles as providing the knowledge available to or used by the individual. Of course, the particular knowledge available to be used in different places, situations and times is always a variable subset of the three categories. It changes continually over time as the knowledge of the individual, profession and broader history of ideas develops.

Higgs and Titchen (1995) use a related approach to make the overall configuration more precisely applicable to professional knowledge contexts (see Fig. 2.2).

They employ a composite set of propositional knowledges (the upper circle), and two forms of non-propositional knowledge, namely professional craft knowledge (arising from professional experience) and personal knowledge (arising from personal experience) (i.e. the lower circles). In this manner, they emphasize how practitioners derive non-propositional knowledge from both personal life experience and work experience, and how they draw on both (as well as on propositional knowledge) in their professional work. (Again this is represented by a variable intersection/knowledge selection.)

It is an important terminological point that Berlin's 'personal knowledge' refers only to experiential knowledge possessed by the individual, while in the Higgs and Titchen model that same concept comprises both personal knowledge

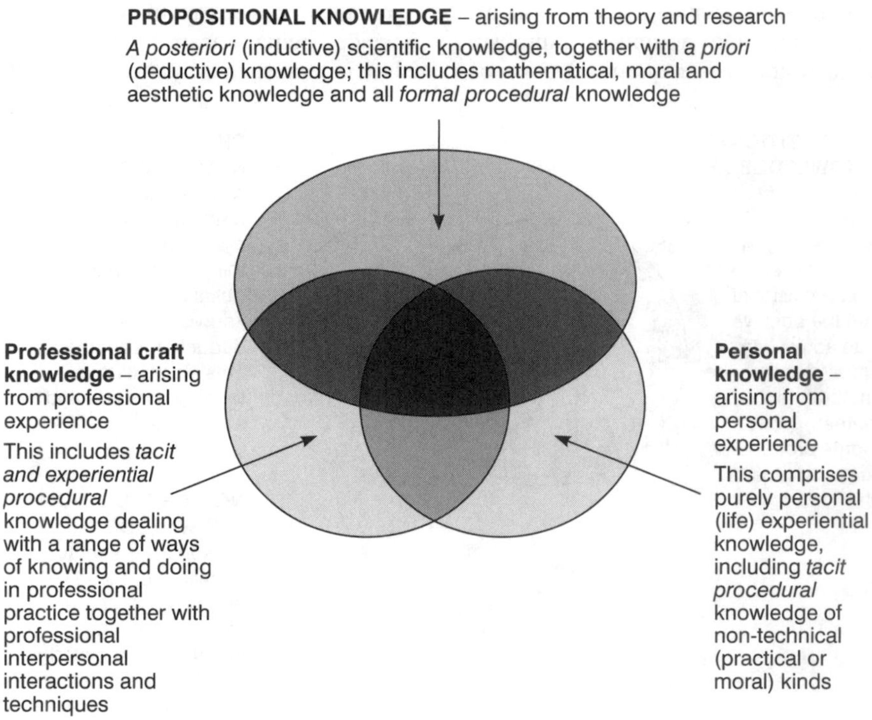

**Figure 2.2** Overlapping knowledge types (after Higgs and Titchen, 1995)

(from life experience) and professional craft knowledge (from work/professional experience).

Whichever model we use to understand knowledge, we commonly see a dynamic relationship between the various knowledges, each one informing the others and being informed by them. In professional practice, whether this occurs in (clinical) practice, research or educational contexts, professionals draw on all their knowledge reserves to inform, guide, direct and (at the end of the day) to justify their practice.

## Knowledge and believability: the 'truth' of the threads and patterns

We must now consider questions concerning verification, falsification and validation, and this is no straightforward matter. Barnett (1990, p. 41) argues that the search for an agreed set of criteria 'which absolutely separate legitimate from non-legitimate knowledge is bound to failure'. However, he contends that it is possible to deal credibly with knowledge and knowledge claims, using a flexible framework comprising the four key elements that are common to all knowledge-oriented activities, i.e. the development of the mind, social interaction, personal commitment, and value implications of knowledge.

In Vico's knowledge framework, a priori or deductive knowledge is held to be true/verified by virtue of its definition or because it follows by logical deductions from some original definition or premise. And, of course, we have to assume that the place where we started represents 'truth' because everything else derives from it.

In contrast, questions of credibility in scientific knowledge have to be answered in a quite different manner. Although the subject of ongoing debate and disputation, the three most widely used tests[16] are:

1 **justification** How soundly is the claimant able to justify what they say they believe? What evidence, for example, can be produced? Can it be demonstrated to be not simply the product of guessing or dreaming?
2 **truth** How well does it correspond with what is independently believed from other sources of perception, awareness and proof? How well does it cohere or stand together as a whole argument or proposition? How well does it serve as a means to other knowledge? How useful is it?
3 **belief** (believability) How convincingly does this knowledge provide a basis for firm conviction and commitment on the part of those who accept it?

When we look at experiential knowledge the question of credibility is even more problematic. However, at the very least, this knowledge would need to both (i) make sense in its own right, and (ii) be compatible or consistent with other knowledge which can be or has been justified. This does not rule out the possibility, however, that experience can present challenges to pre-existent knowledge; hence we must not be over-dogmatic about things in this under-theorized domain.

It is nonetheless important to find ways of testing whatever experiential knowledge (especially professional craft knowledge) comes to be used in professional practice. Every professional has a duty of care to provide quality professional services to clients. Recently this professional responsibility has gained added layers of accountability (often economic) under the banner of evidence-based practice. Ways of testing the credibility of professional craft knowledge (i.e. of converting knowledge claims to knowledge) include systematic observation of, and reflection on, the effectiveness of clinical reasoning and clinical interventions, and presentation of practice knowledge for critical peer appraisal. Further professional craft knowledge can be subjected to theorization and research (within a range of research paradigms, including empirico-analytical, interpretive and critical paradigms) in search of propositional knowledge derivatives.

Perhaps the best-known and most widely used stance towards testing knowledge arising from lived experiences is found in hermeneutics, the science of interpretation (van Manen, 1977, 1990; Audi, 1995). In the approach known as the 'hermeneutic circle', each knowledge claim is tested in relation to connected claims on either side of it (fore and aft), i.e. by asking where the interpretation comes from and where it leads to. At the same time all interpretations are tested against the whole, in the context of the totality or Gestalt of beliefs, which is that web or interconnected network of everything the person holds to be true or correct within that field of experience.

Historical truth is related to this, though of course it builds upon its indispensable scientific ('factual') base (who did what, when, and where, and what happened then). But in interpretive historical work (why did they do it? why did it happen that way?), we incline to believe something because we can imagine it happening. We believe it because it makes experiential sense that such a thing could have been what motivated people in other ages to act as they did. Vico argued that all worthwhile historical knowledge is based on our ability to use 'historical imagination', which itself depends entirely upon the experiential knowledge about life, people and the world that we have accumulated through having been thoughtfully alive.

We see now the importance of the principle of historicism. It requires any profession's knowledge evolution to be interpreted within the context(s) of its time. From Vico's idea of historical knowledge being the result of a process of imaginative interpretation, we can go on to view the evolution of a profession's knowledge base as involving the need to interpret and derive meaning from history to apply to problems and tasks in the present.

## Multiple threads and figures, equal in beauty, strength and value

*Imagine a long-ago scene, the arrival in the great hall of visiting craftspeople to appraise the value of the tapestries and the carpet for the lord of the manor. Imagine too a modern-day valuer assessing the quality of these works. Each would see, through different eyes with different understandings and techniques, the same whole but many and varied threads, modes of weaving, patterns and beauties.*

So too, each appraiser and generator of knowledge weaves his or her own carpets – their unique knowledge bases. So also they each contribute to the greater, evolving tapestry of knowledge, seeing different paths and products of knowing and weaving this knowledge within different frames of reference (see also Eisner, 1993). From a research perspective we could compare the notion of paradigms (representing ways of knowing and crafting knowledge) to the schools and traditions in ancient guilds, which in the same ways served to guide the weavers' hands, intentions and designs. Table 2.2 summarizes the frameworks for knowledge generation, illumination and critique which different paradigms[17] can provide.

From the perspective of experiential learning, Kolb (1984) identified four widely known 'experiential learning strategies' (abstract conceptualization, reflective observation, concrete experience and active experimentation). In one sense these processes can be seen as though in opposition, i.e. strategies we must choose between. But Kolb also saw these processes as contributing as equal partners to one rich learning outcome. (See Fig. 2.3.)

Humans, he said, will progressively and gradually seek to integrate – or in Rawls' (1972) terms, equilibrate[18] – the separate competing strategies into one harmonious outcome. The harmonious outcome achieved by each individual is something that is constantly developing as he/she matures as a learner. At any particular time it is something uniquely different from that of any other person.

**Table 2.2 A framework for research implementation and reporting – dimensions (based on Higgs, 1998)**

| *Research paradigm* | *Research goals* | *Research approach(es)* | *Quality control/review* |
|---|---|---|---|
| Empirico-analytical paradigm | To measure, test hypotheses, discover, predict, explain, control, generalize, identify cause-effect relationships | Experimental method (the scientific method) | Objectivity, validity, reliability |
| Interpretive paradigm | To understand, interpret, seek meaning, describe, illuminate, theorize | Hermeneutics, phenomenology, narrative inquiry, naturalistic inquiry | Trustworthiness, authenticity, credibility, congruence, ethicality |
| Critical paradigm | To improve, empower, change reality or circumstances | Action research/collaborative research, collaborative and planned action to achieve agreed goals, praxis: acting on existing conditions to change them | Trustworthiness, authenticity, credibility, congruence, whether the change action/strategy is deemed to be successful by the actors, whether or not it leads to an improvement in the situation<br>Existing knowledge is refined or elaborated |

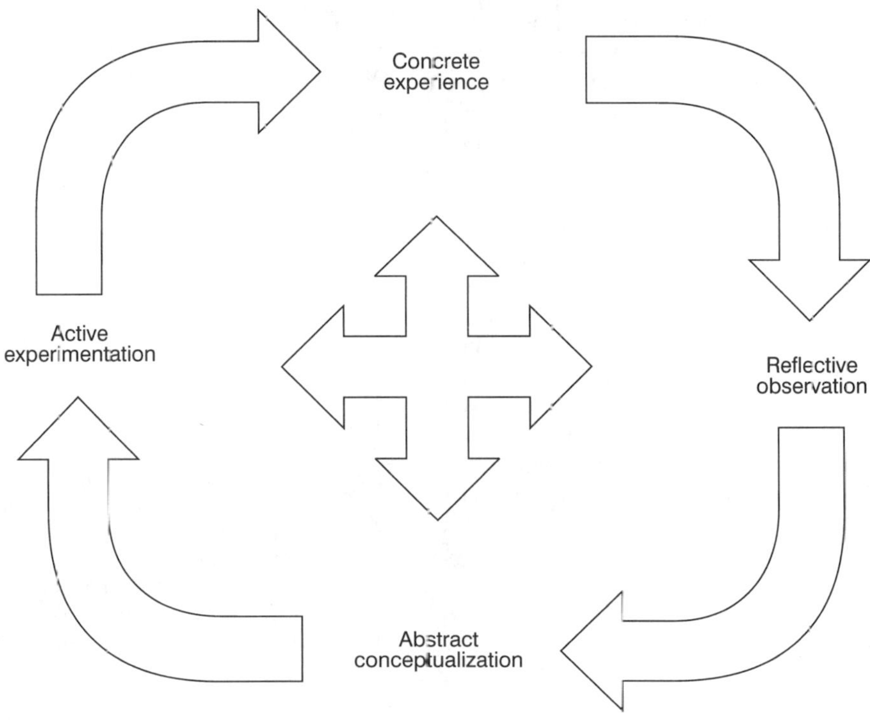


**Figure 2.3** Experimental learning cycle (after Kolb, 1984)

We present knowledge and knowing as the weaving of many threads and figures that are all equal in beauty, strength and value. Each school of practitioners, indeed each practitioner, offers a unique and valuable contribution. Professional practice knowledge (both of the individual and the professional group) needs to draw upon and be enriched by the integration of all these ways of knowing and knowledge outcomes. Professional knowledge needs to draw on the scientific/technical (evidential), the aesthetic, moral and theoretical (intuitive and definitional) and the experiential (phenomenological) realms (see, e.g., van Manen, 1977). All of these together provide the richest possible foundation for quality professional practice. This is in contradistinction to a hard-line bureaucratic view that often masquerades[19] as quality evidence-based practice, but which (unlike our view) focuses exclusively on scientific evidence and demands predictability, uniformity, measurability and cost-efficiency in circumstances which are uncertain, unequal, unpredictable and humanly variable.

In contrast, we espouse a model that supports the blending and valuing of different ways of knowing. This is not to say that all knowledges and approaches to knowledge generation are equal or equally appropriate in all situations. It is not a matter of mere personal preference, as is implied by the doctrine of relativism (i.e. what is true is always relative to the person who thinks it). Rather, we endorse the principle of pluralism, which states that to any significant question there will commonly be more than one correct answer. Pluralism implies that there is likely to be more than one way of being an expert practitioner, and that those several (perhaps many) ways may even be radically different.

The goal for each knower is to make informed and credible choices of strategies for knowing and crafting knowledge. Table 2.2, for instance, provides guidelines for choosing and evaluating different research approaches and products. So too, we need to avoid inferior and unacceptable practices. Pluralism is not the abdication of values. To be a pluralist one is never required to abandon one's capacity for discriminating between clinical/professional actions which are credible or defensible and those which are neither. Without ever abandoning standards, pluralism demands that we embrace a richer view of the world of knowledge than a narrowly conceived evidence-based practice stance would admit.

At any stage, we may aim for a harmonious action outcome in professional practice by relying on our capacity to hear each form of knowledge speak to or dance with the other(s). We look for designs forming in our tapestry as the differently coloured threads weave together. The outcome will not necessarily be predictable or uniform across practitioners. It will be influenced by our stage of development (in terms of knowledge, personal values, reasoning abilities). It will always result in our unique choice and implementation of a chosen, credible, situationally defensible course of action for us, at that time, in that place. Truth may in fact be many things, but those who commit themselves to act upon the full diverse repertoire of the best they know are more likely to be internally coherent, integrated, and undivided, as well as being expert at their jobs.

## Conclusion

Visitors to the great hall see the breadth of knowledge encompassing the history of ideas, and within this, they see practice knowledge, its images, versatility, practicalities, wisdom and beauty. They see the products of the applied skill and imagination of many individuals and groups; a timeless tapestry. And, before they quit the hall, they too leave their mark on the knowledges of time – the carpet of their own weaving.

## Notes

1 Dr Who's TARDIS (Time And Relative Dimension in Space) time machine.
2 See a parallel to this in van Manen (1977, pp. 216–218).
3 See related discussion in van Manen (1977, pp. 215–216).
4 This discussion picks up the following notion: 'Every mode of knowing is participation in the continual creation of the universe – of one's self, of others, of the dwelling places of the world. It is co-creation' (Huebner, 1985, p. 172).
5 In producing this metaphor we recognized the wealth of understanding that can come from the creative arts. As Eisner (1993, p. 7) contends, 'the images created by literature, poetry, the visual arts, dance, and music give us insights that inform us in the special ways that only artistically rendered forms make possible'.
6 See also the notion of education as cultivation, awakening and transformation, in Clandinin and Connelly (1995, p. 82).
7 See also 'Area of Experience: The Knowing Process; Field of Philosophy: Epistemology or Methodology' (Reimer and Wright, 1992, p. xi).
8 Referring to 'Out of experience, concepts (being) . . . formed . . . imaginative distillations of the essential features of the experienced world' (Eisner, 1993, p. 7).
9 A room in which holographic projections can be created and interacted with, to create new experiences.
10 Connelly and Clandinin (1985, p. 180), for instance, argue that 'it is good pedagogical theory to cast teaching and learning acts in the context of alternative epistemologies'.
11 That is, seeking to interpret or find meaning.
12 Hermeneutics is the 'science of interpretation'; hermeneutic thought is significant within social-science and human studies and is at the heart of the interpretive paradigm.
13 A more celebrated but analogous idea, that of knowledge as an ongoing conversation through the ages, was published by philosopher Michael Oakeshot (1962, pp. 197–247) and has been influential in providing the metaphor for many subsequent work in epistemology and education. Chapter 1 also suggests the metaphor of the individual's evolving knowledge as a river, flowing into the sea of our collective knowledges.
14 For example, Eisner (1993, p. 5) argues 'What we think about matters. What we try to do with what we think about matters . . . Education itself is a mind-making process'.
15 'The function of memory is to place us under the influence of the past' (Wollheim, 1979, p. 218).
16 Derived from the entry under 'truth' in Audi's (1995) *Dictionary of Philosophy*, pp. 812–813.
17 These we regard as not discrete or opposing but complementary and potentially overlapping.
18 The principle of dynamic equilibration proposes that, whenever we perceive two or more competing routes or pathways to truth, we consider them as equals.
19 We say 'masquerading', because key enlightened leaders of the evidence-based practice movement expect quality practice to utilize a range of evidence, including the experiential knowledge of patients and clinicians.

## References

Arnheim, R. (1985) The double-edged mind: intuition and the intellect. In *Learning and Teaching the Ways of Knowing. Eighty-fourth Yearbook of the National Society for the Study of Education*, Part II (E. W. Eisner, ed.), pp. 77–96. Chicago: NSSE.

Audi, R. (1995) *The Cambridge Dictionary of Philosophy*. Cambridge: Cambridge University Press.

Barnett, R. (1990) *The Idea of Higher Education*. Buckingham: The Society for Research into Higher Education and Open University Press.

Berlin, I. (ed. H. Hardy) (1979) *Against the Current: Essays in the History of Ideas*. London: The Hogarth Press.

Berlin, I. (1990) *The Crooked Timber of Humanity*. Princeton, NJ: Princeton University Press.

Bruner, J. (1985) Narrative and paradigmatic modes of thought. In *Learning and Teaching the Ways of Knowing. Eighty-fourth Yearbook of the National Society for the Study of Education*, Part II (E. W. Eisner, ed.), pp. 97–115. Chicago: NSSE.

Clandinin, D. J. and Connelly, F. M. (1995) Narrative and education. *Teachers and Teaching: Theory and Practice*, **1**(1), 73–85.

Connelly, F. M. and Clandinin, D. J. (1985) Personal practical knowledge and the modes of knowing: Relevance for teaching and learning. In *Learning and Teaching the Ways of Knowing. Eighty-fourth Yearbook of the National Society for the Study of Education*, Part II (E. W. Eisner, ed.), pp. 174–198. Chicago: NSSE.

Dewey, J. (1960) Qualitative thought. In *On Experience, Nature and Freedom: Representative Selections* (R. J. Bernstein, ed.), pp. 176–198. Indianapolis and New York: Bobbs-Merrill.

Eisner, E. W. (1985) Aesthetic modes of knowing. In *Learning and Teaching the Ways of Knowing. Eighty-fourth Yearbook of the National Society for the Study of Education*, Part II (E. W. Eisner, ed.), pp. 23–36. Chicago: NSSE.

Eisner, E. W. (1993) Forms of understanding and the future of educational research. *Educational Researcher*, **22**(7), 5–11.

Fish, D. and Coles, C. (1998) *Developing Professional Judgement in Health Care: Learning Through the Critical Appreciation of Practice*. Oxford: Butterworth-Heinemann.

Grimmett, P. P. and Mackinnon, A. M. (1992) Craft knowledge and the education of teachers. *Review of Research in Education*, **18**, 385–456.

Higgs, J. (1998) Structuring qualitative research theses. In *Writing Qualitative Research* (J. Higgs, ed.), pp. 137–150. Sydney: Hampden Press.

Higgs, J. and Titchen, A. (1995) Propositional, professional and personal knowledge in clinical reasoning. In *Clinical Reasoning in the Health Professions* (J. Higgs and M. Jones, eds), pp. 129–146. Oxford: Butterworth-Heinemann.

Huebner, D. E. (1985) Spirituality and knowing. In *Learning and Teaching the Ways of Knowing. Eighty-fourth Yearbook of the National Society for the Study of Education*, Part II (E. W. Eisner, ed.), pp. 159–173. Chicago: NSSE.

Kolb, D. A. (1984) *Experiential Learning: Experience as the Source of Learning and Development*. New Jersey: Prentice Hall.

Oakeshot, M. (1962), *Rationalism in Politics and Other Essays*. London: Methuen.

Phillips, D. C. (1985) On what scientists know, and how they know it. In *Learning and Teaching the Ways of Knowing. Eighty-fourth Yearbook of the National Society for the Study of Education*, Part II (E. W. Eisner, ed.), pp. 37–59. Chicago: NSSE.

Rawls, J. (1972) *A Theory of Justice*. Cambridge, MA: The Belknap Press of Harvard University Press.

Reimer, B. and Wright, J. E. (1992) *On the Nature of Musical Experience*. Niwot, CO: University Press of Colorado.

Schön, D. A. (1983) *The Reflective Practitioner: How Professionals Think in Action*. New York: Basic Books.

Stanford, M. (1998) *An Introduction to the Philosophy of History*. Oxford: Blackwell.

Sternberg, R. J. and Caruso, D. R. (1985) Practical modes of knowing. In *Learning and Teaching the Ways of Knowing. Eighty-fourth Yearbook of the National Society for the Study of Education*, Part II (E. W. Eisner, ed.), pp. 133–158. Chicago: NSSE.

van Manen, M. (1977) Linking ways of knowing with ways of being practical. *Curriculum Inquiry*, **6**(3), 205–228.

van Manen, M. (1990) *Researching Lived Experience: Human Science for an Action Sensitive Pedagogy*. London, ON: State University of New York Press & University of Western Ontario.

Wollheim, R. (1979) Memory, experiential memory, and personal identity. In *Perception and Identity* (G. F. Macdonald, ed.), pp.186–276. Ithaca, NY: Cornell University Press.

# 3

# Social and cultural perspectives on professional knowledge and expertise

**Richard Walker**

## Professional knowledge and sociocultural practices

Although professional knowledge may be developed in many ways, as we have seen in this book so far, considerable experience in the practice of the profession (Benner, 1984; Benner et al., 1996) is generally considered essential. Until recently, theories of learning and the development of expertise have given little attention to the place of practice in learning and have therefore been limited in what they can offer the professional or the professional educator by way of understanding the nature and development of professional expertise. Social views of learning, and particularly the sociocultural theory of participation in cultural practices and activities, however, have much to offer those wishing to develop such an understanding. After outlining previous approaches to learning and the development of expertise, this chapter briefly introduces the social explanation of learning and expertise, with special emphasis on the sociocultural practice approach. The chapter concludes by considering some implications of this approach for an understanding of professional knowledge and expertise.

## Learning and the development of expertise

The relationship between theories of expertise and professional practice is complex and involves an intertwining of the two (Benner, 1984; Benner et al., 1996). As the purpose of this chapter is to provide an understanding of theories of learning and expertise and to indicate their relevance for professional education in the health professions, no attempt will be made to consider ways in which professional practice has impacted upon theories of learning and expertise.

Theories of learning and expertise have undergone great change over the last 40 years (Derry, 1992; Mayer, 1992) and are currently in a state of flux, change and contestation. Forty years ago, learning and expertise were explained by the principles of association as advocated by behaviourist psychologists; these principles were considered adequate to explain the learning of human beings as well as other living organisms. These mechanisms of association, explained through theories of conditioning or reinforcement, indicated that learning was under the control of environmental cues and stimuli, and was essentially a passive process. The onset of the cognitive revolution in the 1950s saw a move away from learning viewed as behavioural change to a conception of learning as knowledge acquisition. Learning was now conceived as an information-processing endeavour in which the active learner selected, processed and integrated knowledge acquired from the environment. An extensive literature emanating from this information-processing psychology perspective has examined expertise (Chi et al., 1988; Ericsson and Smith, 1991) in knowledge domains as diverse as medical diagnosis, radiology, engineering, teaching, waitressing and taxi driving. This literature reveals that experts, as a consequence of their considerable experience in a knowledge domain and their strong intention to achieve mastery in the domain, have acquired extensive declarative and procedural knowledge, are capable of self-regulated practice in the domain, and have automatized many of the skills required for successful practice in that knowledge domain. More recently, Alexander (1997) has proposed a model of domain learning which explains the development of expertise through the interplay of various cognitive and motivational psychological constructs.

In the last decade, the constructivist approach to learning, while maintaining the view of learning as an active process, asserts that knowledge is not acquired from the external environment but is constructed from within, as the individual interacts with the external world (Hendry, 1996). Although this more recent learning approach has important implications for pedagogy in professional education, it is broadly compatible with findings of research into expertise derived from information-processing psychology.

These approaches to learning and expertise are typical of traditional psychological conceptions of learning, in that learning is viewed as an individual enterprise and one in which, from the perspectives of both information-processing and constructivist theories, knowledge accumulates or is constructed in the mind of the individual learner. This view, which at best allows a limited role to social and cultural factors in learning and development, has been critiqued by socially oriented theorists of learning (Wertsch, 1985, 1991; Lave, 1988; Rogoff, 1990; Lave and Wenger, 1991; Cole, 1996), resulting in considerable recent theoretical debate (e.g. Anderson et al., 1996; Greeno, 1997; Cobb and Bowers, 1999). Two important issues in this debate have been the nature and existence of symbolic representations of knowledge (Suchman, 1993; Vera and Simon, 1993) and the question of whether knowledge is located in individual minds or distributed across cultural practices and resources (Cobb, 1994). Although they take different positions on these issues, socially oriented theorists are united in claiming that learning is fundamentally a social rather than an individual phenomenon; they argue that all learning must be seen as specific to particular cultural, social and historical contexts.

Socially oriented theories of learning and expertise have their origins in the work of the Russian psychologist Lev Vygotsky, whose work was written in the 25-year period after the Russian Revolution and has been translated and interpreted in the West since the 1960s (O'Connor, 1998). Vygotsky's writing emphasized the role of cultural and social factors in learning. It has given rise to many theoretical variants which share common assumptions concerning the nature of learning and the development of expertise. These differing theoretical approaches have produced a diverse set of terminological labels; socially oriented theories of learning have been labelled as 'social constructivist', 'sociocultural', 'cultural-historical' and 'socio-cultural-historical'. The two emerging subdisciplines of cultural psychology and discursive or narrative psychology also owe much in their theoretical conceptualizations to Vygotsky's writing.

Vygotskian theories (Wertsch, 1985; Palincsar, 1998; O'Connor, 1998) state that individual thought and expertise has its origins in the collective life of the culture and social world of the individual. Vygotsky asserted that knowledge and the higher mental processes (e.g. memory, attention, problem-solving and reasoning) are initially interpsychological and become intrapsychological through collaborative and cooperative activity. That is, knowledge and the higher mental processes are considered to be initially external to the individual, but to be subsequently internalized or appropriated by the individual through processes of social interaction. This process of internalization was not considered by Vygotsky to involve the transmission of knowledge; rather it was seen as a constructive and transformative process. Vygotskian theories, therefore, share with constructivist theories the assumption that learning involves the active construction of knowledge.

According to Vygotskian theories, the internalization of knowledge and higher mental processes is aided by the cultural tools and artefacts of a society, culture or community (Wertsch, 1985; O'Connor, 1998). Such tools and artefacts, which include the language of the society, as well as other psychological and technical tools, are considered to play a mediating role in the development of thought. Language is accorded a central role in the internalization of knowledge in these theoretical approaches, as it is considered by Vygotsky to be the primary mediator of thought. The internalization of knowledge is also assisted by the creation of learning contexts, which Vygotsky called **zones of proximal development**, in which the learner's developing understandings are scaffolded or supported by more able learners or by cultural tools. More able learners may be parents, teachers, mentors, professional colleagues, peers or any of the vast range of more competent others that the individual encounters. Cultural tools, which may range in importance and scope from the new electronic technologies, books and professional journals to coloured stick-it notes, also scaffold learning and are important aids to the development of thought.

Vygotsky argued that language is internalized through the creation of zones of proximal development (Wertsch, 1985) and, once internalized, provides the basic tool of human thought, as well as the basis of the human capacity for self-regulation and self-control. From this perspective, thinking is essentially the process of engagement in an internal conversation or dialogue with oneself; this capacity to talk to oneself also allows people to regulate and control their own behaviour. Vygotskian theory therefore explains the development of metacognitive skills, which include self-regulation and self-reflection, through this process of internalization. Metacognitive processes are central to effective learning and expert performance, as they provide individuals with the capacity to reflect upon and make judgments concerning their learning, performance and behaviour.

The development of expertise is explained in Vygotskian theory (Tharp and Gallimore, 1988) through reference to the notion of the zone of proximal development and the processes of internalization or appropriation. Tharp and Gallimore (1988) have developed a model of expertise centred on the zone of proximal development, which is considered relevant to the development of expertise across the life span. This model suggests that the creation of a zone of proximal development occurs when two or more individuals enter a state of intersubjectivity and begin to negotiate the demands of a task or activity. The more capable of the individuals provides cognitive scaffolding and structuring which allows the less able individual successfully to perform aspects of the task. As the less able individual becomes more competent at the task or activity, they become more able to regulate and control their own learning; thus the individual moves from a phase of assisted or guided regulation to a phase of self-regulation and self-direction of learning. In the professional education context, zones of proximal development may be created in the many situations, such as clinical supervision, where experts work closely with students or less experienced colleagues.

## Communities of practice, learning and expertise

Of all the social approaches to learning, the sociocultural practice approach offers the most exciting and contemporary perspective on the development of professional expertise. Socioculturalist theorists (Lave, 1988, 1991; Rogoff, 1990, 1998; Lave and Wenger, 1991) explain learning and the development of expertise in terms of an individual's enculturation into the cultural practices or activities of their society and, more particularly, into the subcultures or communities of that society. Rogoff (1994, 1998) has defined learning as a process of transformation of participation in communities of practice. From this perspective, expertise develops as an individual gains greater knowledge, understanding and mastery over the practices of the various communities in which the individual participates and works, and into which the individual chooses to enter. As individuals are enculturated into the practices of their society and communities, they are transformed by the experience, and simultaneously may transform the community's practices. For individuals, an important aspect of this transformation is the change in identity which accompanies enculturation into community practices. For communities, transformation of practices is essential for the further development of the community and occurs because individuals do not uniformly adopt the practices of their respective communities; some practices will be actively embraced while others will be resisted or rejected.

Cultural practices have been defined as actions that have a routine or repeated quality to them, a recurrent sequence of activities (Miller and Goodnow, 1995). They are social or cultural actions that are engaged in by many or most members of a cultural group and that carry with them normative expectations about how things should be done. Miller and Goodnow (1995) point out that cultural practices involve values, and that as people adopt the practices, their values develop and change and they develop a sense of belonging and identity within the community. Miller and Goodnow also note that the shared quality of the practices means that they may be sustained, changed or challenged by a variety of people. Finally, Miller and Goodnow suggest that practices do not exist in isolation from each other; cultural practices have their own histories and trajectories and are part of, and linked to, other practices. The members of a culture or society, therefore, participate in many overlapping or connected practices simultaneously. In the health profession context, the importance of these practices is demonstrated in a recent ethnographic study (Ersser, 1997) of the sociocultural practices involved in nursing as a therapeutic activity.

The sociocultural view of the development of expertise as participation in cultural practices recognizes the essentially social nature of learning and development and moves beyond the view, common in socialization theory, of the passive individual shaped by socialization agents such as family, educational institutions, workplace and the media. Rather, the view of the individual is one of an active, constructive and transforming agent who shapes and is shaped by their experience of participation in cultural practices. Furthermore, the acknowledgement in the sociocultural practice approach of normative expectations, goals, values, motives and the social ordering of the society means that many of the traditional concerns of social psychologists (such as interpersonal relations, communication, social behaviour and social influence) are investigated from the sociocultural perspective. This trend in sociocultural research is exemplified by Ersser's (1997) research above and in an article by Renshaw (1998), which examines issues of student resistance to learning in the school context.

The notion of learning and development as transformation of participation in communities of practice has had an important impact on the understanding of learning and development in educational (Derry, 1992; Greeno, 1997) and developmental psychology, and has produced a body of research which challenges many accepted notions of learning and development. Important research from this perspective (Rogoff and Chavajay, 1995), of relevance to all educators, has been conducted in the areas of literacy and mathematics. The work of Cole and his associates (Scribner and Cole, 1981; Cole, 1996) on the nature and impact of literacy practices on cognition, conducted in Liberia, demonstrated that the cognitive effects of literacy were specific and were closely tied to the practices in which they were embedded. Cole showed, for instance, that literacy practices associated with religious practice and involving memorization produced improvements in memory abilities. In the area of mathematics, Lave (1988) demonstrated that American weight watchers, engaged in mathematical practices which were supported by their weight-watching practices and context, did not utilize the methods of abstract mathematical calculation they had been taught in school. For instance, Lave (1988) reported that when preparing a meal where the recipe required 3/4 of 2/3 of a cup, one weight watcher used a measure to obtain 2/3 of a cup, then created a round pancake which was then divided into four quarters, three of which were used in the recipe. Lave (1988) also reported that American grocery shoppers likewise employed mathematical approaches that were supported by the shopping context when comparing the prices of commodities, rather than the mathematical procedures they had learned at school. Somewhat similar findings involving young children selling candy on street corners in Brazil are reported by Nunes (1995); this research shows that the Brazilian candy sellers were able to make quick sophisticated calculations in the context of their selling practices, but were unable to perform the same calculations in a school context.

This and other research from this perspective (Greeno, 1997) suggests that learning is intimately bound up with the cultural practices in which it is embedded, and that consequently such learning is specific rather than general. Furthermore, this research suggests that the transfer or application of learning in contexts different from the learning context cannot be assumed. From the sociocultural practice perspective, transfer of learning is likely to occur to the extent that similar practices exist in the two contexts, and to the extent that these practices are supported by similar contextual resources. Notions of generic skills and of the transfer of generic skills are thus considered problematic from the sociocultural practice perspective. These findings have important consequences for all educational institutions; they highlight the fact that educational institutions have their own cultures and practices, essentially practices associated with learning, and these practices may not necessarily be similar to the practices in which students are required to participate when leaving the institution. Furthermore, accounts of learning and the development of expertise as participation in cultural practices recognize that enculturation into cultural practices takes place through the creation of zones of proximal development. Such accounts also acknowledge that metacognitive processes which are developed and internalized through zones of proximal development, and the reflection inherent in these processes, play an important role in learning and the development of expertise.

The view of learning and development as transformation of participation in communities of practice has probably had a greater impact on the understanding of the development of expertise in contexts other than specifically educational ones. The development of expertise through participation in cultural practices by children, often in countries other than Western ones, has been a significant focus of research over the last decade, as has the development of expertise in the workplace. Both areas of research have emphasized the way in which enculturation into cultural practices for novices is assisted by the structuring activities of experts or more capable others; both areas assign importance to the creation of zones of proximal development in this process and suggest that the notion of apprenticeship is important to an understanding of learning and the development of expertise. Research into the development of expertise in children is typified by Rogoff's work (Rogoff, 1990, 1998), which demonstrates how parents and other experts scaffold the child's participation in cultural activities. Rogoff makes an important contribution to sociocultural theory through her analysis of participation in cultural practices from personal, interpersonal and community perspectives. Research into the development of expertise in the workplace is typified by Lave's work (Lave, 1991; Lave and Wenger, 1991). In their analyses of the development of expertise of midwives, tailors and butchers, for instance, Lave and Wenger (1991) argue that participants move from a position of **peripheral or marginal participation** to a position of **central or legitimate participation**. The continuum from peripheral to central participation provides a useful framework for the analysis of professional expertise.

## Professional knowledge and communities of practice

From the sociocultural practice perspective, the learning of professional knowledge and the development of professional expertise, like other forms of expertise, occurs in the context of an individual's enculturation into particular communities of practice. This process begins during initial professional training, continues as the individual begins to practise in the profession, and further continues during the individual's lifetime of practice in that profession. The process marks the individual's movement from a position of peripheral participation during training and early professional practice to central or legitimate participation in later professional practice.

In relation to initial enculturation into professional practices, problem-based approaches to professional education, now common in the health sciences and other professional education, provide the earliest professional communities of practice. In problem-based learning, students are introduced to the knowledge, skills and practices of their profession as they work on problem scenarios in their courses. In problem-based learning in the health sciences and other professional education, students, working in small groups, are presented with authentic problems from their profession and are required to make judgments and evaluations concerning the information provided. They are required to find relevant disciplinary knowledge concerning each problem scenario, to use this information to make patient diagnoses and to suggest treatment solutions for these diagnoses. During the course of these activities, students are introduced to the clinical reasoning processes that are the basis of practice in the health sciences; simultaneously they are introduced, through textbook accounts, to many of the practices of their profession. In most problem-based learning programmes, such learning experiences are complemented, from an early stage in the programme, by experience in the authentic professional context and by interaction with professionals in the field. Although such experiences are generally brief, they provide students with authentic professional models and a powerful motivation to master the knowledge and skills of their profession and to enter into their chosen community of professional practice.

Problem-based learning programmes in the health sciences and other professions also help students to develop the metacognitive skills of reflection and self-directed learning (Ryan, 1997) required for a lifetime of practice in their profession. While problem-based learning programmes aim to develop self-regulatory skills in learners, there may be many reasons, as Hendry and Walker (1999) discuss, why alignments between teaching and assessment do not produce desired levels of student self-directed learning. In a related vein, the authentic nature of the learning context will influence the learning approaches adopted by health profession students, as Titchen and Coles (1991) demonstrated in a study which showed that physiotherapy students used more desirable learning approaches when they were experiencing the real clinical context or, failing that opportunity, a simulation of the clinical context.

Enculturation into professional practice takes place in many ways once one has completed profession education and entered the profession. This process of professional development can be conceptualized as the entering of the multiple communities of practice associated with the profession, such as professional associations and the like. Professional in-service programmes also introduce practitioners to new aspects of professional practice. Although there has been little research into the processes of professional enculturation from the perspective of the sociocultural theory of learning and expertise, a study by Palincsar et al. (1998) provides interesting insights into the way this process may operate in a professional in-service context, at least in the teaching profession.

This paper describes the creation or birth of a community of practice designed to assist primary school teachers in their teaching of science. The community consisted of two university-based teacher educators and 18 school-based educators who met on a regular basis to assist each other in the understanding and development of inquiry or constructivist approaches to science teaching. The work of the in-service community was based on the following three design principles (Palincsar et al., 1998, pp. 7–10):

- The work of. . . (the) community of practice is the development of teaching practice reflective of a specific orientation to teaching.
- The community of practice relies upon diverse expertise to contribute to the community's intellectual resources.
- Central to the work of this community of practice is the intellectual activity associated with teaching, including planning, enacting and reflecting upon one's teaching.

Thus the aim of the community was to help teachers make changes to their current professional practice and to assist transformations in the classroom cultures of participating teachers. While these points are considered important indicators of the success of the community of practice, the authors do not report on the success of the community in terms of transformations in the classroom cultures of participating teachers. Although this community of practice differs from many others in that it was artificially created, whereas most communities of practice come together and evolve organically, it nevertheless demonstrates the way in which such communities may enculturate individuals into the practices of their profession. The authors clearly consider the community of practice as a success in these terms.

## Conclusion

This chapter has introduced the socially oriented theories of learning and the development of expertise which have attracted considerable attention in educational psychology in recent years. These approaches, and particularly the sociocultural practice theory of researchers like Rogoff (1990, 1998) and Lave (1991), offer much to a contemporary understanding of the nature and development of expertise. Although this work has yet to be applied in any detailed way to an understanding of the development of professional knowledge in the health sciences or in general, it clearly provides a basis for understanding professional development through the course of professional education and subsequent professional practice. This approach, furthermore, helps to explain how people's professional identity and self-reflective and self-directed capacities are formed in the context of their social, cultural and professional practices.

## References

Alexander, P. A. (1997) Mapping the multidimensional nature of domain learning: The interplay of cognitive, motivational and strategic forces. In *Advances in Motivation and Achievement* (M. L. Maehr and P. R. Pintrich, eds), pp. 213–250. Greenwich, CN: JAI Press.

Anderson, J. R., Reder, L. M. and Simon, H. A. (1996) Situated learning and education. *Educational Researcher*, **25**(4), 5–11.

Benner, P. (1984) *From Novice to Expert: Excellence and Power in Clinical Nursing Practice*. Menlo Park, CA: Addison-Wesley.

Benner, P., Tanner, C. A. and Chesla, C. A. (1996) *Expertise in Nursing Practice*. New York: Springer.

Chi, M. T. H., Glaser, R. and Farr, M. J. (eds) (1988) *The Nature of Expertise*. Hillsdale, NJ: Erlbaum.

Cobb, P. (1994) Where is the mind? Constructivist and sociocultural perspectives on mathematical development. *Educational Researcher*, **23**, 13–20.

Cobb, P. and Bowers, J. (1999) Cognitive and situated learning perspectives in theory and practice. *Educational Researcher*, **28**(2), 4–15.

Cole, M. (1996) *Cultural Psychology: A Once and Future Discipline*. Cambridge, MA: Harvard University Press.

Derry, S. J. (1992) Beyond symbolic processing: Expanding horizons for educational psychology. *Journal of Educational Psychology*, **84**(4), 413–418.

Ericsson, K. A. and Smith, J. (eds) (1991) *Toward a General Theory of Expertise: Prospects and Limits.* New York: Cambridge University Press.

Ersser, S. J. (1997) *Nursing as a Therapeutic Activity: An Ethnography.* Aldershot: Avebury.

Greeno, J. (1997) On claims that answer the wrong questions. *Educational Researcher*, **26**(1), 5–17.

Hendry, G. D. (1996) Constructivism and educational practice. *Australian Journal of Education*, **40**, 19–45.

Hendry, G. D. and Walker, R. A. (1999) Course evaluation and regulation of learning: A case study in anatomy. Invited symposium paper presented at the 8th Biennial Conference of the European Association for Research on Learning and Instruction. Goteborg, Sweden, August 24–28.

Lave, J. (1988) *Cognition in Practice*. Cambridge: Cambridge University Press.

Lave, J. (1991) Situating learning in communities of practice. In *Perspectives on Socially Shared Cognition* (L. Resnick, J. Levine and S. Teasley, eds), pp. 63–82. Washington, DC: American Psychological Association.

Lave, J. and Wenger, E. (1991) *Situated Learning: Legitimate Peripheral Participation.* New York: Cambridge University Press.

Mayer, R. E. (1992) Cognition and instruction: Their historic meeting within educational psychology. *Journal of Educational Psychology*, **84**, 405–412.

Miller, P. J. and Goodnow, J. J. (1995) Cultural practices: Toward an integration of culture and development. In *Cultural Practices as Contexts for Development* (J. J. Goodnow, P. J. Miller and F. Kessel, eds), pp. 5–16. San Francisco: Jossey-Bass.

Nunes, T. (1995) Cultural practices and the conception of individual differences: Theoretical and empirical considerations. In *Cultural Practices as Contexts for Development* (J. J. Goodnow, P. J. Miller and F. Kessel, eds), pp. 91–103. San Francisco: Jossey-Bass.

O'Connor, M. C. (1998) Can we trace the efficacy of social constructivism? In *Review of Research in Education*, Vol. 23 (P. D. Pearson and A. Iran-Nejad, eds), pp. 25–72. Washington, DC: American Educational Research Association.

Palincsar, A. S. (1998) Social constructivist perspectives on teaching and learning. *Annual Review of Psychology*, **49**, 345–375.

Palincsar, A. S., Magnusson, S., Marano, N., Ford, D. and Brown, N. (1998) Designing a community of practice: Principles and practices of the GIsML community. *Teaching and Teacher Education*, **14**(5), 5–19.

Renshaw, P. (1998) Sociocultural pedagogy for new times: Reframing key concepts. *The Australian Educational Researcher*, **25**(3), 83–101.

Rogoff, B. (1990) *Apprenticeships in Thinking: Cognitive Development in Social Context.* New York: Oxford University Press.

Rogoff, B. (1994) Developing understanding of the idea of community of learners. *Mind, Culture, and Activity*, **1**, 209–229.

Rogoff, B. (1998) Cognition as a collaborative process. In *Handbook of Child Psychology*, 5th edn, vol. 2 (W. Damon, ed-in-chief; D. Kuhn and R. Siegler, eds), pp. 679–744. New York: Wiley.

Rogoff, B. and Chavajay, P. (1995) What's become of research on the cultural basis of cognitive development? *American Psychologist*, **50**(10), 859–877.

Ryan, G. L. (1997) The development of problem solving and self-directed learning ability in problem based learning. PhD thesis, University of Sydney.

Scribner, S. and Cole, M. (1981) *The Psychology of Literacy.* Cambridge, MA: Harvard University Press.

Suchman, L. (1993) Response to Vera and Simon's situated action: A symbolic interpretation. *Cognitive Science*, **17**, 71–75.

Tharp, R. G. and Gallimore, R. (1988) *Rousing Minds to Life: Teaching, Learning, and Schooling in Social Context.* Cambridge: Cambridge University Press.

Titchen, A. and Coles, C. (1991) Comparative study of physiotherapy students' approaches to their study in subject-centred and problem-based curricula. *Physiotherapy Practice*, **7**, 127–133.

Vera, A. H. and Simon, H. A. (1993) Situated action: A symbolic interpretation. *Cognitive Science*, **17**, 7–48.

Wertsch, J. V. (1985) *Vygotsky and the Social Formation of Mind.* Cambridge, MA: Harvard University Press.

Wertsch, J. V. (1991) *Voices of the Mind.* Cambridge, MA: Harvard University Press.

# 4

# Integrating knowledge and practice in medicine

**Ann Jervie Sefton**

This chapter deals with different aspects of medical knowledge. While some forms of knowledge are learned explicitly from books or classes, others are acquired more by observation, practice, imitation and experience. Effective medical curricula are planned and implemented only by understanding the mechanisms by which the less well identified aspects of medical knowledge are transmitted both inside and outside the formal instructional approach. The boundaries between different sorts of knowledge are ill-defined, making the task of integration challenging. With the possible exception of medical communication, the craft of medicine is less subject to experimental study or documentation than is specific subject knowledge acquired in formal educational contexts. Increasingly, though, medical curricula are being designed to develop a wide range of holistic skills, and other aspects of knowledge are now better identified.

## Different forms of knowledge

There is a large literature on **ways of knowing**, but for the purposes of this chapter it seems appropriate to select one model as a framework for discussion. In distinguishing 'knowing what' and 'knowing how', Ryle (1949) provided a simple dichotomy. For medical education, 'knowing what' equates with book knowledge, and 'knowing how' not only with technical skills but also with aspects of professional clinical behaviours. In neural terms 'knowing how' includes motor (procedural) memory; the rehearsal of skill-based activities involves cerebellar function. 'Knowing what' involves the forebrain areas associated with episodic, priming and somatic memory (Markowitsch, 1995).

Carper (1978) identified four interdependent elements in nursing: empirics (science), aesthetics (art), personal knowledge, and ethics (moral knowledge). Kolb (1984) also defined four experiential subdivisions: concrete experience, reflective observation, abstract conceptualization and active experimentation; however, this categorization is less readily applicable to medical education. Eraut's (1994) five-category model encompasses: propositional, tacit, personal and process knowledge, and know-how. While those divisions have some attraction, the model of Higgs and Titchen (1995), comprising propositional and non-propositional/experience-based knowledge (professional craft knowledge and personal knowledge) provides a simpler and more convenient theoretical structure for this discussion.

As noted by Schön (1987) and later reinforced (Eraut, 1994; Higgs and Titchen, 1995), propositional knowledge has been most highly valued in academic institutions. Thus a hierarchy of esteem has developed, based on the history of ideas, academic values and the extent to which knowledge may be validated (Eraut, 1994), although Schön (1983) drew attention to the gap between research-based knowledge and the knowledge needed for actual professional practice. More recently, however, some Australian universities are stressing the importance of generic skills and knowledge, outside of specific propositional knowledge. These generic attributes are needed by all graduates in order to perform in any workplace. The generic skills overlap with clinical skills specifically expected of a medical professional and include elements both of craft and personal knowledges.

## Knowledge and skills for medical practice

What constitutes essential knowledge for a medical practitioner? Undoubtedly, it is difficult to separate the different subsets of knowledge (Higgs and Titchen, 1995). One model (Norman, 1985) includes:

1 clinical and technical skills, which might be seen largely in the domain of craft knowledge;
2 knowledge and understanding (largely propositional);
3 interpersonal attributes (largely personal);
4 problem-solving and clinical judgment (across all domains).

Many aspects of diagnosis, decision-making and management involve integrating propositional with experience-based knowledge and craft skills. However, the issue is complicated by the variety within medical practice: essential knowledge varies for a general practitioner, a public health officer, a researcher or a specialist. This heterogeneity gives rise to real challenges for medical educators, although much of the differentiation occurs after graduation (Eraut, 1994). Core components, common to most forms of practice, include communication and physical examination. These skills have been learned by example in medical settings over time; more formal and analytical educational approaches are more recent.

A modern professional values lifelong learning; the increase in information and altered patterns of health delivery make such learning imperative for effective medical practice. New curricula prepare students for continuing learning by stressing independence and self-direction across all categories of knowledge. In medical curricula, attention is now being paid to reflection, building on the reflective practitioner model of Schön (1987), which has for rather longer been incorporated into other health professional programmes. A reflective approach, particularly during experiential learning (Eraut, 1994), should encourage students to evaluate their own progress so that later in practice they can identify specific needs for further learning.

Clinical reasoning remains a focus of modern clinical practice (Higgs and Jones, 2000), and newer educational methods, including problem-based learning, support its early introduction (Sefton et al., 2000). A critical component of clinical craft knowledge, clinical reasoning clearly depends on propositional knowledge and is to some extent coloured by personal knowledge. The reasoning process, now better understood (Schmidt et al., 1990; Boshuizen and Schmidt, 1995; Elstein, 1995), is taught explicitly in some medical schools (Sefton et al., 2000). Medical reasoning is a subset of broader critical thinking, which itself can be taught effectively (Halpern, 1998). The early development of students' general thinking skills would not only strengthen clinical reasoning, but also help in understanding and countering the irrational beliefs and flawed reasoning of some students.

Although some formal ethical philosophy is often taught in medical programmes (e.g. Loewy, 1989), a student's learning about ethical thinking and behaviours is strongly influenced by previous beliefs and values, as well as by practices observed in clinical settings. Supervisors and mentors can shape students' approaches to ethical dilemmas by incorporating ethical reasoning within daily practice. A student's maturing approach to ethical problems is as much a part of their craft education as it is of propositional or personal knowledge.

Doctors are autonomous and, at least to some extent, self-regulating. Yet they are accountable to patients, colleagues, employers and society (Eraut, 1994). Although propositional knowledge is a central factor in professional competence, the clinician relies heavily on personal and professional craft knowledge to manage competing role demands and tensions. A related issue is that of professional error, seldom acknowledged and often poorly managed (Leape, 1994). Only recently has the recognition and amelioration of factors that contribute to error been considered in the context of medical curricula. One consequence of such considerations is the establishment of thinking processes and practical procedures both to limit and to acknowledge error; these strategies become part of a changing body of medical craft knowledge.

Another fundamental requirement of health professionals is the capacity to adapt to change, which is occurring at an increasing pace. For example, the increasing emphasis on patient-centred care (Fulford, 1996) gives greater significance to patients' needs and values (Heginbotham, 1996), including cultural considerations (Doyal, 1996). As clinical practice becomes more complex, craft knowledge and behaviours acquired from earlier times may no longer be appropriate. Thus current students may be exposed to clinical supervisors and role models whose practices are inappropriate. Staff development then becomes particularly crucial.

Other changes are equally challenging. In addition to patients' expectations, Towle (1998) highlights an increasing volume of propositional knowledge, changing demographics, new technologies and different patterns of health care as factors influencing practice. Not only are anticipation of and adaptation to change essential personal skills, but appropriate responsiveness represents an important element of craft knowledge. The contemporary delivery of health care sees sicker patients spending less time in increasingly technical hospitals. Thus, strong arguments are mounted to support moving more of medical education to community and ambulatory settings (Moore et al., 1994; Davis et al., 1997), aligning students' developing craft knowledge more closely with likely practice. Towle (1998) draws attention to the implications of ongoing change both for medical curricula and continuing professional education, a call that is equally relevant to other health professions. In particular, change necessitates more flexibility in curricula, a greater emphasis on 'learning to learn' rather than the acquisition of facts or technical skills which themselves are subject to change, and a greater emphasis on informatics as essential craft knowledge.

Information technology is deeply embedded into modern medicine. Students must become effective users of the computers and sophisticated instruments found in practice (Coiera, 1997; Carlile and Sefton, 1998). Although a formal understanding of informatics represents propositional knowledge, the day-to-day use of computers and technology is more appropriately regarded as craft knowledge. Further, increasingly autonomous patients now access information of variable quality on the Internet from medical services, patient support groups and commercial sources. Practitioners need the skills to evaluate such resources critically and offer advice in discussion with patients. Thus, new curricula (e.g. at the University of Sydney) embed the use of computers deeply within the processes of learning across all categories of knowledge (Carlile et al., 1998).

Evidence-based medicine (Sackett et al., 1997) involves locating valid sources of knowledge and evaluating them critically to aid rational decision-making. The separate elements of knowledge generation and evaluation include framing questions, searching databases, and appraising and applying information to specific situations. The steps can be taught explicitly, but students fully embrace the skills only when they are embedded regularly in the practice of respected role models in hospitals and the community. The teaching and role-modelling process undoubtedly contributes to the development of essential craft and propositional knowledge, but penetration into all clinical environments is as yet incomplete.

While individual practice was once the norm, professionals now often work in teams, particularly in the context of patient-centred care (Fulford et al., 1996). Newer medical curricula, particularly those that are problem-based, explicitly value and encourage group cooperation (Kaufman, 1985; Des Marchais, 1991; Tosteson et al., 1994; Sefton, 1995; Henry et al., 1997; Teubner and Prideaux, 1997). Clinical teams may be medical or multiprofessional. In either case, professional boundaries, responsibilities and expertise become issues. Thus medical students learn by observation the different roles of doctors and other health professionals. Bashford (1998) offers an interesting historical perspective on such interprofessional boundaries from the time in the nineteenth century when women sought access to medical education. In particular, she notes the tensions such women faced, including professional, scientific, feminine and middle-class issues, in distinguishing themselves not only from male practitioners but also from the newer, middle-class, trained nurses. Indeed, the only way in which such pioneers could gain the requisite clinical experience was as nurses, putting them into an ambiguous position. Some acute modern observers note parallels among those health professionals (e.g. nurses or therapists) who subsequently enrol in medicine. They provide insights into the conflicts arising from adapting to different roles and conforming to new boundaries, particularly when they continue to work in their original profession during medical training. Although some health professional groups learn together (e.g. Bergdahl et al., 1994), substantial logistic issues and old territorialities impede collaborative teaching that might erode the boundaries.

## Medical curricula and the development of students' knowledge

Historically, the dichotomy between propositional and craft knowledge was more apparent. In medieval times, most practitioners were apprentice-trained as surgeons or apothecaries (Rawcliffe, 1995). At the universities of Oxford and Cambridge, only theoretical subjects, usually theology and philosophy, were taught to student physicians. Relevant medical knowledge was later acquired from a mentor or a continental university. Apart from some surgical procedures and a few effective medicines, the capacity of doctors actively to cure and prevent disease was limited until recently (Thomas, 1995; Porter, 1996). Increasing scientific understanding – propositional knowledge – has shaped clinical behaviours and craft knowledge.

Since the late nineteenth century in Britain and Australia, and since Flexner (1910) in the USA, medical school curricula have been didactic and formal. Hierarchical programmes provided a background in basic and then paraclinical medical sciences, usually before clinical experience commenced. In more recent years curricula became grossly overloaded with new propositional knowledge (Bordage, 1987). Craft learning was delayed and never well integrated; personal knowledge was not generally recognized.

More recently, writers of influential reports have challenged that traditional view of medical education (Association of American Medical Colleges, 1984; Walton, 1990; Towle, 1991; General Medical Council, 1992). Some schools had, however, already established different programmes (Neufeld and Barrows, 1974; Barrows and Tamblyn, 1980; Kaufman, 1985; Henry, 1994) and many have followed since. The dominant educational philosophy of many innovative medical programmes is constructivism (Tinkler, 1993), with a commitment to the values of problem-based, self-directed, active learning. Cooperative learning in small groups provides a mechanism for students to construct their own understanding in a medical context (e.g. Des Marchais, 1991; Tosteson et al., 1994; Sefton, 1995; Henry et al., 1997; Teubner and Prideaux, 1997).

For curricular design the taxonomy of Bloom (1965) has been influential. Bloom's first domain of knowledge includes largely propositional **knowledge** at different levels, although the hierarchy has been questioned (Eraut, 1994). The **skills** domain in medicine traditionally includes communication and clinical examination. One vital skill is clinical reasoning, which depends on good clinical knowledge (including propositional and professional craft knowledge) as expertise is developed (Schmidt et al., 1990; Boshuizen and Schmidt, 1995; Elstein, 1995; Sefton et al., 2000), indicating some blurring of Bloom's categories. Some elements of reasoning (such as critical self-reflection) are learned experientially as craft knowledge when teaching actually models clinical behaviour (Kassirer, 1983). The third domain, **attitudes**, is more problematic, since it has been argued that a proper educational concern is to encourage appropriate professional behaviours, not to mandate particular personal attitudes. Nevertheless, students' learning will always be influenced substantially by their backgrounds, expectations, aspirations and cultural values.

Newer medical programmes frequently include early clinical exposure. When there are opportunities to interact with patients in clinical or community settings, rather than in skills laboratories, students develop elements of personal as well as craft knowledge. Such experiential learning reinforces the development of clinical reasoning (Sefton et al., 2000) and enhances the validity of problem-based tutorials (Henry et al., 1997). Clinical experiences strongly motivate students, although if visits are merely token and unrelated to concurrent learning, the value is reduced. The use of simulated or standardized patients, helpful for developing practical skills (Barrows, 1993), is less valuable for enriching understanding of broader aspects of patient care and health delivery.

Early hospital-based or community-based experiences provide opportunities to integrate the different forms of knowledge. They reflect, however, apprentice-based educational models in which the quality of the individual contact with mentors is variable and unregulated. To counteract this unpredictability, staff development is now taken seriously and high-quality, structured and reliable experiences can be provided for medical students (Weinholtz and Edwards, 1992; Newble and Cannon, 1994). The need for all teachers to commit to new educational principles of mutual respect, support, and student-directed learning is increasingly accepted. Staff development sessions to discuss critical incidents now encourage debriefing after difficult clinical or educational situations.

In educational institutions generally, the hierarchy of different forms of knowledge has been reinforced with assessments which emphasize propositional knowledge. Students sensibly target their efforts in order to optimize their grades and qualify for practice (Newble and Jaeger, 1983; Ramsden, 1992). A student's perception of the amount of time needed in private study appears to determine the relative values placed on different kinds of knowledge. Medical teachers have been concerned to develop and assess clinical competence (Neufeld and Norman, 1985; Newble, 1992) as one element of professional craft knowledge. Nevertheless, the emphasis often remains on the assessment of propositional knowledge, with clinical skills allocated lower weightings. Some other aspects of craft and personal knowledge, essential for making clinical and ethical decisions, are less easily assessed and may be relatively neglected both by students and staff.

## Conclusion

How students learn propositional knowledge and related skills like clinical reasoning has been extensively studied. By contrast, the ways in which students acquire professional craft and personal knowledge are less scrutinized and documented. Nevertheless, the performance of a competent professional requires an integration of all three forms of knowledge. Better means of analysis and interpretation of personal and professional craft knowledge will lead to a better understanding of the whole of a medical student's learning. Only then can we develop effectively integrated methods of teaching and learning across the components of knowledge.

## References


Association of American Medical Colleges (1984) *Physicians for the Twenty-First Century.* Washington, DC: Association of American Medical Colleges.

Barrows, H. (1993) An overview of the uses of standardised patients for teaching and evaluating clinical skills. *Academic Medicine*, **68**, 443–453.

Barrows, H. S. and Tamblyn, R. M. (1980) *Problem-Based Learning: An Approach to Medical Education.* New York: Springer.

Bashford, A. (1998) *Purity and Pollution.* London: Methuen.

Bergdahl, B., Koch, M., Ludvigsson, J. and Wessman, J. (1994) The Linköping medical programme: A curriculum for student-centred learning. *Annals of Community-Oriented Education*, **7**, 107–119.

Bloom, B. S. (1965) *Taxonomy of Educational Objectives – the Classification of Educational Goals.* New York: Longman Green.

Bordage, G. (1987) The curriculum: overloaded and too general? *Medical Education*, **21**, 183–188.

Boshuizen, H. P. A. and Schmidt, H. G. (1995) The development of clinical reasoning expertise. In *Clinical Reasoning in the Health Professions* (J. Higgs and M. Jones, eds), pp. 24–32. Oxford: Butterworth-Heinemann.

Carlile, S. and Sefton, A. J. (1998) Medical education for the information age. *Medical Journal of Australia*, **168**, 340–343.

Carlile, S. C., Barnet, S., Sefton, A. J. and Uther, J. (1998) Medical problem-based learning supported by intranet technology: A natural student-centred approach. *International Journal of Medical Informatics*, **50**, 225–233.

Carper, B. A. (1978) Fundamental patterns of knowing. *Advances in Nursing Science*, **1**, 13–23.

Coiera, E. (1997) *Guide to Medical Informatics, the Internet and Telemedicine.* London: Chapman & Hall.

Davis, W. K., Jolly, B. C., Page, G. G., Rothman, A. I. and White, B-A. (eds) (1997) *Moving Medical Education from the Hospital to the Community.* Ann Arbor: University of Michigan Medical School.

Des Marchais, J. E. (1991) From traditional to problem-based curriculum: How the switch was made at Sherbrooke, Canada. *Lancet*, **338**, 234–237.

Doyal, L. (1996) Needs, rights and the duty of care towards patients of radically different cultures. In *Essential Practice in Patient-Centred Care* (K. W. M. Fulford, S. Ersser and T. Hope, eds), pp. 198–209. Oxford: Blackwell Science.

Elstein, A. S. (1995) Clinical reasoning in medicine. In *Clinical Reasoning in the Health Professions* (J. Higgs and M. Jones, eds), pp. 49–59. Oxford: Butterworth-Heinemann.

Eraut, M. (1994) *Developing Professional Knowledge and Competence.* London: The Falmer Press.

Flexner, A. (1910) *Medical Education in the United States and Canada.* New York: The Carnegie Foundation.

Fulford, K. W. M. (1996) Concepts of disease and the meaning of patient-centred care. In *Essential Practice in Patient-Centred Care* (K. W. M. Fulford, S. Ersser and T. Hope, eds), pp. 1–16. Oxford: Blackwell Science.

Fulford, K. W. M., Ersser, S. and Hope, T. (eds) (1996) *Essential Practice in Patient-Centred Care.* Oxford: Blackwell Science.

General Medical Council (1992) *Tomorrow's Doctors.* London: General Medical Council.

Halpern, D. (1998) Teaching critical thinking for transfer across domains. *American Psychologist*, **53**, 449–455.

Heginbotham, C. (1996) Patient-centred management: Patient-centred care through continuous quality improvement. In *Essential Practice in Patient-Centred Care* (K. W. M. Fulford, S. Ersser and T. Hope, eds), pp. 121–136. Oxford: Blackwell Science.

Henry, R. L. (1994) Implementation of a philosophy at Newcastle, Australia. *Annals of Community-Oriented Education*, **7**, 79–92.

Henry, R., Byrne, K. and Engel, C. (1997) *Imperatives in Medical Education.* Newcastle, NSW: University of Newcastle, Faculty of Health Sciences.

Higgs, J. and Jones, M. (eds) (2000) *Clinical Reasoning in the Health Professions*, 2nd edn. Oxford: Butterworth-Heinemann.

Higgs, J. & Titchen, A. (1995) Propositional, professional and personal knowledge in clinical reasoning. In *Clinical Reasoning in the Health Professions* (J. Higgs and M. Jones, eds), pp. 129–146. Oxford: Butterworth-Heinemann.

Kassirer, J. P. (1983) Teaching clinical medicine by iterative hypothesis testing: Let's preach what we practice. *New England Journal of Medicine*, **309**, 921–923.

Kaufman, A. (1985) *Implementing Problem-Based Education: Lessons from Successful Innovations*. New York: Springer Publishing Company.

Kolb, D. A. (1984) *Experiential Learning: Experience as the Source of Learning and Development*. Englewood Cliffs: Prentice-Hall.

Leape, L. L. (1994) Error in medicine. *Journal of the American Medical Association*, **272**, 1851–1857.

Loewy, E. H. (1989) *Textbook of Medical Ethics*. New York: Plenum Medical Book Company.

Markowitsch, H. J. (1995) Anatomical basis of memory disorders. In *The Cognitive Neurosciences* (M. S. Gazzaniga, ed.), pp. 765–779. Cambridge, MA: MIT Press.

Moore, G. T., Innui, T. S., Ludden, J. M. and Schoenbaum, S. C. (1994) The 'teaching HMO': A new academic partner. *Academic Medicine*, **8**, 595–600.

Neufeld, V. and Barrows, H. (1974) The McMaster philosophy: An approach to medical education. *Journal of Medical Education*, **49**, 1040–1050.

Neufeld, V. R. and Norman, G. R. (eds) (1985) *Assessing Clinical Competence*. New York: Springer.

Newble, D. and Cannon, R. (1994) *A Handbook for Medical Teachers*, 3rd edn. Dordrecht: Kluwer Academic Publishers.

Newble, D. I. (1992) Assessing clinical competence at the undergraduate level. *Medical Education*, **26**, 504–511.

Newble, D. I. and Jaeger, K. (1983) The effects of assessment and examinations on the learning of medical students. *Medical Education*, **17**, 165–171.

Norman, G. R. (1985) Defining competence: A methodological review. In *Assessing Clinical Competence* (V. R. Neufeld and G. R. Norman, eds), pp. 15–35. New York: Springer.

Porter, R. (ed.) (1996) *The Cambridge Illustrated History of Medicine*. Cambridge: Cambridge University Press.

Ramsden, P. (1992) *Learning to Teach in Higher Education*. London: Routledge.

Rawcliffe, C. (1995) *Medicine and Society in Later Medieval England*. Stroud, UK: Alan Sutton Publishing Company.

Ryle, G. (1949) *The Concept of Mind*. London: Hutchinson.

Sackett, D. L., Richardson, W. S., Rosenberg, W. and Haynes, R. B. (1997) *Evidence-Based Medicine: How to Practice and Teach EBM*. New York: Churchill Livingstone.

Schmidt, H. G., Norman, G. R. and Boshuizen, H. P. A. (1990) A cognitive perspective on medical expertise: Theory and implications. *Academic Medicine*, **65**, 611–621.

Schön, D. A. (1983) *The Reflective Practitioner: How Professionals Think in Action*. New York: Basic Books.

Schön, D. A. (1987) *Educating the Reflective Practitioner: Towards a New Design for the Teaching and Learning Professions*. San Francisco: Jossey-Bass.

Sefton, A. J. (1995) Australian medical education in a time of change: A view from the University of Sydney. *Medical Education*, **29**, 181–186.

Sefton, A., Gordon, J. and Field, M. (2000) Teaching clinical reasoning to medical students. In *Clinical Reasoning in the Health Professions* (J. Higgs and M. Jones, eds), 2nd edn, pp. 184–190. Oxford: Butterworth-Heinemann.

Teubner, J. and Prideaux, D. (1997) An innovative medical school. *Journal of Higher Education Policy and Management*, **19**, 21–26.

Thomas, L. (1995) *The Youngest Science*. Harmondsworth: Penguin Books.

Tinkler, D. E. (1993) A 'constructivist' theory of acquisition, and its implications for learner-managed learning. In *Learner Managed Learning* (N. J. Graves, ed.), pp. 132–148. Leeds: World Education Fellowship.

Tosteson, D. C., Adelstein, S. J. and Carver, S. T. (1994) *New Pathways to Medical Education*. Cambridge, MA: Harvard University Press.

Towle, A. (1991) *Critical Thinking: the Future of Undergraduate Medical Education*. London: The King's Fund.

Towle, A. (1998) Changes in health care and continuing medical education for the 21st century. *British Medical Journal*, **316**, 301–304.

Walton, H. J. (1990) Statement on medical education in Europe. *Medical Education*, **24**, 78–80.

Weinholtz, D. and Edwards, J. (1992) *Teaching During Rounds*. Baltimore, MD: The Johns Hopkins University Press.

# 5

# The nature of professional craft knowledge

**Angie Titchen and Steven J. Ersser**

## Introduction

Professional craft knowledge is often tacit and unarticulated and sometimes intuitive. This knowledge is brought to bear spontaneously in the care of patients, and guides day-to-day actions in the clinical area (Brown et al., 1988). It underpins the practitioner's rapid and fluent response to a situation. Short-term, taken-for-granted goals are achieved by strategies that take account of, and show sensitivity to, the multiplicity of aspects of the situation. The practitioner reacts to the whole situation and makes highly skilled judgments, often without being conscious of a deliberate way of acting.

Since professional craft knowledge is frequently tacit and is embedded in practice, it is important for us to understand its nature if we are to access it, study it, develop it further and make it available for others to acquire expertise and improve their practice. This is what this chapter and Chapter 7 are all about. In this chapter, we reveal more about the nature of professional craft knowledge by looking critically at the way health care researchers and theorists currently use established epistemological terminology to describe the nature of knowledge relevant to professional action. However, in developing this critique, we discover an epistemological mess, which we attempt to unravel by introducing into health care the term 'professional craft knowledge', a term coined in education by Brown and McIntyre (1993). We also draw some conclusions about the shortcomings of contemporary understandings of epistemological concepts and typologies relevant to professional craft knowledge, which lead us into our discussions in Chapter 7.

Before beginning our survey of how the professional literature addresses epistemological concepts relevant to the concept of professional craft knowledge, we would like to point out that we undertake this analysis from the perspective of health professional researchers and scholars examining philosophical ideas, and not as philosophers. Debate about an appropriate epistemology for practice disciplines is an evolving one and we seek to contribute to this debate.

## Analysis of epistemological concepts and typologies relevant to professional craft knowledge used in the health care literature

Epistemology is a term referring to the theory of knowledge, encompassing philosophical problems concerned with the origin and structure of knowledge (Rawnsley, 1998), as well as claims to its validity. The literature provides discussion of a range of epistemological concepts that are helpful in describing, explaining and analysing the different types of knowledge relevant to professional health care practice, including:

1. practical knowledge
2. knowing-in-practice
3. experiential knowledge
4. aesthetic knowledge
5. intuitive knowledge
6. ethical/moral knowledge

7 embodied knowledge
8 personal knowledge
9 propositional/empirical knowledge
10 scientific knowledge

The first eight terms are often considered to be non-propositional in nature, whilst the last two are propositional in nature. Our analysis of the non-propositional concepts is summarized in Table 5.1 (terms 9–10 have been considered in earlier chapters and are not included here).

There are variations in the literature in the way epistemological concepts are applied. Although it is useful to examine variation as well as uniformity, variation can cause confusion, as reflected in the number of related terms cited in Table 5.1. Often terms are not clearly differentiated, and their subtlety may not be understood by the reader. In addition, terms 2–8 above are not mutually exclusive; for example, personal knowledge can also be intuitive or embodied, and the terms, 'practical knowledge' and 'knowing-in-practice' encompass all the other terms (i.e. terms 3–8). Nevertheless, revealing these variations can help to convey the potential usefulness of some terms in characterizing professional craft knowledge.

## Overall critique

In this analysis, we have drawn most heavily on the work of nursing theorists and researchers because it is nurses who have been most active in exploring the epistemological basis of their practice. However, we have a concern that Carper's (1978) seminal and influential work may have been accepted uncritically in the nursing profession and possibly in other health care professions that are starting to take an interest in epistemology. Carper's paper does not provide methodological details of how she derived her ways of knowing from a conceptual and syntactical analysis of nursing knowledge, so it is not possible to judge the validity of her analysis. There was also very little empirical research available at that time from which she could derive the non-propositional patterns of knowing, i.e. personal, aesthetic and ethical. In addition, we find that her description of aesthetic knowledge lacks clarity.

Whilst this examination of health care literature shows that there is current recognition that many of the epistemological terms overlap in complex ways, we have three further areas of concern. First, the use of a large number of the terms in health care literature creates a confusion that makes it difficult for the practitioner and the researcher to relate the knowledge generated in a particular study to that uncovered in another. For example, in a review of research exploring the expressive elements of nursing (Titchen, 2000), only MacLeod (1990) was noted to consider the possible relationships between the different types of knowledge. Furthermore, confusion may exist because the terminology appears sometimes to be determined in different ways according to the nature of the knowledge (e.g. intuitive knowledge as understanding without a rationale), its substance (e.g. ethical knowledge), the way it is generated (e.g. practical knowledge derived through experience), or the way it is known (e.g. intuitive knowledge known through the senses or 'gut feeling'). Third, there appears to be a broadly held assumption that only propositional and scientific knowledge are propositional in expression.

In response to the first two concerns, Titchen (2000) adopted the metaphor of professional craft knowledge in health care as a carrier for these complex concepts and their relationships, devising an analytical framework for examining professional craft knowledge, which we present in Chapter 7. Below, Titchen justifies her use of a metaphor rather than an analytical term and explains why the above terms (and others) were rejected.

## The metaphor of professional craft knowledge

Consensus on a term that captures the diverse and dynamic nature of the knowledge accrued through experience is important for effective communication and understanding among practitioners, researchers and educators. Many terms seem to fall short of capturing the nature of such knowledge. Carper's (1978) 'patterns of knowing' (aesthetic, ethical and personal) put artificial and fixed boundaries around knowledge, while her patterns underplay practical experience. The term 'practical knowledge' (Benner, 1984) avoids parcelling up knowledge and emphasizes practical experience, but fails to convey the interpersonal and the aesthetic connotations. Although MacLeod's (1990) term 'knowing-in-practice' includes the imbuing of practical knowledge with theoretical knowledge, and as such, is the most suitable analytical term, it still seems to miss the personal, interpersonal and aesthetic connotations or 'feel'.

**Table 5.1 Epistemological concepts relevant to the study of professional craft knowledge**

| *Epistemological concept* | *Citation example* | *Related philosophical /social-scientific citations* | *Commentary* |
| --- | --- | --- | --- |
| **1. Practical knowledge**<br>*Descriptor(s)*<br>'Knowing how' to perform a task or operation or to exercise practical skill. Developed through skill acquisition (Burnard, 1992). | Benner (1984) describes six areas of practical knowledge, e.g. paradigm cases and maxims.<br>Burnard (1992) discusses relationship to health care curriculum. | Ryle (1949).<br>Polanyi (1958)<br>Heron (1981) | *Nature*: Non-propositional; may be embodied (i.e. known by the body and not the mind) or represented in the mind.<br>*Derivation*: Knowing through engaging in action and through experience which reaches consciousness (i.e. when preconceived notions are turned around).<br>*Interrelated concepts*: Terms 3–8.<br>*Critique*: After Habermas (1972), this term is used to describe a type of propositional knowledge, generated through research and scholarship. This duplication of terms causes confusion. In addition, the descriptors in use are skills-based and so downplay the practical strategies that professionals create to realize theoretical ideas and research findings in their practice. In other words, the term polarizes practical and theoretical knowledge. |
| **2. Knowing-in-practice**<br>*Descriptor(s)*<br>As above, plus:<br>Practical know-how is imbued with theoretical knowledge. | MacLeod (1990) concludes that theoretical knowledge is contextualized and transformed by means of practitioners' practical knowing.<br>Street (1992) demonstrates that the product of this transformation is perceptual knowing which is temporal and context-specific. | None<br>MacLeod (1990) invented the term within her study. | *Nature:* Non-propositional; may be embodied or represented in the mind.<br>*Derivation*: Knowing through engaging in action/practising/from experience without reaching consciousness.<br>*Interrelated concepts*: Terms 3–8.<br>*Critique*: No longer polarizes practical and theoretical knowledge. |
| **3. Experiential knowledge**<br>*Descriptor(s)*<br>Knowledge derived through direct encounter with something: a subject, person or thing, an observation of events. | Burnard (1992)<br>Ersser (1997) | Heron (1981)<br>Kolb (1984) | *Nature*: Non-propositional knowledge about an instance or encounter; does not necessarily involve action.<br>*Derivation*: Emphasis is on acquaintance through sense data and not other sources (memory, introspection).<br>*Interrelated concepts*: A precursor to skill/action-related practical knowledge. Overlaps with knowing-in-practice. Burnard (1992) says experiential knowledge is synonymous with Polanyi's (1958) concept of personal knowledge and tacit knowledge. Relates to Russell's (1980) idea of knowledge by acquaintance with anything of which we are aware, without the intermediary of any process of interference or any knowledge of truths. Distinguished from knowledge of things that are known through description or articulation.<br>*Critique*: Interrelationships with above terms often not recognized. Difficult to access in research designs which depend on practitioners articulating what they know of the encounter. |

*continued*

**Table 5.1 (continued)**

| *Epistemological concept* | *Citation example* | *Related philosophical /social-scientific citations* | *Commentary* |
|---|---|---|---|
| **4. Aesthetic knowledge**<br>*Descriptor(s)*<br>Concern with the particular, form and style.<br>Professional artistry. | Carper (1978) focuses on significance of behaviour, the uniqueness of the particular situation and a variety of modes of perception.<br>Fish and Coles (1998) refer to:<br>• Knowing how to make professional judgments and improvise in uncertain and messy situations, where neither ends nor specific means can be pre-specified.<br>• Using practical principles, not competencies or skills that can be predetermined.<br>Aldridge (1991)<br>Ersser (1997)<br>Titchen (2000) | Schön (1983)<br>Eisner (1985) | *Nature*: Non-propositional knowledge.<br>*Derivation*: Paying attention to something by using all the senses, artistic perception searches for qualities, patterns, plays with alternatives, using imagination, recognizing significant features, discriminating subtleties (Eisner, 1985). Occurs through engagement with the other and the situation and also through critical reflection upon practice. Critical appreciation (awareness of assumptions underlying the situation), value considerations, improvisation, inquiry into action.<br>*Interrelated concepts*: Manley (1991) indicates that this is related to Benner's (1984) practical knowledge. Vaughan (1992, p. 8) relates aesthetic knowledge to intuitive knowledge, describing it as 'that intuitive act that makes the expert practitioner behave in an unexpected way from time to time'.<br>*Critique*: Aesthetic knowledge appears to be the mediator between propositional, practical and personal knowledges, i.e. knowing how to: (a) mediate the use of applied science and technique in the messy world of practice through professional judgment and realizing practical principles, and (b) use the whole self in care (e.g. engagement, comportment, humour, feelings). |
| **5. Intuitive knowledge**<br>*Descriptor(s)*<br>Understanding or belief without rationale.<br>'Gut feeling'. | Agan (1987)<br>Benner and Tanner (1987)<br>Paul and Heaslip (1995) | Russell (1980) | *Nature*: Non-propositional knowledge.<br>*Derivation*: Through the senses and through engagement and attunement to the patient and the situation.<br>*Interrelated concepts*: Agan (1987) describes 'intuitive knowing' as a dimension of the art of nursing.<br>*Critique*: Ayer (1973) argues that there is no reason why one's intuition should be trusted unless the hypothesis is found to agree with observable evidence. However, Benner (1984) and others have found that nurses frequently know intuitively when something is wrong with their patients before there is any observable evidence. Easen and Wilcockson (1996) argue that intuition is presented in the literature in ways that lack clarity and coherence. They see it best understood as a rational process that has a rational basis. |
| **6. Ethical/moral knowledge**<br>*Descriptor(s)*<br>Knowledge of right and wrong.<br>Focusing on moral obligation and what ought to be done in the clinical situation and managing value conflict. | Carper (1978)<br>Fjelland and Gjengdal (1994, p. 20) conclude that 'good nursing also depends on what is morally right'. The authors discuss the place of ethics as a theoretical foundation for nursing. | Hobbes (Kavka, 1986)<br>Hume (1977)<br>Kant (1949)<br>Goldman (1988) | *Nature*: May be non-propositional or propositional. Formalized as ethical theory.<br>*Derivation*: The development of a sense of morality is a feature of a person's psychological and social development. It can be derived experientially through observing others putting beliefs and values into action in their practice.<br>*Interrelated concepts*: Moral knowledge requires both personal knowledge and practical knowledge, e.g. knowing how to: |

| | | | |
|---|---|---|---|
| **6. Ethical/moral knowledge** *(continued)* | | | • Live out one's beliefs and values of what is right and good in practice<br>• Deal with value conflict<br>• Recognize incongruence between one's espoused values and values-in-action, and challenge others' incongruences.<br>*Critique*: Facilitating the acquisition of moral knowledge from a critique of everyday practice may be a neglected area in the development of expertise, since curricula in the health care professions tend to focus on the application of ethical theory to ethical dilemmas such as those around abortion and euthanasia. |
| **7. Embodied knowledge**<br>*Descriptor(s)*<br>Based on Savage's (1995) work:<br>Knowing by the body and not the mind; reinforces the unity of body and mind, the physical and the existential; non-intellectual in nature.<br>Benner and Wrubel (1989, p. 409) refer to the concept of 'embodied intelligence' – 'the body itself is a knower and interpreter'. | Benner and Wrubel (1989)<br>MacLeod (1990)<br>Lawler (1991)<br>Savage (1995)<br>Ersser (1997)<br>Titchen (2000) | The body is seen as moving with intention in a meaningful world, what Merleau-Ponty (1962) termed 'bodily intelligence'. | *Nature*: Non-propositional. Not represented in the mind.<br>*Derivation*: Derived through the senses and by being there, immersed in the world of practice.<br>*Interrelated concepts*: Background concept – embodiment: derived from the 'person as embodied' concept used in Heideggerian phenomenological philosophy. In contrast to the Cartesian notion of the body as a possession and the dualism of mind and body, the phenomenologist views being-in-the-world as 'embodied' (Leonard, 1994). It is assumed that our common practices are based on shared embodied perceptual capacities (Benner, 1985).<br>Drawing on Savage (1995), such knowledge is related to intuitive and experiential knowledge.<br>*Critique*: Savage (1995) argues that embodied knowing does not fit with Carper's (1978) taxonomy of patterns of knowing in nursing. Difficulty in making a distinction between embodied knowledge and knowledge that was once represented in the mind and has then, with time and experience, become unconscious. |
| **8. Personal knowledge**<br>*Descriptor(s)*<br>Understanding and evaluating self in context of caring for patients.<br>Self-awareness. | Carper (1978)<br>E.g. therapeutic use of self concept (Balint, 1957; Ersser, 1997; Titchen, 2000). | Polanyi (1958) | *Nature*: Non-propositional knowledge.<br>*Derivation:* Through critical reflection upon self in the context of one's own life experiences and practice.<br>*Interrelated concepts*: Intuitive knowing is an aspect of personal knowledge (Agan, 1987). Manley (1991) and Burnard (1992) consider this synonymous with experiential knowledge; i.e. one encounters oneself.<br>*Critique*: Although personal knowledge would appear to be synonymous with experiential knowledge, the latter is not dependent on the former, because it would seem possible to come to know something by direct encounter, in a way that does not require self-knowledge. |

Alternatives used in other professional contexts are also unsatisfactory. In education, 'procedural knowledge', or 'theory-in-use' (Biggs and Telfer, 1987), has been used, but, whilst appearing to be analytically useful, it does not convey the above connotations either. 'Experiential knowledge' (Heron, 1981; Kolb, 1984) is too narrow as it reflects only how the knowledge is generated. In other professional contexts, such as engineering, architecture and town planning, Schön's (1983) term 'professional artistry' comes nearer to expressing the above desired connotations, but the concept 'artistry' might be construed as the peak of practice and not as occurring in ordinary everyday work. Borrowing from education, Titchen adopted the rhetorically useful metaphor 'professional craft knowledge', used by Brown et al. (1988). Whilst recognizing that it might not be the best analytical term because of its broader focus, it seems best able to convey the above connotations and provide a container for the kinds of knowledge with which this book is concerned.

The word craft implies work in which performance is improved through experience. It also provides the connotation of aesthetics within ordinary, everyday work and gives a sense of practitioners knowing their way around their world; knowing what to do, what they are trying to achieve, and what the outcomes might be in a particular case or situation, as well as knowing how and when to do it. The term 'craft' could, however, be seen as denigrating health care professions if taken out of the context of professional knowledge as a whole. Knowledge within a craft can be conceptualized as bits and pieces of information acquired through experience, including a system of trial and error (Tom, 1984). This is counterbalanced by the terms professional and knowledge. Professionalism provides the context (with its inherent standards and accountability) in which this craft knowledge is being generated, used and critiqued. Thus it becomes professional craft knowledge that is embedded within the framework of the profession's knowledge base.

We return now to our third area of concern, i.e. the assumption that professional craft knowledge is always non-propositional in its expression.

### Expression of professional craft knowledge in a propositional form

From the foregoing review of epistemological concepts, it is apparent that professional craft knowledge bears a direct relationship to the non-propositional categories within the various typologies presented. However, professional craft knowledge can also be expressed propositionally, in the sense that, in accessing and using their professional craft knowledge in the course of their work, practitioners employ working hypotheses. These hypotheses are likely to operate when practitioners are examining, in a literal technical sense, the relationship between ends and means, or intervention and outcome in professional work. Based on Benner's (1984) and our own research (Ersser, 1997; Titchen, 2000), we argue that one way in which practitioners develop professional craft knowledge and expertise is through testing and refining propositions, hypotheses and principle-based expectations in their actions and experiences in clinical practice. It should be noted that such professional craft knowledge is distinct from propositional knowledge derived through research and scholarship because there is no attempt to generalize beyond the individual's or a group of colleagues' practice.

## Conclusion

In this chapter we have made a case for using the term 'professional craft knowledge' to encompass the epistemological concepts and their relationships that make up practical know-how or professional wisdom. We believe that questions remain regarding the defining properties of the knowledge structures, their interrelationship and how they function in the process of knowing.

We have demonstrated that contemporary accounts of non-propositional knowledge within the health care literature are problematic due to: (i) a profusion of terms which are not clearly differentiated or related to each other; (ii) the possibility that their subtlety may thus be lost; and (iii) a possible lack of recognition that professional craft knowledge is sometimes expressed propositionally. With the metaphor of professional craft knowledge as a term which captures the diverse, complex and dynamic nature of knowledge derived from practice, the way is more open to reaching some sort of consensus on terms and meanings in the health professions. Consensus should facilitate effective communication and further knowledge development. We address the above problems further in Chapter 7 by offering two analytical frameworks for the examination of professional craft knowledge.

## References


Agan, R. D. (1987) Intuitive knowing as a dimension of nursing. *Advances in Nursing Science*, **10**, 63–70.

Aldridge, D. (1991) Aesthetics and the individual in the practice of medical research: Discussion paper. *Journal of the Royal Society of Medicine*, **84**, 147–150.

Ayer, A. J. (1973) *The Central Questions of Philosophy*. Harmondsworth: Penguin.

Balint, M. (1957) *The Doctor, His Patient and the Illness*. London: Pitman.

Benner, P. (1984) *From Novice to Expert: Excellence and Power in Clinical Nursing Practice*. London: Addison-Wesley.

Benner, P. (1985) Quality of life: A phenomenological perspective on explanation, prediction and understanding in nursing science. *Advances in Nursing Science*, **8**, 1–14.

Benner, P. and Tanner, C. (1987) Clinical judgement: How expert nurses use intuition. *American Journal of Nursing*, **87**, 23–31.

Benner, P. and Wrubel, J. (1989) *The Primacy of Caring: Stress and Coping in Health and Illness*. Wokingham: Addison-Wesley.

Biggs, J. B. and Telfer, R. (1987) *The Process of Learning*, 2nd edn. Sydney: Prentice Hall.

Brown, S. and McIntyre, D. (1993) *Making Sense of Teaching*. Milton Keynes: Open University Press.

Brown, S., McIntyre, D. and McAlpine, A. (1988) The knowledge which underpins the craft of teaching. Paper presented to the Annual Meeting of the American Education Research Association, April 5–9th. Edinburgh: Scottish Council for Research in Education.

Burnard, P. (1992) Learning nursing knowledge. In *Knowledge for Nursing Practice* (K. Robinson and B. Vaughan, eds), pp. 172–186. Oxford: Butterworth-Heinemann.

Carper, B. A. (1978) Fundamental patterns of knowing. *Advances in Nursing Science*, **1**, 13–23.

Easen, P. and Wilcockson, J. (1996) Intuition and rational decision making in professional thinking: A false dichotomy? *Journal of Advanced Nursing*, **24**, 667–673.

Eisner, E. (1985) *The Art of Educational Evaluation: A Personal View*. London: The Falmer Press.

Ersser, S. J. (1997) *Nursing as a Therapeutic Activity: An Ethnography*. Aldershot: Avebury.

Fish, D. and Coles, C. (1998) *Developing Professional Judgement in Health Care: Learning Through the Critical Appreciation of Practice*. Oxford: Butterworth-Heinemann.

Fjelland, R. and Gjengdal, E. (1994) A theoretical foundation of nursing as a science. In *Interpretive Phenomenology: Embodiment, Caring and Ethics in Health and Illness* (P. Benner, ed.), pp. 3–25. Thousand Oaks, CA: Sage.

Goldman, A. H. (1988) *Moral Knowledge*. London: Routledge.

Habermas, J. (1972) *Knowledge and Human Interest*. London: Heinemann.

Heron, J. (1981) Philosophical basis for a new paradigm. In *Human Inquiry: A Source Book of New Paradigm Research* (P. Reason and J. Rowan, eds), pp. 19–35. Chichester: Wiley.

Hume, D. (1977) *Treatise of Human Nature* (Introduction by A. D. Lindsay). London: Dent.

Kant, I. (1949) *Fundamental Principles of Metaphysical Morals* (trans. T. M. Abbott). Indianapolis: Bobbs-Merrill.

Kavka, G. (1986) *Hobbesian Moral and Political Theory*. Princeton, NJ: Princeton University Press.

Kolb, D. A. (1984) *Experiential Learning: Experience as the Source of Learning and Development*. Englewood Cliffs, NJ: Prentice Hall.

Lawler, J. (1991) *Behind the Screens: Nursing, Somology and the Problem of the Body*. Edinburgh: Churchill Livingstone.

Leonard, V. W. (1994) A Heidegerrian phenomenological perspective on the concept of person. In *Interpretive Phenomenology: Embodiment, Caring and Ethics in Health and Illness* (P. Benner, ed.), pp. 43–63. Thousand Oaks, CA: Sage.

MacLeod, M. (1990) Experience in everyday nursing practice: A study of the experienced ward sister. DPhil thesis, University of Edinburgh.

Manley, K. (1991) Knowledge for nursing practice. In *Nursing: A Knowledge Base for Practice* (A. Perry and M. Jolley, eds), pp. 1–27. London: Edward Arnold.

Merleau-Ponty, M. (1962) *Phenomenology of Perception* (trans. C. Smith). London: Routledge.

Paul, R. W. and Heaslip, P. (1995) Critical thinking and intuitive nursing practice. *Journal of Advanced Nursing*, **22**, 40–47.

Polanyi, M. (1958) *Personal Knowledge: Towards a Post-Critical Philosophy*. London: Routledge & Kegan Paul.

Rawnsley, M. M. (1998) Ontology, epistemology and methodology: A clarification. *Nursing Science Quarterly*, **11**, 2–4.

Ryle, G. (1949) *The Concept of Mind*. Harmondsworth: Peregrine.

Russell, B. (1980) *The Problems of Knowledge*. Oxford: Oxford University Press.

Savage, J. (1995) *Nursing Intimacy: An Ethnographic Approach to Nurse-Patient Interaction*. London: Scutari Press.

Schön, D. A. (1983) *The Reflective Practitioner: How Professionals Think in Action*. London: Temple Smith.

Street, A. F. (1992) *Inside Nursing: A Critical Ethnography of Clinical Nursing Practice*. Albany: State University of New York Press.

Titchen, A. (2000) *Professional Craft Knowledge in Patient-Centred Nursing and the Facilitation of its Development* (DPhil thesis, University of Oxford). Oxford: Ashdale Press.

Tom, A. R. (1984) *Teaching as a Moral Craft*. London: Longman.

Vaughan, B. (1992) The nature of nursing knowledge. In *Knowledge for Nursing Practice* (K. Robinson and B. Vaughan, eds), pp. 3–19. Oxford: Butterworth-Heinemann.

# 6

# Professionalization and professional craft knowledge

**Barbara Richardson**

It is salutary to remember that professions are structures of privilege. They are socially sanctioned through an interaction of political and economic power with public consensus and there are no minimal conditions for them (Popkewitz, 1994). A profession is regarded as a special kind of occupation that embodies a promise of service to the community and has sustained a dominant position in the labour market (Wolinsky, 1993). It is autonomous and self-directing, whereas an occupation does not have a capacity to organize for collective validation or control of work practices and is governed and controlled by others (Collins, 1990). A profession stands as the most reliable authority and source of knowledge about the nature of the reality it deals with and assumes a cloak of extreme trustworthiness to society (Popkewitz, 1994). Many occupations strive to become professions, and their members adopt the manner of professionals in the conduct and organization of their work in a dynamic process of professionalization, in which they seek the crucial characteristics recognized of a profession (Volmer and Mills, 1966). This chapter examines the nature of professionalization in the emerging health professions and considers what happens to knowledge in the attempts made to transform from an occupation to a profession. The focus of the chapter is on the health professions. The key arguments, however, transcend professional boundaries.

## Becoming a profession

The move from an occupation to a profession is determined by both a service ideal and the extent of autonomy from government regulation (Friedson, 1970, cited in Palmer and Short, 1994). Autonomy in professional practice is achieved through a gradual acceptance of educational requirements, licensing procedures, codes of ethics, and peer control generated through the formation of professional associations. It is thought that within any labour segment only one occupation may achieve such organized autonomy (Friedson, 1970, cited in Wolinsky, 1993) and in health care this was traditionally granted to medicine (Palmer and Short, 1994). Other occupational groups, such as occupational therapy, physiotherapy, speech and language therapy, and nursing, are regarded by some as semi-professions because they do not have so much control over their affairs. These non-medical health professions aspire to the levels of autonomy, pay and status of the medical profession and have attempted to emulate medicine by claiming privileges of professional reward based on organization into professional associations, an autonomous expertise, and specialized knowledge (Palmer and Short, 1994).

A specialized body of knowledge in itself may be insufficient to gain the prestige and reward of a profession, as witnessed by the comparatively undifferentiated status of engineers and mechanics, who provide invaluable services to society (Collins, 1990). The extent of the education necessary to learn professional skills and the regulation of the supply of skilled practitioners are important factors in creating the status of elitism and the mystery of the knowledge base of professional services (Collins, 1990). Professional knowledge is socially organized and controlled through a university system of education which historically has sharply distinguished facts from values in an embodiment of positivism (Sullivan, 1994) and which gives access to 'wider bases of social power' (Johnston, 1972, in Palmer and Short, 1994). Traditionally, gentlemen of independent means have accessed the learned professions of medicine, divinity and law (Palmer and Short, 1994) and the resulting hierarchy of social class background and (male) gender in gaining the leading jobs has determined the organization and structure of the health services and society generally. Many fledgling, and often predominantly female, health professionals such as occupational therapists, nurses and physiotherapists became 'hand maidens of the doctors' (Palmer and Short, 1994, p. 162) in order to receive their patronage and seek a professional status through medicine. Until comparatively recently, this medical dominance of most allied health care occupations effectively subjected them to close supervision and work under medical prescription (Friedson, 1975, cited in Larkin, 1993), which involved a subservience and obedience to the positivist medical model of health care (Miles-Tapping, 1985). The knowledge base and professionalization of the allied health professions and nursing has been strongly influenced by this medical model framework and also by statutory registration. Registration has led to 'uniform standards of professional practice, improved career mobility for health professionals and more comprehensive, reliable data about these occupational groups for the purpose of workforce evaluation and planning' (Palmer and Short, 1994, p. 135). The scientific, positivistic framework has resulted in a neglect of development of the professions' individual bodies of professional craft knowledge, with such knowledge being regarded as 'pre-knowledge' in a setting which recognizes only propositional (or science/theory-generated) knowledge.

## Professionalization and professional craft knowledge

Professional craft knowledge arises from an awareness of cues from the physical, geographical and chronological location of a health care event, which, together with expectations of the patient and others, define or situate action. In professional practice, the propositional knowledge contained in learned texts is integrated with the procedural knowledge of direct application of techniques and approaches in health care interventions, into knowledge which is unique to a profession through an interpretation of professional purpose in a specific health setting. The experiential knowledge gained from practical doing is an integral part of professional knowledge (Richardson, 1999), which leads to a 'know-how' of the situation (Schön, 1991).

An interplay between the cognitive understandings of practice of individuals in a professional group and their tacit acceptance of certain values and assumptions in day-to-day and minute-to-minute social exchanges will influence the ways in which they apply their knowledge to patients and to their interactions with others in health care. The cognitive, conative and affective behaviour of professionals will be defined in a typical way which is identified with the professional group, for example medicine, social work or physiotherapy (Greenwood, 1966), and will strongly influence the development of their professional craft knowledge. Pursuit of professionalization through a continual refinement of practice will be enacted at both occupational and individual levels in the transition from occupation to profession. The socialization of a group's members to the level of professional status achieved and desired and to the contexts in which the profession operates will manifest itself through the tacit and informal modes of communication of the professional culture.

A professional culture of accepted codes of practice in the workplace will sanction and normalize the professional behaviour within the social group in which the self becomes embedded (Popkewitz, 1994). The emerging health professions facilitated their earlier attempts at professionalization by embracing a positivist knowledge base at the expense of acknowledgement of their professional craft knowledge. This masculinization of knowledge resulted in a greater value being placed upon the propositional, science knowledge and technical rationality of the medical profession than upon the practical rationality (Sullivan, 1994, p. 171) of health care, which became unspoken through the process. Cant and Higgs (1999) suggest that some health care professions, particularly nursing and occupational therapy, have largely reversed this early trend through widespread rejection of the medical model and through a research focus on people-centred, holistic health care and a greater focus on wellness models of health and health care.

A normative model of professionalization in which characteristics of professions are considered to be externally imposed upon occupations has predominated over a symbolic interactionist view of 'situational flexibility and self-creation of identities' (Collins, 1990, p. 13) in which a symbiotic relationship between professional craft knowledge and professional practice expertise is seen to be generated from the social and professional practices within the profession. Today much of health care work is centred on the management of chronic disability that is not amenable to cure (Levine, 1993) and that does not fit with a medical model of care. Changes in health policy and practice (e.g. a greater emphasis on prevention and health, rather than on cure and illness) now offer an increasing opportunity for the full potential of practical rationality. Practical reasoning in health care is made explicit through 'restoring human lives with histories, needs, fears and purposes' rather than through treating technical problems (Sullivan, 1994, p. 186).

## The changing focus of health care knowledge

Major redefinitions of health care now aim for health promotion and client-focused rehabilitation which enables a satisfactory level of well-being and quality of life for individuals with chronic disease. An ethos of the primacy of the user and the enabling function of health care workers is underpinned by a concept of empowering and enabling people to assume responsibility for their health. A health promotion approach is more realistic for health maintenance, longitudinal care, and education for self-care management to enhance quality of life and functional performance (Inui et al., 1998) than therapeutic interventions which aim for short-term changes in clinical signs. In many countries where there has been a crucial shift of the management of health care to self-governing health care trusts and primary care trusts, it is increasingly questioned whether health care outcomes emphasizing collaborative client-centred practice and a paradigm of teamwork fit with an economic rationalization approach (Hensel and Dickey, 1998) and the professional–patient relationship orientation of traditional professional work. The modes of practice which were acceptable in a predominantly acute care setting under medical patronage are now being challenged by a competitive provider-and-purchaser health care market that is governed by the needs of the clients and controlled by allocation of resources.

If health care professionals work only from a scientific knowledge base then their perception of the problems of their practice, the methods they use to solve these problems and the criteria they use to evaluate progress will focus only on prevention of disease and objectively measurable outcomes of interventions. This approach may have little relevance to the needs of clients of health care who wish to manage their quality of life and health in their own homes. Modes of care that focus on enhancing health and assessing health outcomes in people-oriented ways are needed. As Fulford (1996, p. 1) argues, 'the movement towards patient-centred health care is now well established'; for the foreseeable future, demands for health care will continually change as the needs of the community and individuals within it become more defined and local purchasers of health care services come to new ways of interpreting health care and refining their services.

Policies of skill mix and reallocation of tasks aim to ensure a more equitable use of labour and to provide cost-effective care in a 'contract culture' which embodies expectations of professional accountability, evidence-based practice, team working and a quality of care. Such policies encourage partnerships and dialogue that stress the practical nature and responsibility of doing, and the need to strengthen an informed synthesis of professional thinking with ethical concern (Sullivan, 1994) in dealing with individuals and their lives. The current climate of health care thus favours a rediscovery of practical reasoning that is more intuitive, aware and responsive to assessment of individual needs. The wise professional judgments which define the expert practitioner are based on professional craft knowledge, which is drawn from the experiential knowledge of how to go about health care in particular contexts. Competence has been defined as a combination of attributes such as the knowledge, abilities, skills and attitudes underlying specific aspects of successful professional performance (Gonczi et al., 1990, in Palmer and Short, 1994). However, expertise requires more than technical competence. Expertise can only be achieved in embodied, practically engaged know-how; it cannot be reduced to specified rules and procedures, because experts operate holistically (Sullivan, 1994).

## Development of professional craft knowledge today

The value of treatments which do not follow a medical model of care can no longer be denied. Current health care policies demand a broader notion of professional knowledge to match the different approaches to care needed to accomplish an ambulatory health care mission (Inui et al., 1998). Diverse sources of reflective, tacit and interpretive knowledge are needed in a professional knowledge base, which will underpin the range of skills needed by practitioners to achieve expertise in the heterogeneous settings of health care today. There is an opportunity to reaffirm the unambiguous specialist knowledge and expertise of individual professions, but the maintenance of independent lifestyles and improvement in the quality of life and health of individuals requires participation in teamwork. Collaboration of professional ideas in task-centred care through team working can be seen as an attempt to break down professional boundaries. As Bordage et al. (1998) point out, there is a crucial need to develop process knowledge of ways in which individual practitioner creativity is harnessed to solve individual client problems within the context of working in a multidisciplinary team. This will ensure that development within these contexts avoids a disruption of professional knowledge building, which will ultimately weaken or limit the evolution of the profession's knowledge base.

In the past there has been a lack of articulation of professional knowledge in education programmes for the emerging health professions, and a few well-defined models of practice have been presented as the totality of their professional knowledge. An incomplete understanding of the knowledge gained from practice has been left largely unchallenged in an uncritical culture. Professional craft knowledge becomes elaborated through a cycle in which problems of practice are acknowledged to test the adequacy of the theory underlying practice and models of practice. Working within a positivist paradigm has limited reflection by the allied health professions on the nature of their practice and the underlying professional knowledge base, and has limited the modification and articulation of theory which will continually challenge and question the underlying epistemology of practice (van Gigch and Pipino, 1986). Further development of the knowledge base of these professions requires reflection on practice and its theoretical and epistemological basis.

The positivist medical model of professional expertise is based on a technical rationality which depends upon a prior agreement about 'ends' (Sullivan, 1994, p. 168). It ignores the problem-setting aspects of actual experience and the more feminine characteristics of intuition and caring, which are relevant to a social model of health care. Many general practitioners who are expected to take a lead in the new approaches to health care are lacking in management skills and are still operating within the disease orientation of the medical model (May and Robinson, 1995). Different knowledge bases can be used to identify clinical problems and to generate relevant methods of practice to solve them. As it becomes more incumbent upon individual professions to ensure that they maintain a high profile within local scenarios of health care, the emerging health professions may no longer wish to rely on the paternalistic patronage of the medical profession but rather may want to declare the contribution of their practice drawn from their own professional craft knowledge base.

## Deprofessionalization and the future of professional craft knowledge

In any health care profession, deprofessionalization can occur through loss of prestige and trust or an erosion of special knowledge (Haug, 1973, in Wolinsky, 1993). It can also occur through intent. In Australia and Sweden, for instance, nurses have recognized the potency of research knowledge as a source of power which can develop and legitimize their professional craft knowledge (Elzinga, 1990). They have abandoned professionalism for trade unionism as a means of being heard, and this has resulted in significant moves of nursing education from hospital to university settings. Increasing educational levels in the general population are making medicine less mysterious and more open to challenge, while an increasing medical specialization in some aspects of 'hi-tech' health care has created a dependency on other colleagues such as engineering experts (Haug, 1973, in Wolinsky, 1993). The changing status of medical practitioners and the move away from the handmaiden image by nurses and the allied health professions have combined to effect a general diminishing of the authority of medicine. As stated by Haug (1973, in Wolinsky, 1993, p. 15), the 'authority-based superordinate role of physicians vis-à-vis patients no longer holds as widely'. An unquestioning adherence to the medical model is challenged as the value of other types of knowledge is recognized. Deprofessionalization can be identified in a range of developments today, which include the growing power of a more sophisticated public and the influence of women, minorities and consumer groups (Levine, 1993), but all professions work under public scrutiny and all can be susceptible to changes in status.

Deprofessionalization strategies germane to the health professions can also be identified in government regulatory policies. A shift in political influence and technology within and between occupations can be influenced by the extent of service provision or access to it through education and health care financing policies. Such a shift can be witnessed in contemporary tensions being played out between opposing professional clinical specialists in medicine, nursing and physiotherapy in some accident and emergency departments, rheumatology clinics and community health units. A move to establish competency standards at occupational and industrial levels and their application to vocational education and training in Australia and Britain (Mitchell et al., 1998) may further threaten an autonomy of practice for some emerging health professions. There is increased pressure for universities to fill seats, but an 'attention to the most easily described and measured competency standards, particularly for professional practice, may result in a lack of attention to the less tangible but nevertheless highly valued outcomes of higher education' (Palmer and Short, 1994, p. 138) and lead to increases in numbers of therapists, to the extent that the value of their work is diminished by a surplus of less able workers.

Despite health services management comprising only about 3 per cent of the health workforce, that field exercises a degree of influence over the operations of the health care system that is significantly greater than its relatively small size might suggest (Palmer and Short, 1994). The power of health administrators is increasing (Palmer and Short, 1994) and is manifest, for instance, in an increasing reliance on competency standards. These standards can be used to change perspectives on the knowledge bases of professional work and the identification of problems and problem-solving strategies. However, within the broad agenda of professional education competency standards may simply underpin a move towards reprofiling health care tasks to professional or occupational groups with lower (and less expensive) levels of expertise. Data suggest that less than 37 per cent of practitioners of the professions allied to medicine feel that they are able to provide a satisfactory service (Chartered Society of Physiotherapy, 1995).

The paradox which exists between academic and practical knowledge cannot be ignored. The academic knowledge base that creates a profession can also lead to its downfall. This may be particularly true now for many of the emerging health professions who have accepted the patronage of medicine and an associated positivist knowledge base. For some professions, such as physiotherapy and podiatry, private practice can give greater recognition of individual expertise and greater potential for developing professional craft knowledge. A trend for masculinization within these professions and for more male entrants to migrate to higher paid jobs in the most lucrative areas of private practice, such as sports medicine and spinal manipulation (Palmer and Short, 1994), may also foster professionalization by offering and defining a valued service to the community. However, these trends may equally work against increasing a professional craft knowledge base if they are not coordinated with systematic research to further explore its scope and development.

## Conclusions

The initial role accepted by the professions allied to medicine of the subordinate and ancillary handmaidens of medicine, was typically shaped by passivity, subservience and the selfless devotion of the middle-class feminine professions (Turnbull, 1994) in the late nineteenth and early twentieth centuries. Now, definitions of health care have changed and the move to primary care is offering significant changes in the role and dominance of health care professions. There is a growing influence of women and consumer groups, who recognize the more humane issues of nurture, care and support (Sidell, 1995). A move from role-focused to task-centred working will provide an opportunity for recognition of individual practitioners' creative efforts and of the practical expertise of individual professions. Physiotherapists, for example, can claim to be the most reliable authority on mobility needs for independent living, which clearly does not fall within medical jurisdiction. However, the challenge is now to consider the ethics of professional practice and the need to engage in moral and civic purposes (Sullivan, 1994) as befits mature professions. Without a strong culture of reflective expert practice, the development and dissemination of expert professional craft knowledge, which is essential to that process, will be inhibited (Sullivan, 1994). Professions will flourish only if their decision-making is open to inspection and evaluation (Friedson, 1990). The development and debate of the professional craft knowledge base of practice is the key to the future of professionalization, which will ensure the effectiveness of each health care profession.

## References


Bordage, G., Burack, J. H., Irby, D. M. and Stritter, F. T. (1998) Education in ambulatory settings: Developing valid measures of educational outcomes and other research priorities. *Academic Medicine*, **73**(7), 743–750.

Cant, R. and Higgs, J. (1999) Professional socialisation. In *Educating Beginning Practitioners: Challenges for Health Professional Education* (J. Higgs and H. Edwards, eds), pp. 46–51. Oxford: Butterworth-Heinemann.

Chartered Society of Physiotherapy (1995) *Professional Allied to Medicine and Related Grades of Staff PT 'A' Council, Staff Side Evidence*. London: Chartered Society of Physiotherapy.

Collins, R. (1990) Changing conceptions in the sociology of the professions. In *The Formation of Profession, Knowledge, State and Strategy* (R. Torstendahl and M. Burage, eds), pp. 11–23. London: Sage Publications.

Elzinga, A. (1990) The knowledge aspect of professionalization: The case of science-based nursing education in Sweden. In *The Formation of Profession, Knowledge, State and Strategy* (R. Torstendahl and M. Burage, eds), pp. 151–173. London: Sage Publications.

Friedson, E. (1990) Centrality of professionalism to health care. *Jummetrics Journal*, **30**(4), 431–445.

Fulford, K. W. M. (1996) Concepts of disease and the meaning of patient-centred care. In *Essential Practice in Patient-Centred Care* (K. W. M. Fulford, S. Ersser and T. Hope, eds), pp. 1–16. Oxford: Blackwell Science.

Greenwood, E. (1966) Elements of professionalization. In *Professionalization* (H. M. Vollmer and D. C. Mills, eds), pp. 15–19. Englewood Cliffs, NJ: Prentice Hall.

Hensel, W. A. and Dickey, N. W. (1998) Teaching professionalism: Passing the torch. *Academic Medicine*, **73**(8), 865–870.

Inui, T. S., Williams, W. T., Goode, L. et al. (1998) Sustaining the development of primary care in academic medicine. *Academic Medicine*, **73**(3), 245–257.

Larkin, G. V. (1993) Continuity in change: Medical dominance in the United Kingdom. In *The Changing Medical Profession, an International Perspective* (F. W. Hafferty and J. B. McKinlay, eds), pp. 81–91. Oxford: Oxford University Press.

Levine, S. (1993) Some problematic aspects of medicine's changing status. In *The Changing Medical Profession, an International Perspective* (F. W. Hafferty and J. B. McKinlay, eds), pp. 197–208. Oxford: Oxford University Press.

May, A. and Robinson, R. (1995) Mapping the Course. *Health Service Journal*, **105**(5442), 22–24.

Miles-Tapping, C. (1985) Physiotherapy and medicine: Dominance and control? *Physiotherapy Canada*, **37**(5), 289–307.

Mitchell, L., Harvey, T. and Rolls, L. (1998) Interprofessional standards for the care sector – history and challenges. *Journal of Interprofessional Care*, **12**(2), 157–168.

Palmer, G. R. and Short, S. D. (1994) The health workforce. In *Health Care and Public Policy* (G. R. Palmer and S. D. Short, eds), pp. 134–177. South Melbourne: Macmillan Education Australia.

Popkewitz, T. S. (1994) Professionalization in teaching and teacher education: Some notes on its history, ideology and potential. *Teaching and Teacher Education*, **10**(1), 1–14.

Richardson, B. (1999) Professional socialisation and professionalisation. *Physiotherapy*, **85**(9), 461–467.

Schön, D. A. (1991) *The Reflective Practitioner*. London: Temple Smith.

Sidell, M. (1995) *Health in Old Age*. Buckingham: Open University Press.

Sullivan, W. M. (1994) *Work and Integrity*, pp. 159–190. New York: Harper Business.

Turnbull, G. I. (1994) Dialogue, educating tomorrow's colleagues: The physiotherapist in the university system. *Physiotherapy Canada*, **46**(1), 9–14.

van Gigch, J. P. and Pipino, L. L. (1986) In search of a paradigm for the discipline of information systems. *Future Computing Systems*, **1**(1), 71–91.

Volmer, H. M. and Mills, D. L. (eds) (1966) Editor introduction. In *Professionalization* (H. M. Volmer and D. L. Mills, eds), pp. i–ix. Englewood Cliffs, NJ: Prentice Hall.

Wolinsky, F. D. (1993) The professional dominance, deprofessionalization, proletarianization, and corporatization perspectives: An overview and synthesis. In *The Changing Medical Profession, an International Perspective* (F. W. Hafferty and J. B. McKinlay, eds), pp. 11–24. Oxford: Oxford University Press.

# 7

# Explicating, creating and validating professional craft knowledge

**Angie Titchen and Steven J. Ersser**

## Introduction

So far in this book, the key role of professional craft knowledge in the development of expertise has been stated. Such knowledge is an important source of evidence for use in effective clinical decision-making, alongside research-based evidence and patients' experiences. However, its often tacit nature and the difficulty that experts can have in bringing this kind of knowledge to the surface make it less available for acquisition by less experienced practitioners, or for convincing colleagues that they need to act quickly before empirical evidence is available to warrant action (cf. Benner, 1984). If we use the metaphor of an iceberg to describe the current explication (i.e. articulation and analysis) of professional craft knowledge, only the tip of the iceberg is available for critical, public scrutiny and for its acquisition by others in their development of expertise. This chapter focuses, therefore, on how more of the iceberg can be revealed, better understood and communicated by practitioners, educators and researchers. This is important because learners need to be able to access professional craft knowledge so that they can develop expertise. Practitioners, educators and researchers need to be able to make this knowledge available to learners. In addition, practitioners need to be able to explicate their professional craft knowledge so that they can justify the need for colleagues to act in a particular case, regulate their own practice through critical review of their whole professional knowledge base, and contribute to generating knowledge of the field by engaging in critique, debate, contestation and validation of professional craft knowledge with other practitioners, practitioner-researchers and researchers.

The chapter continues the analysis of professional craft knowledge begun in Chapter 5. There we examined relevant epistemological concepts and typologies presented in the health care literature. Here we show how professional craft knowledge can be:

- Analysed using two analytical frameworks.
- Articulated, critically reviewed, generated and validated by individual practitioners and their peers through critical reflection on practice. There is no attempt to generalize beyond the individual's or group's practice.
- Disseminated by a group and then critiqued, debated and validated consensually with another group. Like ripples caused by throwing a stone into a still pool, an ever-widening group of professionals responds to the explicated knowledge, which is transformed as it moves outwards, again through the processes of critique, debate and consensual validation. As the ripples increase in size and the processes are conducted rigorously and systematically, the explicated knowledge becomes potentially transferable to other settings and patient populations, if rich descriptions of the practices and contexts are provided.

Making professional craft knowledge more available in the above ways relates to a tradition in critical social science, where knowledge can be generated through group debate and critique by expert practitioners. Some of this professional craft knowledge may be slowly transformed into propositional knowledge, if it can be expressed propositionally in the first place, whilst the rest will be made more available in some other form (discussed later in this chapter). Researchers, using more conventional empirical research approaches, may also attempt this transformation by accessing it at any point within the ripples of the pool. A variety of procedures may then be undertaken to strengthen the generalizability of this knowledge beyond the study settings. Discussion of such procedures is, however, beyond the scope of this chapter.

In this chapter, we offer a strategy through which professional craft knowledge can be made more explicit and available to others through analysis and consensual validation:

- for practitioners to help them develop their own and others' expertise and to generate clinical knowledge;
- for educators to help them understand how an expert's professional craft knowledge can be accessed and share that understanding with their students;
- for practitioner-researchers and outsider researchers to help them develop appropriate research methods for accessing practitioners' embedded knowledge.

We offer the strategy with full awareness that much of the body of professional craft knowledge (the 'iceberg') cannot be expressed in words or in formal propositional statements. We propose that there are other avenues for expressing the ineffable, such as the creative arts (see Higgs and Titchen, 2001), but do not explore them here.

## A developmental strategy for making professional craft knowledge more explicit

The strategy consists of analysing practice knowledge (i.e. both propositional and professional craft knowledge) and then articulating, sharing, critically reviewing, creating and validating professional craft knowledge (expressed in both propositional and non-propositional forms). These processes are not necessarily sequential or mutually exclusive. For example, the process of sharing and critically reviewing professional craft knowledge often results in the creation or refinement of such knowledge and validation by others.

The values underpinning the strategy are:

- Critical exploration of an individual's or a group's knowledge is important because knowledge can only be viewed as knowledge if understanding gained from experience or from learned theory is tested.
- There is value in, and need for, the knowledge used by an individual or a group to be critiqued by self/selves and made available to the field for further critique and for informed use by others.
- Professionals are responsible for generating knowledge and contributing knowledge of the field.

### Analysing practice knowledge

As argued in Chapter 5, the analysis of practice knowledge is a key activity for practitioners and educators as well as for researchers and scholars, because if we understand how different types of practice knowledge are derived or generated, then we are likely to be better able to access them in others. We will be able to talk about these types of knowledge in a systematic way, so as to develop an epistemology for practice that better represents experts' knowledge. Furthermore, health professionals are increasingly exposed to studies of practitioners' professional craft knowledge, but very little work has been undertaken to develop frameworks to analyse them. Without such frameworks, it is difficult for professionals fully to:

- examine the knowledge that underpins expert practice – either their own or others;
- critique and evaluate their practice in terms of their whole practice knowledge base as they develop expertise;
- acquire and create craft knowledge consciously from their practice;
- develop shared understandings with colleagues about their professional craft knowledge;
- begin to develop potentially transferable clinical knowledge with other expert practitioners.

Building on Chapter 5, we offer two analytical frameworks (albeit ones that are still in the developmental stage) that could be used to help health professionals examine and evaluate accounts of professional craft knowledge derived from reflections explored, for example, in clinical supervision or research studies.

**Table 7.1 Analytical framework for examining professional craft knowledge. Adapted from Titchen (2000)**

**Characteristics**

- Discourse of the particular.
- Highly specific and situated.
- Contextual, relational, interpretive.
- Taken-for-granted, considered commonplace and not worth mentioning.
- Invisible because it is tacit, embedded in clinical practice and difficult to articulate fully (so that it can never be made completely formal, explicit, general and objective).

It may also be:

- Intuitive.
- Embodied (known by the body and not the mind).
- Perceptual.
- Invisible because people do not want to talk about it (because of taboo).
- A process of encountering in which there is mutual respect for the other.
- An involvement of feelings and commitment and integrity.
- Propositional in expression.

**Focus**

Focus may be on the:

- Personal (in relation to self in the context of practice).
- Interpersonal.
- Aesthetic.
- Ethical.
- Practical.

**Generation**

- Personal knowledge of self-and-other constructed through reflection, synthesis of perceptions, and connecting with what is known.
- Practical knowledge derived through practice.
- Knowing-in-practice derived through practice and through the transformation of theoretical knowledge.
- Critical dialogue with practice experiences.
- Acquisition may be unconscious or deliberate.
- Creation of professional craft knowledge cannot be separated from acquiring, learning and using it.

**Philosophical concern**

Professional craft knowledge can be described from different philosophical perspectives – as having an epistemological concern (i.e. a concern with cognitive knowledge that is represented in the mind) and/or an ontological concern (i.e. a concern with the non-cognitive, embodied knowing of being human and being-in-the-world). Both concerns have cultural and existential dimensions.

*Epistemological concern*

- Cultural knowledge (norms or ways of thinking and behaving and rules of conduct – held in the mind, but often not verbalized.
- Existential knowledge (conscious 'lived experience').

*Ontological concern*

- Cultural knowing (non-verbalized shared meanings in shared background practices which give shape to social life).
- Existential knowing (being, or non-cognitive immersion in the everyday world).

It is important to recognize that the cultural and existential dimensions of each concern are not distinctive; one is likely to imbue the other. For example, within cultural norms, there may be shared meanings in shared background practices and vice versa, and within existential knowledge the conscious and unconscious may coexist.

Concrete examples of these philosophical concerns and dimensions are given in the text in relation to ways in which beginning practitioners can acquire the professional craft knowledge of using the body in patient care.

### *Two analytical frameworks*

The nature of craft knowledge can be examined from four aspects: characteristics, focus, generation and philosophical concern (see Table 7.1).

The current health care literature outlines a number of complex relationships between epistemological concepts used to portray professional craft knowledge (see Chapter 5). We suggest that the key differentiating feature between the different types of professional craft knowledge is the way in which they are generated, which is, in turn, influenced by whether there is an ontological or epistemological concern. By understanding how such knowledge is derived and its associated philosophical concern, we will know where to look for it and how to access it in others.

For example, if beginning practitioners wish to acquire aesthetic knowledge that is derived through the senses and located in the body rather than the mind (professional craft knowledge with an ontological concern), then they would focus on the senses and the wisdom of the body. Within this example, if they wanted to learn how to create a healing environment through their own comportment, then they must become more aware of how their own bodies are behaving, being and perceiving, as they go about their everyday work; and they must compare that with experts' bodies and comportment in similar situations. They might observe and question expert practitioners. That is, they would try to raise experts' consciousness of the wisdom in their own bodies (embodied knowing). They would help them to articulate the cultural and existential knowing (see Table 7.1) that they share with other experts, but which they never explicate to each other because they do not need to. It is so obvious and ordinary to them that it is transparent and not worth mentioning 'because everyone knows that'. The beginning practitioner facilitates this articulation by pointing out specific behaviours, postures, pacing and so on, and questioning the expert about it (Titchen, 2000; see Table 7.2).

They might also ask experts to share what they know about how they use their bodies in relation to specific instances. As this kind of professional craft knowledge has an epistemological concern (because it is represented in the expert's mind), the beginning practitioner seeks to enter into the expert's inner world of consciousness. The expert might reveal the cultural knowledge or norms of expert nurses about use of their bodies in patient care, and/or their existential knowledge (see Table 7.1) about consciously using their bodies in certain ways, such as intentionally keeping still in order to convey to a patient their focused attention, or deliberately pacing their speech patterns and body movements to energize or calm patients. By accessing knowledge with both ontological and epistemological concerns, less experienced practitioners would be able to identify their own learning needs (by comparing their practice with that of the expert) and to test out this new knowledge in their own practice. Merely asking expert practitioners what it is they do, without having observed them in action and asked specific questions about what has been noticed, the beginning practitioner is less likely to access in-depth professional craft knowledge. Put very simply, the beginning practitioner must ask what seem to be 'stupid' questions about the observation, to help experts to state the obvious and to get at their taken-for-granted or unconscious professional craft knowledge, perhaps similar in a way to the 'why' questions of small children.

**Table 7.2 Guidelines for helping experienced practitioners to articulate their professional craft knowledge. Adapted from McAlpine et al. (1988)**

After observing the experienced practitioner in the clinical setting, an opportunity is sought to talk with the practitioner, as soon as possible after the observation, using the following guidelines:

- Focus questions to the practitioner on the events just observed.
- Avoid framing questions in a generalized form.
- Concentrate on what has gone well during the observation period and avoid adverse criticism of the practitioner.
- Aim to probe and find out what the practitioner has done in achieving success.
- Enquire about how the practitioner made various judgments.
- Phrase questions in open rather than closed ways.
- Be supportive and willing to accept the practitioner's responses.
- Allow plenty of time for the practitioner to respond to questions.

Figure 7.1 shows how the epistemological concepts relate in terms of both the way in which the knowledge is generated and the philosophical concern.

The figure shows how the different types of professional craft knowledge are created and how the umbrella terms 'practical knowledge' and 'knowing-in-practice' are informed by the other types of knowledge. These other types of knowledge appear to be prerequisites for practical knowledge and knowing-in-practice. Titchen's (2000) research indicates that these two umbrella terms encompass knowing how to use, synchronize and interplay the different types of knowledge and how to transform generalizable propositional knowledge for use in the particular case. The metaphor of professional craft knowledge holds all these concepts usefully together, not analytically but connotatively. The connotation of the term conveys the practical know-how, know-what, know-where and know-when involved in the complex process of simultaneously learning-using-creating professional craft knowledge, a process also described by Eraut (1994).

## The frameworks in use

Ersser (1997) undertook an interpretative study of the therapeutic effect of nursing, based on diary and interview accounts of nurses and patients, focusing on the relationship between nursing action and its consequences for patients. The aim was to examine the therapeutic nature of nursing by trying to access rarely explicated cultural knowledge, employing ethnographic research methods. Cultural knowledge, derived through socialization, is shared by social groups and gives shape to social life and action. It is by nature tacit because it reflects what are often taken-for-granted cultural rules. The study highlighted nurses' beliefs in the therapeutic significance of the interplay between the nurse's expressive-personal (presentational and relating) actions, such as the use of gesture and timing employed in everyday nursing encounters, and those technical-instrumental actions (specific actions), such as helping a person to bathe or eat. An interpretive research strategy was used to reveal beliefs about embedded concepts and propositions that link nursing action to

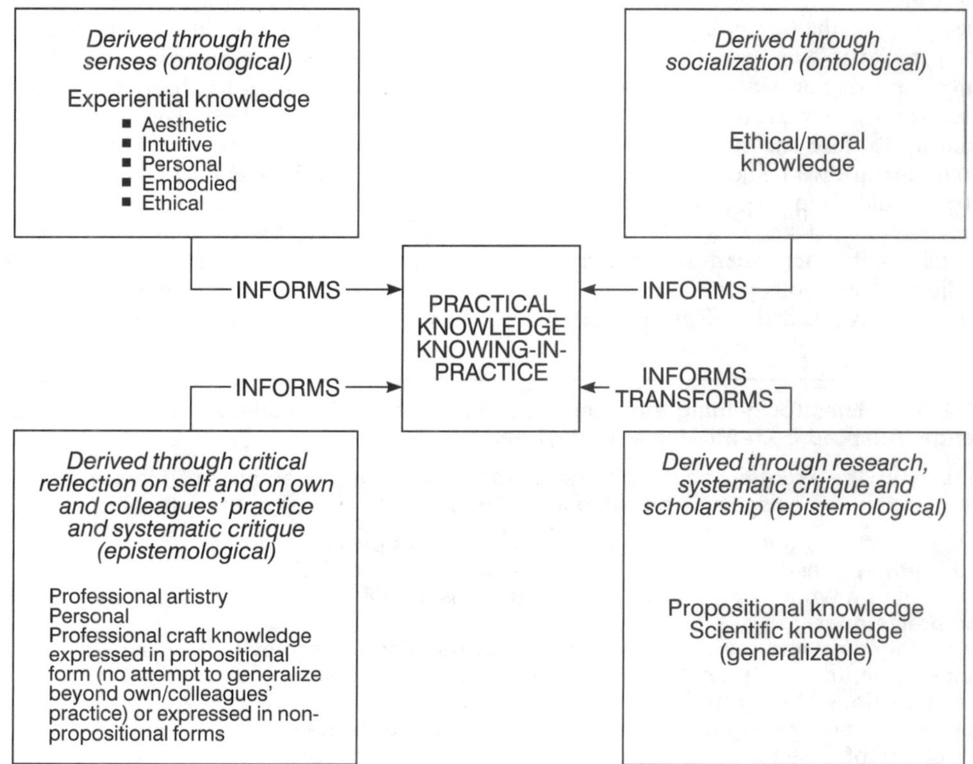


**Figure 7.1** Relationships between epistemological concepts used in the health care literature

patient outcome. In doing so, an attempt was made to identify therapeutic factors that may have been overlooked in established theorized accounts of nursing. It became evident during the research process that ethnographic techniques could help to stimulate critical reflection by individuals and groups. The accounts reveal the nurses' cultural knowing-in-practice, depicting the subtle and artistic ways in which they integrate their knowledge of self and that derived from experience, with knowledge of a moral and scientific nature.

Titchen (2000) developed a methodology designed to uncover both the epistemological and ontological dimensions of the professional craft knowledge embedded in the practice of a nurse who was expert in patient-centred nursing. She explored how this expert acquired, used and created this knowledge. The nature of professional craft knowledge, as summarized in Table 7.1, was found to be supported when Titchen examined the expert's knowledge. In addition, new insights and understandings about the professional craft knowledge used in patient-centred health care and in facilitating learning from clinical practice were gained (see Chapters 9 and 10). Another key finding is that this knowledge can be acquired and created, not only through experience, but also through the educational strategy of critical companionship.

'Critical companionship' accepts the premise that the epistemological dimension of craft knowledge can be seen to be constructed, rather than discovered. The research has indicated that making the cognitions of an expert patient-centred nurse or facilitator of learning accessible to less experienced nurses gives them the opportunity to create unique constructions or interpretations of their own experiences. In addition, what is being learned and the relationships between elements of such knowledge are tested and refined, both against the nurse's own prior knowledge and experience, and also against external knowledge (including the professional craft knowledge of others and research-based and theoretical knowledge). Revealing the ontological dimension of craft knowledge through interpretation provides similar opportunities. Critical companions help nurses to personalize ideas and to self-direct the creation and testing of new craft knowledge through metacognition and deliberative reflection upon, and theorization of, their practice. Thus through scrutiny by others, reflection, concrete experience and active experimentation, nurses demonstrate the validity of their craft knowledge in a particular situation.

(Titchen, 2000, p. 166)

Reflective practitioner accounts, such as those from the *Journal of Clinical Nursing*, can be examined using the two analytical frameworks. The following examples illustrate this:

1 Miller (1992, p. 296) was shocked to discover that 'despite being saturated with the theory of patient-centred care, I found that I had actually been practising task-centred nursing, the theory of which I condemned as an anathema'. Miller gained this personal knowledge through critical reflection.
2 Wade (1992, p. 295) found, through taking oral histories of older women, that they have the capacity to be active participants in their care and 'have a role to play in helping nurses to develop age-appropriate practice'. Wade appeared to be creating ethical knowledge through critical reflection on experience and the literature. This knowledge enabled her to defy established passive stereotypes of older women. She also created and expressed professional craft knowledge in propositional form by hypothesizing that the coping skills and adaptive qualities of older women would enable them to take an active part in decision-making about their health care.
3 Through critical reflection on her feelings, Adair (1992) surfaced personal, aesthetic and embodied knowledge that was embedded so deeply in her practice that only when she left her clinical practice to become a researcher did she become aware of this professional craft knowledge. Examining the source of her feeling of loss, she began to realize that touch within the nurse–patient relationship is therapeutic not only for the patient, but also for the nurse.
4 From her own and colleagues' observations of the impact on patients of different kinds of wound dressings following hip surgery, Mortimer (1992, p. 233) proposed a link between the use of a particular type of dressing and increased haemorrhage risk. By sharing her observations with colleagues, Mortimer's experiential knowledge (in propositional form) prepared the way for a more systematic collection of data which increased the validity of this knowledge by making it available for public scrutiny.

## Articulating, sharing, critically reviewing, creating and validating professional craft knowledge

As mentioned earlier, the processes of articulating, sharing, critically reviewing, creating and validating professional craft knowledge are not necessarily sequential or mutually exclusive.

### *Articulating*

The articulation of professional craft knowledge can be achieved by systematic recording and description of significant practice experiences that illustrate expertise, a breakdown in performance, or the ordinariness of everyday practices. Records and descriptions could be obtained through reflective diaries, story-telling, clinical supervision, preceptorship and action learning sets, learning portfolios generated in work-based learning activities, interviews, observing, listening and questioning (see Table 7.2 and Chapter 10), drawings, mind maps, concept maps and creative arts media.

Some professional craft knowledge can be expressed in propositional statements, practical principles and maxims, whilst some will be expressible only through, for example, recorded observations of practice (e.g. detailed fieldnotes, audio and videotape, photographs), practice stories and creative arts media.

These ways of accessing and articulating professional craft knowledge will only work effectively if a health care, educational or research organization demonstrates the cultural norms, values, shared meanings, beliefs and attitudes of a learning culture. These norms could be incorporated into the system as follows:

- clinical practice is seen as a source of learning;
- professional craft knowledge is considered as important as propositional knowledge in the development of expertise;
- opportunities to reflect are built into the working day;
- 'time out' is provided in a variety of forms;
- practitioners' time spent in the above activities is considered to be time well spent;
- a climate of high challenge/high support is valued by all members of the organization;
- facilitation is offered within trusting relationships.

### *Sharing and critically reviewing*

Once articulated, the knowledge is collaboratively and critically reviewed by the practitioner and appropriate others, for example professional peers and educational colleagues within in-service education programmes (see Titchen, 2000), clinical supervisors or critical companions (see Chapter 10), preceptors, mentors or action-learning-set facilitators and peers.

This process enhances the development of expertise by offering an opportunity for others to judge a practitioner's rational and intuitive judgments and to examine the interplay between them and different types of knowledge. The process also facilitates one of the key characteristics of expertise, i.e. the ability to bring one's judgments and practice knowledge under a process of critical control, involving self-regulation, self-evaluation and 'a disposition to learn from colleagues' (Eraut, 1994, p. 155). It also opens up possibilities for validation and the creation of new professional craft knowledge.

### *Creating*

New, potentially transferable knowledge is created from systematic documentation and critical review of expert practice through a social process, a process of being with others (De Geus, 1997), including:

- Critical dialogue and debate with critical companions, clinical supervisors, etc.
- Pointing out and naming new knowledge (creating concepts and categories).
- Developing new shared language and practical principles, defining terms, making interpretive frameworks or world views explicit and sharing meanings and understandings with colleagues within and without the organization.
- Establishing relationships between concepts, looking for causal relationships – this is professional craft knowledge expressed in propositional form.
- Developing 'aggregate' stories of patients' and experts' experiences of particular interventions, in particular situations, including outcomes for the patient. We propose that such 'aggregate' stories are fictional, but are based on themes developed systematically and rigorously from expert practitioners' stories. ('Aggregate' stories could be developed by practitioners themselves or by researchers.) These stories could be

carriers for professional craft knowledge expressed in both non-propositional and propositional forms.

Titchen (2000) found that the expert she studied developed generalizations and consciously extended and deepened her understanding of the practical principles that she had created, to realize theoretical principles in her practice. This process was achieved through continual comparison, noticing the effects of her actions and conducting a 'dialogue' with her practice (cf. MacLeod, 1990) and by building up a repertoire of cases from which to draw in relation to a current case (cf. Benner, 1984). On the other hand, Tanner et al. (1993, pp. 278–279) conclude that the nurse gets to know many particular patients with similar illnesses over time, which 'allows the nurse to learn common issues and important qualitative distinctions within particular patient populations . . . In turn, knowing a patient population sets up a context for knowing variations and particularity within that population'. This finding suggests that experts search consciously for, and make sense of regularities and differences in practice as they seek to generalize their professional craft knowledge within their own practice. These findings could be used by those who help less experienced professionals to create professional craft knowledge to promote the latter's understanding and accomplishment of these complex activities.

### *Validating*

New and existing professional craft knowledge created and articulated as above could be validated through:

- Critical dialogue and seeking consensual validation in one-to-one relationships with preceptors, critical companions, peers in the workplace, etc., and documenting the process and outcome.
- Progressing to seeking validation with a group of colleagues within the organization.
- When consensual validation is reached locally within the organization, broadening the process to include other groups of practitioners, educators and researchers in ever-widening arenas. Thus the local consensus becomes the stone that is thrown into the professional pool and causes ever-widening ripples. For example, the local group joins a group from a neighbouring health care organization and achieves consensus. Together, they stimulate debates in regional and national professional forums or clinical specialist groups which, in turn, present at research conferences, write papers for publication, run national/international consensus conferences and use the Internet. If a wider consensus is reached, then practitioners have transformed this professional craft knowledge to propositional knowledge.

## Conclusions

In this chapter we have addressed the epistemological inadequacies in the health care literature identified at the end of Chapter 5. Terms have been clearly differentiated and some of their relationships to each other have been clarified so as to retain subtlety. We have argued that professional craft knowledge can be expressed propositionally, as well as non-propositionally, and have explored what this means in terms of developing expertise and clinical knowledge development. The ways and settings in which professional craft knowledge can be articulated, shared, reviewed critically, created and validated have been outlined. These processes have been examined from the point of view of developing practitioners' expertise and practitioners' contribution to developing an epistemology for professional practice.

We have shown how these processes could help less experienced practitioners to access experts' professional craft knowledge and how they could develop the attributes of expertise. We conclude that professional craft knowledge is derived not only through practice, but also through critical reflection, critique and debate. Practitioners need help with these processes for the development of expertise and for clinical knowledge creation to occur most effectively; a 'companionship' model can be used. Companionship is about engaging in a trusting relationship, high challenge/high support, and critical dialogue, journeying together and paying attention to the human aspects and lived experiences of developing expertise and clinical knowledge (Titchen, 2000). Companionship can be offered by clinical supervisors (see Chapters 10 and 16), facilitators (see Chapter 22), research supervisors (see Chapter 25) and educators (see Chapter 21), as well as by preceptors, practice developers, action-learning-set facilitators and so on.

We have presented ways in which practitioners could contribute to the development of potentially transferable knowledge by seeking consensus on professional craft knowledge (expressed both propositionally and non-propositionally) and on transforming some of it to propositional knowledge. This articulated and validated knowledge would provide other practitioners with systematic evidence, based on professional craft knowledge, that could be used for clinical decision-making alongside other sources of evidence, such as research findings and patient experiences. This explication of professional craft knowledge would bring more balance to the contemporary evidence-based health care movement and would build on, rather than downplay, a significant aspect of clinicians' expertise.

## References

Adair, L. (1992) Clinical notes: touch and the nurse. *Journal of Clinical Nursing*, **1**, 4–5.

Benner, P. (1984) *From Novice to Expert: Excellence and Power in Clinical Nursing Practice*. London: Addison-Wesley.

De Geus, A. (1997) *The Living Organisation*. Boston: Longview Publishing.

Eraut, M. (1994) *Developing Professional Knowledge and Competence*. London: The Falmer Press.

Ersser, S. J. (1997) *Nursing as a Therapeutic Activity: An Ethnography*. Aldershot: Avebury.

Higgs, J. and Tichen, A. (eds) (2001) *Professional Practice in Health, Education and the Creative Arts*. Oxford: Blackwell Science.

MacLeod, M. (1990) Experience in everyday nursing practice: A study of 'experienced' ward sisters. Doctoral thesis, University of Edinburgh.

McAlpine, A., Brown, S., McIntyre, D. and Hagger, H. (1988) *Student-Teachers Learning From Experienced Teachers*. Edinburgh: The Scottish Council for Research in Education.

Miller, A. (1992). Clinical notes: from theory to practice. *Journal of Clinical Nursing*, **1**, 295–296.

Mortimer, H. (1992) Clinical notes: Wound dressing use in theatre following hip surgery and haemorrhage risk. *Journal of Clinical Nursing*, **1**, 233.

Tanner, C. A., Benner, P., Chesla, C. and Gordon, D. R. (1993) The phenomenology of knowing the patient. *IMAGE: Journal of Nursing Scholarship*, **25**, 273–280.

Titchen, A. (2000) *Professional Craft Knowledge in Patient-Centred Nursing and the Facilitation of Its Development*. DPhil thesis, University of Oxford; Oxford: Ashdale Press.

Wade, L. (1992) Clinical notes: learning from older women. *Journal of Clinical Nursing*, **1**, 295.

# Section Two

# Professional craft knowledge and expertise

# 8

# Professional expertise

**Joy Higgs and Christine Bithell**

Professional expertise is a goal of health care professionals and an expectation of health care consumers. But what is professional expertise in the health sciences? In this chapter we explore this topic from two perspectives: historicism and dimensions of expertise. We seek to move beyond our inherited framework of expertise to examine current and future expectations of expertise.

## What is expertise? An historicism perspective

Chapter 2 introduced the concept of historicism (see Stanford, 1998), which refers to the need for phenomena to be understood within their historical and cultural contexts. In addition, we need to recognize that the ideas of 'expert' and 'expertise' are socially constructed; these terms have meaning because we assign definitions or constructions to them. Thus they have meaning within the context in which they are used, and meanings change as societal values and beliefs evolve. Within this framework 'expertise' has undergone a significant transition over time and place. Historical, cultural, social and language constructions can serve as lenses to help us understand the concepts of professionalism and expertise. For instance, we can explore expertise through examination of the origins of experience, professionalization, models of practice, ethics, practice settings, consumerism and social responsibility.

### *Origins of expertise in experience*

The word 'expert' appears to have been adopted into English from Old French in the sixteenth century as an adjective derived from the Latin *experiri* meaning 'to test'. In this early usage (c. 1612) expertise meant something which has been tried or proved by experience. Gradually it acquired meaning as a noun which identified someone who has been trained by practice, or become skilled in a craft or profession (c. 1672) and later incorporated the sense of public recognition as one whose special knowledge or skill causes him/her to be an authority or a specialist (c. 1825) (*The Shorter Oxford English Dictionary*, 1973, p. 706).

The emphasis on experience as the core of expertise is reflected in contemporary definitions of experts. In today's society an expert could be broadly considered to be a person with a highly developed specialist skill or knowledge, 'someone who is skilled in any art or science; a specialist' (*Chambers Concise Dictionary*, 1991), 'a person who has extensive skill or knowledge in a particular field' (*New Collins Dictionary and Thesaurus*, 1987, p. 349). Although the most recent dictionary definitions are more compressed, emphasizing skill, knowledge and specialization, they maintain implicitly the earlier strands of meaning which include the development of expertise through training, extensive experience and practice within a specialized and perhaps narrowly focused field.

## *Professionalization and professionalism*

Our second lens through which to view expertise is professionalization. The process of professionalization is the historical and political emergence of occupational groups as professions. This process is one of the key features of today's society, involving the establishment of formal entry qualifications based upon education and examination, the development of regulatory bodies which can admit and discipline members, and a degree of state-guaranteed monopoly rights (Bullock and Trombley, 1988, p. 684). The behaviour of members of a profession is managed by regulatory authorities operating within the legal-judicial system and by peer expectations through professional associations (Cant and Higgs, 1999).

Within the context of professionalization, expertise connotes the possession of an exclusive body of knowledge, and a highly developed level of skill which for the most part is not shared with, or taught to, patients or other non-professionals. Expertise carries with it a high level of status and privilege, and an expert's judgments are held to be incontestable by others of lesser status. Experts are likely to be recognized as outstanding by their peers in terms of knowledge, skills and performance (see, e.g., Benner, 1984; MacLeod, 1990; Conway 1996), and may be regarded as pioneers or 'gurus' with a particular approach to knowledge or theory. The individual professional's moral and ethical accountability to patients is fulfilled by them meeting patients' and the community's expectations that experts will provide the best quality of service in the field, through the possession of outstanding specialized knowledge and skill. The profession is responsible for regulation of practice and setting practice standards; this is accomplished through systems of peer review and disciplinary sanctions. In the UK, however, professional self-regulation is under considerable fire at the moment, with consultations occurring concerning the involvement of the public in regulation of the professions (i.e. stake-holder evaluation) (see Davies, 2000).

Professionalization, as an historical process, reflects an aspiration of emerging professions to attain the privilege, status and self-regulation of the established professions, particularly medicine. In the traditional medical model, the relationship between the health professional and the client is one of inequity, in which the client fulfils the subordinate role of patient. The more powerful professional is the provider of services that are assumed to be beyond the client's ability to evaluate. Clients are expected to place their trust in the professional's judgment and follow the prescribed treatment. In return, the professional undertakes to act within a code of practice that demands that the patient will be provided with the highest standards of health care available.

## *Evolving models of professional practice and expertise*

While professionalization refers to the development of a group, professional socialization illustrates the development of individuals as they become members of a profession. Throughout history, a range of models have been employed to provide a vehicle for professional socialization and a frame for practice.

The transition of health professionals from the master-apprentice era to autonomous competent professionals is discussed by Higgs and Hunt (1999). They identify the following models which reflect trends in notions of practice, education and expertise, but which may well continue to exist concurrently in different contexts:

### *The apprenticeship model*

This system evolved during an era when practice knowledge was acquired on the job, was closely guarded within the professions and was handed on to learners in individual or small group tuition. Society largely accepted, unquestioningly, the power of the professionals. Here the expert began as an apprentice, and learned in the workplace at the feet of the master. The focus of the apprenticeship system was on the practical knowledge, craft and art of the practice role of the health care worker. Expertise arose as a product of the quality of the master's competence, tuition and feedback and the work-based experience of the learner.

### *The health professional model*

This arose early in the twentieth century. It involved a shift from the earlier apprenticeship model's artistry and craft knowledge and expertise to clinical-technical competence supported by a more scientific knowledge base within the context of professionalism (i.e. a responsibility for knowledge generation and quality regulation). This was a time of knowledge expansion and development of societies. Professionalization flourished, bringing the dual blessings of professional responsibility for service quality and professional self-interest. Expertise in this model is typified by the diagnosis and disease management roles of the physician.

*The clinical problem-solver model*
This was a response to the knowledge and technology explosions and the concomitant threat of obsolescence in the mid- to late twentieth century. While problem-solving was a necessary and desirable competence for health professionals to acquire, the deliberate de-emphasis on knowledge, in contradistinction to the previous reverence for knowledge accrual, needed to be reconsidered when the central link between reasoning/problem-solving and knowledge was (re-)discovered. The expert in this model demonstrates skills of self-directed learning, clinical problem-solving and thinking skills. In today's educational and practice models, which focus on clinical problem-solving, the importance of domain-specific knowledge is manifest in curricula and practice.

*The competent clinician model*
This emerged with government and community emphasis on competencies in the 1970s and 1980s as part of the worldwide interest in accountability and cost-effectiveness. Expertise became synonymous with cost-efficiency, cost-effectiveness and demonstrable competencies. At its worst this model leads to an overvaluing of specific, measurable, technical competencies. Holistic and person-centred care can, however, be articulated and implemented in competency approaches.

*The reflective practitioner model*
This sought to reduce the theory–practice gap (Schön, 1983). Expertise in this model involves an advanced degree of higher level cognitive skills, particularly reflection-in-action. Schön (1988) argues that outstanding practitioners do not have more professional knowledge, but more wisdom, talent, intuition and artistry. Reflection and reflective practice are key dimensions of professional expertise. However, reflection needs to be part of an overall approach which encompasses knowledge and technical ability, as well as interpersonal and cultural competence.

*The scientist-practitioner model*
This emerged in the second half of the twentieth century during a period of considerable reflection on professional credibility, particularly concerning the scientific basis for health care (Michels, 1982). Expertise became synonymous with scientific rigour and evidence-based practice. With this trend come questions concerning the nature of acceptable evidence in support of practice and the need to seek evidence beyond science (Jones and Higgs, 2000).

*The interactional professional model*
This model (Higgs and Hunt, 1999) identifies the need for health professionals to be client centred and to be equipped with generic skills (including skills in communication, problem-solving, evaluation and investigation, self-directed learning and interpersonal interaction) to enable them to engage in lifelong learning, research, professional review and development, and responsible, self-critical autonomous professional practice. In addition, they need to be able to interact effectively with their context, to be competent professionals, situational leaders, interdependent team members, and reflective practitioners capable of substantiation of their actions.

## Ethical aspects of health care

Another lens which illuminates the concept of practice expertise is professional ethics. Health care can be critiqued on many grounds, including effectiveness, cost-efficiency, patient satisfaction (with process and outcomes) and best practice standards. Further, the ethics of health care provision need to be included in our evaluation of expertise. Benner and Wrubel (1989), for instance, demonstrate that expertise is related to the primacy of caring realized through a genuine engagement and connection with the patient and family. Kitson (1993) presents a conceptual framework of caring, in an historical sense, in which 'caring as an ethical position' is identified as the most contemporary conceptualization of caring. The orientation of this ethical model of caring is the contextualization of caring practices, relationships characterized by mutuality and trust, confidentiality and respect for persons and mutual realization and empowerment. White (see Chapter 18) also addresses the central importance of ethical competence in clinical decision-making and practice. The expert must demonstrate sound ethical behaviour as well as competence. This is of particular relevance to today's societies, in which health care consumers are increasingly well informed about clinical practice, and the mystique and unassailable stance of the traditional health professional are no longer tenable.

### *Medical and other models of health care*

While all models or approaches to health care aspire to promote ethical behaviour, health care occurs in a number of different practice contexts such as medical care, rehabilitation and health promotion. To conceptualize expertise we need to understand the frame of reference within which the expert is operating. Rothstein (1999, p. xiv), for instance, argues, 'The traditional notions of healing and comfort were conceived in a time when the health professional (i.e. physician) was deemed all-knowing and all-powerful – the very means to healing and comfort from the suffering caused by injury or illness'. From further back in time, of course, traditional healers (e.g. medicine men and women) held equally powerful positions in their communities (Sigerist, 1967).

In contrast, the rehabilitation professions arose 'in a different time and place: partially in the ravages of war, when the human will to survive and thrive was far more central an agent of healing and comfort than the availability of health professionals or health care technology . . . The ideas of what it meant to cure and comfort had to be expanded, and the rehabilitation professions were one healthy offspring of the mating of tradition with these new social forces' (Rothstein, 1999, p. xiv).

Nursing, like the rehabilitation professions, needed to follow a different (but complementary) path to medicine. Rolfe (1996, p. 9) describes the traditional nursing model as being 'supplementary and subservient to medicine' and valuing of 'caring-as-duty' (Kitson, 1993, p. 38). The evolution of nursing as a profession has seen challenges to the medical model and scientific rationality. The role of the nurse evolved from the nurse-technician to the nurse-practitioner. The foundations for a new paradigm of nursing, argues Rolfe (1996, p. 44), lie in 'the model of nursing praxis and the role of the nurse-practitioner'. Other authors in the nursing context emphasize a future for nursing which combines the recognition of nursing expertise with patient-centred care (Fulford et al., 1996; Binnie and Titchen, 1999; see also Chapter 12), the 'caring-as-ethical position' (Benner and Wrubel, 1989; Kitson, 1993, p. 41) and a humanistic existentialist knowledge base (Conway, 1996).

The traditional model of health care in Western medicine has been interpreted in different ways across the professions and still influences notions of expertise. For example, in her study of 35 nominated expert nurses, Conway (1996) identified four embodiments of expertise that develop according to the world view of the nurse and the culture in which the nurse works: technologist, traditionalist, specialist and humanistic existentialist. She established that each type of expert developed distinct knowledge bases. For example, traditionalists are task-focused, 'preoccupied with "getting the work done" and managing care with scarce resources' (Conway, 1996, p. 15). Medically focused, they operate as overseers of other nurses' work and as doctors' assistants.

Today we could consider the various health professions to fall within several different models of health care: the medical (or illness) model, the wellness model, the model of social responsibility and the rehabilitative model. We would expect experts within these models to demonstrate (primarily) cure, enhancement of quality of life, service to society and restoration of independence/function, respectively. The community also looks to complementary health professions (e.g. naturopathy) for services, particularly holistic health care, which are seen to be lacking or limited in mainstream medicine (Bridgman, 2000). We cannot comprehend or seek expertise without understanding the contexts, goals and standards inherent in these models. In addition, expertise requires an understanding of the way each model creates the frame of reference for knowledge generation, the practice epistemology of the profession.

### *Consumerism*

As part of our contextual understanding of professionalism and professional expertise, the recent trend in consumerism warrants consideration, since it affects how we view the expertise we purchase. Consumerism has become a significant influence across health care systems of developed countries, under pressure from overstretched resources and demands for the highest standards of clinical effectiveness (e.g. Department of Health, 1997). Consumerism in developed countries is also driven by societal forces such as a more educated and articulate society, and lay pressures on governments in relation to state health services. Increasing uptake of health insurance and the ability to access private health care also increase the pressure on health professionals to adopt work practices which conform to this model of commodified health care and purchasable health.

Consumers tend to seek out experts in all service industries, whether as computer programmers, car mechanics or health professionals. Their expectation of experts in any field is that they will carry out their work effectively and successfully. This is not dissimilar to the expectation within the professionalization model of professional practice and expertise, but has an added dimension of economic effectiveness. A consumerist culture or a valuing of consumerism in health care demands highly effective practitioners, able to make efficient and accurate diagnoses/treatment decisions and deliver a high standard of treatment, with a successful and timely outcome wherever possible.

In a market context, the expert provides a higher level of service and competence which the consumer chooses to purchase. Expert health professionals are now expected to provide an excellent service that gives value for money. Within a consumerist model of health care, expertise, whether in the form of services and skills or information, becomes a commodity. A commercial relationship between the professional and the client develops in which it is important that the client's expectations are met as far as possible. This potentially (more) equal and empowering relationship involves a degree of consumer choice and negotiated action on the part of the professional, who is accountable to the consumer or client. In state-funded health systems the identity of the consumer is more complex, but the relationship is still clear. Health professionals are accountable for the provision of expertise, effectiveness and value for money to the purchaser of their services, whether it is the state or the individual. However, commercialized health care also brings its own side-effects such as litigiousness, defensive practice, and even the abandonment of altruism or selfless care.

### *Social responsibility*

In contrast with the notion of health as a dehumanized commodity as reflected in the consumerism approach, the social responsibility model views health care as an expectation of society. In educating health professionals (and other tertiary graduates) for social responsibility we aim to prepare them 'to take a leadership role in the intellectual, cultural, economic and social development of the nation' (Higher Education Council, 1992, p. 12). The social responsibility model is particularly clear in professions such as nursing or social work, whose primary purpose entails a service orientation towards meeting the needs of the sick and underprivileged (Eraut, 1994). Expertise includes having the skills and knowledge to determine the needs of the recipients of care. Accountability for high standards of professional behaviour is directed to the state or the employer as well as to the client. The expectation held of expert practitioners is that they will make the right decisions in complex individual circumstances and provide optimal services to clients within available resources.

### *Summary*

In reflecting on the evolution of the professions and the context in which this evolution has occurred, it is evident that the ways in which society and the professions have viewed and interpreted expertise over time are deeply embedded in the ways the professions are conceptualized, practised and managed. This is the historicism principle in action. We cannot view expertise as a single, unchanging or universal concept or model. Instead, we ask the questions:

- What does a society expect of those on whom it bestows the label 'expert'?
- How do members of a particular profession define and judge their experts?
- What are the desired goals or characteristics to which each professional in a given context should aspire in the journey towards expertise?

## What is expertise? Dimensions of expertise

Just as the concepts of expert and expertise vary, so too we find numerous ways of describing the dimensions or characteristics of expertise. Dictionary definitions, for instance, emphasize the knowledge and skills of experts. *The Shorter Oxford Dictionary* (1973) defines expertise as 'the quality or state of being an expert', which may also be reified to the special skill, knowledge or judgment possessed by an expert (*Webster's Third New International Dictionary*, 1966, p. 800). Delitto et al. (1989) describe professional experts as people who are very skilled or highly trained and informed in their field. Generally the accolade carries with it the expectation that the expert professional is one of the best in the field.

Beyond these definitions, various researchers and scholars have examined the characteristics of experts more deeply. Jensen et al. (1999), for example, conducted grounded theory research in physiotherapy and identified four dimensions of expertise:

- Knowledge, including deep level declarative knowledge, a large dimension of practice-based (procedural) knowledge.
- Clinical reasoning and judgment, including practical reasoning, a central focus on patients, and moral, deliberative practice.
- Reflection or metacognitive skills (planning, monitoring and self-evaluation).
- Skill acquisition within a frame of intense, focused practice, high motivation and internal drive.

Jensen's model exemplifies the fundamental elements of expertise required for action at the cutting edge of clinical practice. The expert uses these abilities to engage intensively with the task, role and people that comprise clinical practice. Educational preparation faces the challenge of preparing graduates with beginning-level abilities in each of these areas and the capacity to continue to enhance these abilities towards the goal of expert performance.

Similarly, Higgs and Hunt (1999) argue that a comprehensive range of competencies is required by health professionals to meet the emerging challenges and expectations of the health care system. They endorse seven broad competencies of health professionals: technical competence, interpersonal competence, capacity to be problem-solvers and change agents, professional responsibility, interaction, social responsibility and situational leadership. These competencies characterize 'the interactional professional' and illustrate the complex array of skills and knowledge required to address the situational and human variabilities which characterize soft system[1] health care arenas. Experts need to demonstrate superior performance in all of these areas.

Another approach to examining the dimensions of expertise is through cognitive psychology, which uses the term 'expertise' to denote the superior **performance** of experts (Ericsson and Smith, 1991, p. 2), thus drawing attention to the requirement for the knowledge and skills of the expert to be in some way overt. In this way the expert's knowledge and skills are open to public scrutiny and the judgment of others. Cognitive psychologists have studied experts in a wide variety of different fields since the 1960s. The reasoning strategies and decision-making of experts in such diverse fields as chess, computer programming, physics, sports, musical performance and clinical medicine have been tested under experimental conditions, simulations and observation of real practice situations. From an analysis of numerous studies Glaser and Chi (1988, pp. xvii–xx) have identified seven generic characteristics of experts:

- Experts excel mainly in their own domains.
- Experts perceive large, meaningful patterns in their domain.
- Experts are fast. They are faster than novices at performing the skills of their domain and they quickly solve problems with few errors.
- Experts have superior short-term and long-term memory.
- Experts see and represent a problem in their domain at a deeper (more principled) level than novices; novices tend to represent a problem at a superficial level.
- Experts spend time analysing a problem qualitatively.
- Experts have strong self-monitoring skills.

Moving from a cross-disciplinary, psychological perspective on experts to the specific expected characteristics of expert health professionals, Higgs and Jones (2000) have added the following to the characteristics developed by Glaser and Chi (1988):

- Experts value the participation of relevant others (clients, caregivers, team members) in the decision-making process.
- Experts utilize high levels of metacognition in their reasoning.
- Experts recognize the value of different forms of knowledge in their reasoning and use this knowledge critically.
- Experts are patient-centred.
- Experts share their expertise to help develop expertise in others.
- Experts are able to communicate their reasoning well and in a manner appropriate to their audience.
- Experts demonstrate cultural competence in their reasoning and communication.

This set of characteristics was established in discussion of reasonable expectations that the community may have of experts. It reflects the changing views the community holds of the nature of health and the role of health care systems in health maintenance and promotion.

Another way of thinking about expertise is to consider it as a goal to seek to attain rather than simply as a state which has or has not been achieved. People could then be considered to have more or less expertise in given fields. Viewing expertise in this way allows a developmental process to be considered. Investigators in Maastricht have explored the development and changing form of knowledge structures which occurs as medical students and junior doctors acquire expertise through education and training (Schmidt et al., 1990). Through numerous experiments, the Maastricht team was able to specify how cognitive structures, which embodied the different ways that biomedical and clinical knowledge was represented in the minds of students and doctors, changed with increasing experience.

Cognitive structures, variously labelled schemata or scripts, have been postulated to explain the way that knowledge clusters and operates in domain-specific memory organization. The term 'schema' is used to denote the essential features of memory in a particular category (Anderson, 1990). Schemata enable information about category membership to be received and organized. Thus clinical information which is derived from examining a patient can be organized and developed into clinical decisions about the patient's diagnosis and what kinds of treatment to initiate. The concept of a 'script' was introduced by Schank and Abelson (1977) in postulating the existence of a mental framework which can be used to organize particular sequences of common and familiar knowledge or actions. Scripts develop as a result of personal experience, the linkages between the knowledge in the script being made because of their occurrence within the same event or time span. Scripts contain mechanisms for recognizing repeated or similar sequences. Once sequences are recognized as similar, unspecified detail implicit in a situation can be 'filled in' or assumed from previous knowledge of a similar situation (Schank and Abelson, 1977, p. 19).

Through work carried out with medical students, Schmidt and Boshuizen (1993) proposed a theory of expertise development in medicine which describes how expertise develops as a progression through four consecutive stages.[2] Memory is a major source of difference influencing diagnostic expertise in people of differing expertise. Further, each stage is distinguished by functionally different cognitive structures within which knowledge is stored and used in different ways.

- In *Stage 1*, students develop elaborate networks of pathophysiological knowledge which they use to explain the causes or consequences of disease. These knowledge networks are typically lengthy, drawing extensively on the preclinical medical curriculum in terms of explanatory information.
- *Stage 2* involves the truncation of these elaborate explanations into more clinically based explanations of a patient's signs and symptoms. The more often students make these direct lines of reasoning between clinical presentations and diagnostic categories and explanations, the more the concepts cluster together and links can be made between the beginnings and ends of lines of reasoning (Boshuizen and Schmidt, 1995). This is termed knowledge compilation (Schmidt et al., 1990). All information remains accessible if needed but does not appear to be accessed routinely. Boshuizen and Schmidt (1992) hypothesize that the individual's biomedical knowledge becomes encapsulated within clinical knowledge. Experiments have demonstrated that it could be retrieved when necessary but was normally integrated into clinical knowledge.
- In *Stage 3*, clinical education and knowledge transformation evolve through experience and increasing exposure to clinical situations. The network of knowledge developed earlier becomes transformed into 'an illness script', which is a means of cognitively storing information for subsequent use. The script, in the medical context described by Boshuizen and Schmidt (1995), has three components: enabling conditions of the disease such as medical, hereditary, environmental and social or personal information; the cause or 'fault' of the disease in the pathophysiological sense; and the consequences of the fault in the form of signs and symptoms. Illness scripts are activated as further encounters with clinical cases occur; they guide the physician through the examination and diagnostic process.
- In *Stage 4*, as doctors develop more and more illness scripts, these scripts are transformed from rather general information structures into more 'instantiated' or specific scripts in which expert physicians are able to recall the details of individual patient's clinical presentations many years after the encounter. In this way the increasing organization of clinical knowledge and experience stored in the memories of experts can be explained, and expertise in rapid and accurate diagnosis can be interpreted as a form of 'pattern matching' with former similar patients.

***Summary***

The dimensions of expertise are multiple, complex and interactive. In their patient-centred clinical reasoning model, Higgs and Jones (2000) propose that clinical expertise should be viewed as a continuum along multiple dimensions. Figure 8.1 illustrates dimensions/continua of clinical expertise, including clinical outcomes, attributes such as professional judgment, clinical reasoning, technical clinical skills, communication and interpersonal skills (to involve the client and others in decision-making and to consider clients' perspectives), a sound knowledge base, as well as cognitive and metacognitive proficiency.

## Conclusions

Society seeks a high standard of service from those it designates as experts. However, differences in emphasis emerge when the social constructs of expert and expertise are viewed through the lens of different models of health care provision. In this chapter we have considered a number of such lenses including professionalization, consumerism, social responsibility, traditional models of health care and emerging patient-centred approaches. The relationship between clients and clinicians is changing. The authority of expert opinion in health care is no longer unchallenged, as health care systems worldwide undergo radical change, paternalistic cultures giving way to consumerist, evidence-based, negotiated and partnership models of health care delivery. In addition, the role of the stakeholder as invited guest and political agent in health care evaluation and regulation is increasingly a reality of current health care systems.

We have emphasized, in this chapter, that expertise in the health sciences has multiple interpretations depending on context (including culture and professionals' world views) and time, and that clinical expertise has multiple dimensions.

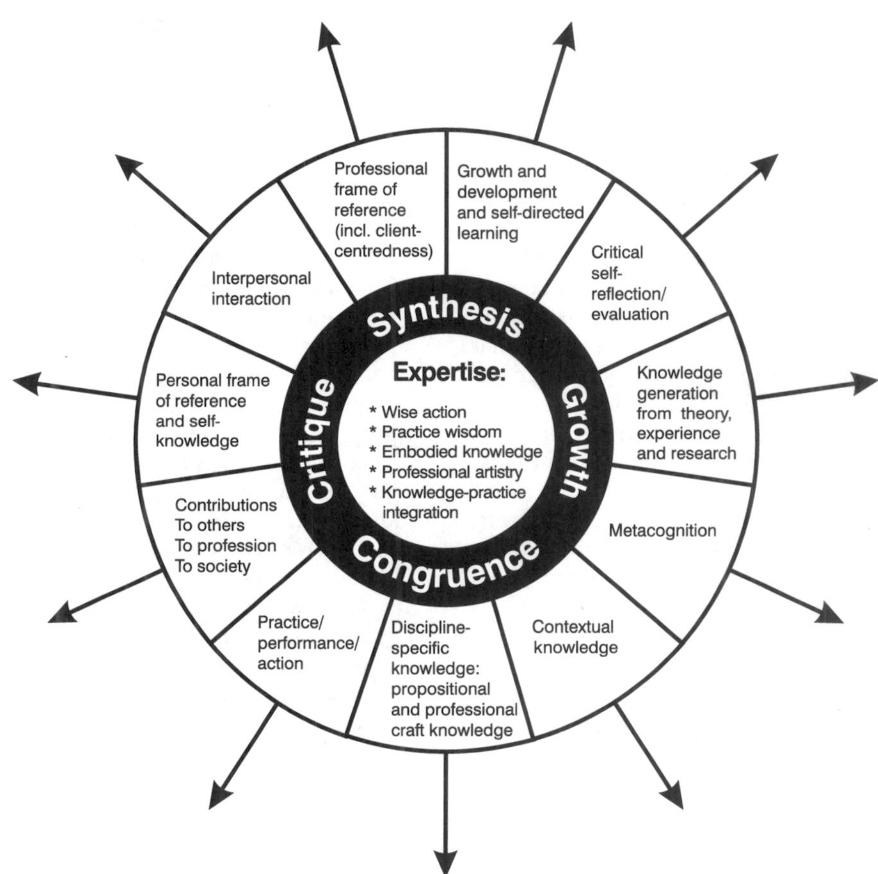


**Figure 8.1** Dimension of practice expertise – multiple continua

These dimensions critically include a sound knowledge base and clinical reasoning skills, to which are added attributes such as professional judgment, technical skills, communication and other interpersonal skills which enable clients' and carers' perspectives to be included in decision-making (Higgs and Jones, 2000). Moreover, experts have something else to offer. Beyond 'more knowledge', 'more skill' and so on, experts have the capacity to achieve a rare blend of practice synergy between wise action/practice wisdom, embodied knowledge, professional artistry, and knowledge–practice integration (see Fig. 8.1). Their performance is the epitome of higher level achievements of critique, synthesis, growth and congruence between the numerous dimensions which comprise expertise. Yet even while we accord experts these accolades, we remember the argument that expertise is a goal, a journey rather than an arrival; perhaps then we should call these people 'more expert', and remember the need for continual growth, critical evaluation and development needed along each dimension continuum.

Returning to the central theme of this book (the multiple forms of knowledge which comprise practice knowledge), professional craft knowledge (particularly deep, discipline-specific clinical knowledge) has been identified as crucial to clinical expertise. When we consider the soft science contexts which comprise health care settings, and the cycle of health care models which began in the valuing of experience-based knowledge and moved to the pre-eminence of scientific knowledge, it is refreshing to see the emergence in recent years of a more mature valuing of both of these knowledges, along with personal knowledge. In this evolution we see the recognition and realization of expertise as a blend of art, craft, science and humanity. Herein lies the future of professional expertise, as inclusive, not limited. We need all the talents and options at our disposal to engage fully with the challenge that is quality, people-oriented health care.

## Notes

1 Soft or purposeful systems are those in which goals may be unrecognizable and outcomes ambiguous. Hard or purposive systems, by comparison, are those with clear goals and/or predictable outcomes (Checkland, 1981).

2 Readers may wish to compare this model with the five Benner–Dreyfus stages in development from novice to expert (Benner, 1984).

## References


Anderson, J. R. (1990) *Cognitive Psychology and Its Implications*, 3rd edn. New York: W. H. Freeman & Co.

Benner P. (1984) *From Novice to Expert: Excellence and Power in Clinical Nursing Practice*. London: Addison-Wesley.

Benner, P. and Wrubel, J. (1989) *The Primacy of Caring: Stress and Coping in Health and Illness*. Wokingham: Addison-Wesley.

Binnie, A. and Titchen, A. (1999) *Freedom to Practise: The Development of Patient-Centred Nursing*. Oxford: Butterworth-Heinemann.

Boshuizen, H. P. A. and Schmidt, H. G. (1992) On the role of biomedical knowledge in clinical reasoning by experts, intermediates and novices. *Cognitive Science*, **16**, 153–184.

Boshuizen, H. P. A. and Schmidt, H. G. (1995) The development of clinical reasoning expertise. In *Clinical Reasoning in the Health Professions* (J. Higgs and M. Jones, eds), pp. 24–32. Oxford: Butterworth-Heinemann.

Bridgman, K. E. (2000) Rhythms of awakening: Re-membering the her-story and mythology of women in medicine. PhD thesis, University of Western Sydney, Hawkesbury, Sydney.

Bullock, A. and Trombley, S. (assisted by Eadie, B.) (1988) *The Fontana Dictionary of Modern Thought*, 2nd edn. London: Fontana.

Cant, R. and Higgs, J. (1999) Professional socialisation. In *Educating Beginning Practitioners: Challenges for Health Professional Education* (J. Higgs and H. Edwards, eds), pp. 46–51. Oxford: Butterworth-Heinemann.

*Chambers Concise Dictionary* (C. Schwarz, ed.) (1991) Edinburgh: Chambers.

Checkland, P. B. (1981) *Systems Thinking: Systems Practice*. New York: John Wiley & Sons.

Conway, J. (1996) *Nursing Expertise and Advanced Practice*. Dinton: Quay Books.

Davies, C. (2000) *Stakeholder Regulation: A Discussion Paper*. London: Royal College of Nursing.

Delitto, A., Shulman, A. D. and Rose, S. J. (1989) On developing expert-based decision-support systems in physical therapy: The NIOSH low back atlas. *Physical Therapy*, **69**, 554–558.

Department of Health (1997) *The New NHS: Modern, Dependable*. Cm 3807. London: The Stationery Office Ltd.

Eraut, M. (1994) *Developing Professional Knowledge and Competence*. London: Falmer.

Ericsson, A. and Smith, J. (eds) (1991) *Toward a General Theory of Expertise: Prospects and Limits*. New York: Cambridge University Press.

Fulford, K. W. M., Ersser, S. and Hope, T. (1996) *Essential Practice in Patient-Centred Care*. Oxford: Blackwell Science.

Glaser, R. and Chi, M. T. H. (1988) Overview. In *The Nature of Expertise* (M. T. H. Chi, R. Glaser and M. J. Farr, eds), pp. xvi–xxviii. Hillsdale, NJ: Lawrence Erlbaum Associates.

Higgs, J. and Hunt, A. (1999) Redefining the beginning practitioner. *Focus on Health Professional Education: A Multi-disciplinary Journal*, **1**(1), 34–48.

Higgs, J. and Jones, M. (2000) Clinical reasoning in the health professions. In *Clinical Reasoning in the Health Professions*, 2nd edn (J. Higgs and M. Jones, eds), pp. 3–14. Oxford: Butterworth-Heinemann.

Higher Education Council (1992) *Achieving Quality*. Canberra: National Board of Employment, Education and Training, Australian Government Publishing Service.

Jensen, G. M., Gwyer, J., Hack, L. M. and Shepard, F. (eds) (1999) *Expertise in Physical Therapy Practice*. Boston: Butterworth-Heinemann.

Jones, M. and Higgs, J. (2000) Will evidence-based practice take the reasoning out of practice? In *Clinical Reasoning in the Health Professions*, 2nd edn (J. Higgs and M. Jones, eds), pp. 307–315. Oxford: Butterworth-Heinemann.

Kitson, A. L. (1993) Formalizing concepts related to nursing and caring. In *Nursing: Art and Science* (A. L. Kitson, ed.), pp. 25–47. London: Chapman & Hall.

MacLeod, M. (1990) Experience in everyday nursing practice: A study of 'experienced' ward sisters. Doctoral thesis, University of Edinburgh.

Michels, E. (1982) Evaluation and research in physical therapy. *Physical Therapy*, **62**(6), 828–834.

*New Collins Dictionary and Thesaurus* (W. T. McLeod, ed.) (1987) London: Collins.

Rolfe, G. (1996) *Closing the Theory–Practice Gap: A New Paradigm for Nursing*. Oxford: Butterworth-Heinemann.

Rothstein, J. (1999) Forward II. In *Expertise in Physical Therapy Practice* (G. M. Jensen, J. Gwyer, L. M. Hack and F. Shepard, eds), pp. xvii–xx. Boston: Butterworth-Heinemann.

Schank, R. C. and Abelson, R. (1977). *Scripts, Plans, Goals and Understanding*. Hillsdale, NJ: Erlbaum.

Schmidt, H. G. and Boshuizen, H. P. A. (1993) On acquiring expertise in medicine. *Educational Psychology Review*, **5**, 205–221.

Schmidt, H. G., Norman, G. R. and Boshuizen, H. P. A. (1990) A cognitive perspective on medical expertise: Theory and implications. *Academic Medicine*, **65**, 611–621.

Schön, D. A. (1983) *The Reflective Practitioner: How Professionals Think in Action*. London: Temple Smith.

Schön, D. A. (1988) From technical rationality to reflection-in-action. In *Professional Judgement* (J. Dowie and A. Elstein, eds), pp. 60–77. Cambridge: Cambridge University Press.

Sigerist, H. (1967) *A History of Medicine*, vol. 1: *Primitive and Archaic Medicine*. Oxford: Oxford University Press.

Stanford, M. (1998) *An Introduction to the Philosophy of History*. Oxford: Blackwell.

*The Shorter Oxford English Dictionary* (C. T. Onions, ed.) (1973) 3rd edn, vol. 1. Oxford: Clarendon Press.

*Webster's Third New International Dictionary* (P. R. Gove, ed.) (1966) London: G. Bell & Sons.

# 9

# Skilled companionship in professional practice

**Angie Titchen**

Working within close professional–patient relationships, patient-centred practitioners collaborate with patients and families to promote healing and health or a supported death. However, the knowledge underpinning the strategies that practitioners use to achieve these outcomes is poorly understood, possibly because this knowledge remains largely tacit and embedded in practice. This chapter reports on a study (Titchen, 2000) that uncovered professional craft knowledge in patient-centred nursing. This case study of an expert, patient-centred nurse, working in a busy, acute medical ward is concerned with explicating the nature of professional craft knowledge in patient-centred practice. It is proposed that the findings transfer to other health care professions.

The **skilled companionship** framework generated in this study comprises two domains of practical know-how: the **relationship domain** and the **rationality-intuitive domain**. Each domain describes several processes (concepts), and practical strategies for realizing them in patient care. Overarching these two domains is the **therapeutic use of self domain**. Professional artistry is discerned in the complex balancing of these domains and in managing the fine interplay between intuitive and rational judgment and between theoretical and professional craft knowledge. The concepts of each domain and their associated practical strategies are presented and illustrated through stories. These findings elaborate concepts already identified in previous empirical research, add practical detail to the strategies that realize them, in addition to articulating new concepts and strategies. It is argued that professional artistry is the hallmark of professional expertise. The implications of skilled companionship for professional education and the development of expertise are considered.

## Introduction

This study (Titchen, 2000) attempted to make sense of patient-centred nursing from the perspective of qualified nurses, in an attempt to redress a gap in the empirical research literature. The context of the work was a major practice development project in an acute medical unit in a large, general hospital, where Alison Binnie (AB), a recognized expert in patient-centred nursing, and I (AT) helped to transform a traditional nursing service to a patient-centred one (Binnie and Titchen, 1999). In this study I was concerned with gaining an understanding of the nature of experts' professional craft knowledge of patient-centred nursing. From this understanding, a conceptual framework was generated and grounded in rich, contextualizing data.

I designed the case study using ideas from two distinctive, but complementary, traditions of sociological phenomenology and hermeneutic phenomenology. Data were gathered over two years using participant observation, in-depth interviews, storytelling and review of documentation. They were analysed using an approach devised from both phenomenological traditions and the findings were tested against the empirical research literature which examines the expressive elements of nursing (as opposed to the instrumental or technical elements).

The research revealed professional craft knowledge about the helping relationship between a nurse and patient. A theorized account of this knowledge is offered in the form of a metaphor and a conceptual framework for patient-centred nursing. The framework is supported by 31 nursing studies investigating expertise, the lived experience of nursing, nurse–patient relationships, and the provision of comfort and patient education. Within the limited space of this chapter, it is not possible either to present this supporting research or to ground the framework fully in data. Interested readers, therefore, are referred to the original report to judge for themselves the trustworthiness and transferability of the findings.

## Skilled companionship as a metaphor for patient-centred health care

**Skilled companionship** was first described by Campbell (1984), as imagery for a nurse accompanying and assisting a patient on a healing journey. It implies being together for the duration of the journey and parting at the end, each going their separate way.

AB: Being effective, being therapeutic as a nurse means, for me, helping a patient to move from an unsatisfactory or problematic position to a more positive and healthy one. It means accompanying and assisting a person in the transition from pain to comfort, from fear to confidence, from distress to coping or from loss to adjustment. Alistair Campbell's (1984) notion of the nurse as a skilled companion who accompanies a person on a journey until he is ready to go his own way, has been helpful and influential here. Campbell describes this companionship as a 'delicately balanced relationship' in which the nurse's sensitive presence, her willingness to recognise the nature of the patient's very personal journey and share in it, is as important as the practical or technical skill she may use to smooth his path.[1]

In this study, I developed the imagery of skilled companionship to create a metaphor for patient-centred nursing. The metaphor is imbued by three theoretical perspectives. The first is located in **humanistic existentialism** and is particularly influenced by the work of Rogers (1983). The second is **spiritual** in nature, elaborating on the ideas of Campbell (1984). It does not lie within a particular religion or doctrine. It refers to the transcendental, symbolic acts of caring for others and unconditional, moderated love. The third perspective is **phenomenological** in that the skilled companion is concerned with addressing patients' lived experiences of their illness and health care (Benner and Wrubel, 1989).

The conceptual framework of skilled companionship delineates the practical know-how of the skilled companion. It shows, both conceptually and practically, how practitioners are likely to form, sustain and close a 'delicately balanced relationship' (Campbell 1984, p. 51) and how they think, feel and act within the relationship, as a professional and person.

## The conceptual framework

The conceptual framework is set out in eight concentric circles (see Plate 2 at the front of Section 3, p. 119).

The innermost circle denotes the skilled companionship (professional–patient) relationship. Radiating out is the **relationship domain** with its four process concepts:

- mutuality or 'working with' the patient;
- reciprocity or 'reciprocal closeness and giving and receiving';
- particularity or 'knowing the patient';
- graceful care or 'using all aspects of self'.

These concepts, first described by Campbell (1984), are now found to stand in a prerequisite relationship with each other, mutuality being the most dependent. In other words, mutuality cannot be effectively put into practice if the other concepts are not fully realized in practice.

The next circle represents the **rationality-intuitive domain** and its three process concepts:

- intentionality or 'I made a conscious decision to. . .';
- saliency or 'knowing what matters';
- temporality or 'time, timing, anticipating, pacing'.

These concepts comprise a set of practical tools which enable the companion to put the relationship domain into action. The rationality-intuitive domain is prerequisite for the relationship domain.

Moving out, the next circle contains the **strategies** that realize the concepts within the professional–patient relationship. (While I present the seven process concepts, available space allows presentation of only some of the strategies that put them into action.)

The outermost circle contains the **aspects of being human**, with which we are all familiar in our everyday lives. The small arrows attached to the outer circle indicate the **antennae** through which skilled companions sense what is happening within themselves, within the relationship and outside in the clinical context. The larger, dotted arrow symbolizes the pathway or movement of skilled companions as they take themselves into the relationship. Within this pathway, the overarching **therapeutic use of self domain** is represented. In this domain, in any number of ways, the relationship and rationality-intuitive domains configure, interplay and are imbued by the aspects of being human. The dotted lines illustrate how, on the way into the relationship, appropriate strategies, associated with each concept, are 'picked up' and employed to enable use of self as a person in the context of helping a patient on their particular journey.

## The relationship domain

Rather than presenting the concepts of the relationship domain in prerequisite order, I start with particularity because this is where Alison starts in her work with patients. I then move towards the centre, presenting the concepts and strategies of reciprocity and mutuality before moving out to graceful care.

### Particularity: 'knowing the patient'

Particularity is getting to know and understand the unique details of a patient, within both the context of a specific illness situation and the context of the person's life. The particulars relate to two broad categories of knowing:

1 The patient's responses, physical functioning and body typology.
2 The patient's feelings, behaviours, perceptions, beliefs, imaginings, expectations, memories, attitudes, meanings, self-knowledge, knowledge about and interpretations of health and illness, current experience of illness and what is happening, responses to illness, needs, concerns, and significant social relationships, life events and experiences.

Both these kinds of knowing are gained through an involved (rather than detached) understanding and stance. Practitioners appear to acquire the first category of knowing primarily through an immediate grasp of the patient's situation and responses. This understanding is directly apprehended and may remain largely ineffable (Tanner *et al.*, 1993). Apprehension appears to occur through practitioners' attunement to their patients and their situations and perceptual knowing.

The second category of knowing can be acquired through individualistic, interpersonal, patient-centred assessment in which there is not only an understanding of the patient and the patient's responses as a person, which can be directly observed and/or sensed perceptually by the professional, but also a deliberate, conscious accessing of patients' stories from their own perspective. This latter understanding is indirectly apprehended; that is, it is known only in as far as the other is prepared to share and communicate.

#### *'Who is this person and where are they at?': acquiring knowledge of the particular through a patient-centred assessment*

Alison saw each patient as different, 'special', and needing to be nursed accordingly. Providing care that was individually tailored to the patient's needs meant that patients had to be carefully assessed.

AB: For me, assessing a new patient is an infinitely variable interpersonal process; not a predetermined procedure. The process is adapted according to the patient's condition and how he responds to me, and according to other demands within the ward. But in some way or other, I spend time being with the patient and, at some stage, his family too. I listen to his story, as he presents it, encouraging or empathising in whatever way seems helpful at the time. I try to discover 'where he is at' and what his perceptions and concerns are. As I listen, my nursing observational skills are at work, partly at a rational, partly intuitive level. I pick up cues that my professional knowledge enables me to recognise as significant and worthy of further exploration. As the conversation proceeds, or maybe at a later stage, I ask questions that arise from the patient's story or from what I have observed or sensed. In this way, I begin to get to know the patient and his family and build a relationship with them.

In the following story, establishing some sense of Peter and Mary's life together, Alison described how she attempts to see patients and their relatives through their own eyes, as well as through the eyes of a professional nurse.

Mary had been admitted to the ward with a severe subarachnoid haemorrhage. She had had a haemorrhage 14 years before which had left her quite disabled. Over the years, she had developed ways of dealing with her disabilities and had managed to lead a happy and successful family life.

**Establishing some sense of Peter and Mary's life together**

AB: Mary was unconscious when she was admitted and her husband, Peter, and 12 year old son, Richard, were with her and were very distressed. I invited Peter into the office to talk. First of all, I established some sense of Mary's life and their life together. When we first went into the office I wanted to let him decide what he wanted to talk about. We sat down and I was silent. I wanted to let him talk and then pick up any cues. He started off by talking about practical things. He said that he wouldn't be able to sit at the bedside all the time, but he didn't want the nurses to think that he wasn't a caring husband; he was. He felt that he wanted to retain memories of Mary as she was, not as a body lying in the bed dying. I told him there would be absolutely no pressure from the nurses and that he should decide the best way for him.

Peter's mother died recently and he told me that he had spent many hours at her bedside watching her die, and that this had coloured his memories of his mother so that he wasn't able to remember her the way she used to be. I said that I understood how he wanted and needed to protect himself against distorting memories of his wife ... I suggested that he bring in a photograph of Mary and put it on the locker to keep her image fresh in his mind.

... He told me how he had been through all this before ten years ago, when she had had the first haemorrhage. He had stayed by the bedside then because he found that he was useful to the nurses. I asked him, 'Was it helpful for you?'. He replied, 'No'. What I was trying to find out was whether he wanted to participate in her care. I established that he didn't want to be involved in the practical things, that it wouldn't be helpful for him.

... I encouraged him to talk about all the family. I wanted to establish his support network. I found out that her family were not very close. I asked him whether there was somebody around for him to talk to and he said, 'Do you mean somebody to talk to like I am talking to you now?'. He said that there were friends who lived over the road and that he had used them before for support. What I was trying to do here was to help him to establish, in his own mind, what support he needed, what his support networks were and how he could use them.

... Peter does not want any heroic treatment that was going to prolong Mary's life in this state for another two or three days. I said, 'I completely understand'.

In this story, Alison reveals how she uses silence to enable people to raise the issues that concern them. Having listened to Peter's concern about 'distorting memories of his wife', she then asks questions that establish that he does not wish to participate in her care. We also see examples of her empathetic understanding of Peter needing 'to protect himself against distorting memories'. In addition, the story shows that it is patients' own stories that structure the conversation and set the agenda in the initial assessment. Skilled practitioners are open both to patients' interpretations and needs, as they see them, and to their own interpretations of patients' experiences and assessment of needs and future possibilities. They use knowledge of the particular to learn more about the patient and to develop each unique relationship sensitively and appropriately. This knowing attunes them to the person and to the situation that they are to work with, which leads us to the second strategy that facilitates particularity.

***'Starting where the patient is at and moving on in the journey': particularizing general knowledge to design, give and evaluate personalized care***

Alison believes that starting 'where the patient is at' requires being with patients. 'You've really got to engage with the patient' (Titchen, 2000, p. 82), to be 'tuned in to the patient's senses'. The next story shows how she tunes in and uses knowledge of the particular to help the patient to move on. Both categories of knowing (i.e. knowing the patient's responses and feelings) are used by the professional to particularize general theoretical and research-based knowledge (Benner et al., 1996) and practical principles (which are part of the practitioner's professional craft knowledge). This particularized knowledge may then be used alongside imagination, in a complementary way, to design, give and evaluate personalized care.

**Tim and the orange**

AB: The patient had been in hospital feeling unwell and with rather vague symptoms, profuse sweating, fevers, vomiting, diarrhoea and had had a whole battery of tests that hadn't produced any answers. Not surprisingly, he was getting rather low in spirits . . . At 11 a.m. one morning, a nurse asked me if I would go and spend some time with him, because she didn't know what to do with him; he didn't want to get out of bed. I remember going into his room and finding him lying dishevelled, unshaven, hot and sweaty in a very crumpled bed. He looked lethargic and miserable. I sat on his bed with him for a few minutes, not saying very much at all, just with my hand on his hand. I could feel inside of me quite a strong desire to get him out of bed, get him in the bath, washed and get his bed freshened up and I knew if we could do all that, he would feel better. I also knew that if I suggested such a line of activity he would resist strongly because it wasn't at all what he was feeling like. So I just sat and waited for some initiative to come from him.

After a period of silence, he said, 'Do you know what I have been dreaming about? I've been dreaming about a fresh orange; I want to suck on a fresh orange' . . . (So I got an orange from the kitchen) and brought it back, peeled and nicely presented, cut up into small segments. He said he thought that he was allergic to oranges and it would probably make him sick, but it was what he wanted more than anything else. I thought that it wouldn't matter too much if it did make him a bit sick if he . . . could recognise, that I was trying to respond to his needs, as he saw them.

So I sat on the bed with him as he sucked away on his orange. He told me that he hadn't eaten anything for four days and that he thought it had something to do with why he was feeling so weak and lethargic. There were very few things that he fancied to eat and very few things that didn't make him feel sick or have diarrhoea. While I listened to him and we talked together gently, he did come up with a few suggestions of things he might be able to tolerate . . . Limited though they were, we did manage to find out a number of things he could cope with . . .

Having started at a point where he was at, wanting an orange, I gently built up some trust and confidence with him and felt able to tentatively suggest that he might like to have a bath. He said that he felt that he couldn't cope, that he wouldn't have the energy; so I suggested taking him in a wheelchair and sitting him on a seat in the shower. He said that he would try that. So I did exactly that . . . really freshened him up, helped him to shave, change, gave him fresh sheets . . . He was very weak and he did find it very tiring, but he really felt better afterwards, he felt much more positive and was very pleased to have made the effort.

My interpretation of this story is that Alison was valuing and building on Tim's knowledge of his own body, so that she could attend to the particularity of his needs. She was aware that in order to respond creatively, rather than predictably, she needed information from her patient about what would help restore his strength at his own pace. She knew that merely imposing her own professional (and therefore, general) knowledge of what would help would be unsuccessful. So she waited until they had addressed his primary concern – having an orange – before gently putting forward suggestions based upon her professional knowledge.

Another interpretation concerns the time and attention demanded of professionals when they use knowledge about illness and health which is based on generalizations in their encounter with the individual case. Alison attended to and made time for this encounter in a busy ward, by prioritizing and 'focusing down in detail on certain things' (Titchen, 2000, p. 83). This story supports, in a practical way, Campbell's (1984) assertion that the encounter requires moving away from accepting sameness and predictability in work to seeking the new and different. By responding in an unorthodox way to Tim's desire for a fresh orange, Alison was able to develop an understanding of his unique world and, by using that understanding in combination with her professional knowledge, to work out with him a few things that he could eat.

In her work with Peter, Alison particularized her general knowledge about the importance of closing relationships with her knowledge of him to terminate the relationship in a caring way.

**Closing the relationship**

Mary died a few hours after Alison had talked with Peter. The next day, Peter made an appointment to come and see her.

AB: His main purpose was to thank me and he gave me a hug when he arrived. He just kept on going on about how grateful he was, but his gratitude was overwhelming. He kept going back to wanting to thank me, but I was more interested to be clear that he was all right and to close the relationship . . . I did think about asking him to come back, but decided against it as he is a man about my age and I think it could be difficult if he becomes over-attached to all this and the hospital. I know he has other people now – his sister, father and his neighbour.

### Reciprocity: 'reciprocal closeness and giving and receiving'

Building on Marck's (1990) definition, reciprocity is a mutual, collaborative, probabilistic, educative and empowering exchange of feelings, thoughts, knowledge, interpretations and actions between the practitioner and patient. This exchange occurs during the development of the relationship and in the realization of particularity, mutuality and graceful care. It is an exchange for the purposes of mutual benefit and enhancement of the human outcomes of the relationship for all concerned. There is a recognition that the closeness of the relationship is negotiated by the professional and patient and that both are recipients of gifts of care, concern, satisfaction and wisdom.

Peter and Tim both benefited from Alison's care and Alison gained the satisfaction of knowing that she had helped each of them to move on. In addition, reflecting on her work with Tim helped her to understand better the nature of skilled companionship and of the professional craft knowledge embedded in her practice.

### Mutuality: 'working with'

Mutuality is the working together of the professional and the patient and family in a genuine partnership. Professionals offer their expertise as a resource to maximize patients' control in their own care and recovery, and to help them and their families deal with the consequences of illness and find their own solutions. The practitioner realizes mutuality by:

1 Helping patients and families understand the illness, what is happening and what is going or is likely to happen.
2 Sharing responsibility with them for defining problems, making choices and decisions about care and enabling them to make informed, independent decisions.
3 Involving patients in care and in professional discussion.
4 Accepting and thus legitimizing families' desire to participate in care and then giving them explicit permission to participate.
5 Helping patients and families to work together.

In Alison's view, the 'Tim and the orange' story captures the essence of how she **works with** her patients, by responding to their needs as they see them, rather than imposing on them what she feels is best. Offering acceptable help to the patient required a meeting of the patient's world with her own. This means that the world of the patient has first to be accessed and then accepted, which, according to Campbell, is restorative:

> . . .we feel cared for when *our* need is recognized and when the help which is offered does not overwhelm us but gently restores our strength at a pace which allows us to feel part of the movement to recovery. Conversely, a care which imposes itself on us, forcing a conformity to someone else's ideas of what we need, merely makes us feel more helpless and vulnerable.

(Campbell, 1984, pp. 107–108)

There is, therefore, a possibility that the special knowledge of practitioners can be used as a form of domination, if they impose what they think is best for the patient. We get a sense that Tim experienced a restoration of strength because help was designed and paced with knowledge which he offered, suggesting that Alison avoided such domination by curbing her 'strong desire' to get him out of bed and to freshen him up. Professional knowledge in patient-centred health care is, therefore, a negotiable resource for patients, rather than a source of power and control.

#### *'Involving patients and families': legitimizing and facilitating active involvement and choice*

Seeing patients as active partners in care suggests an egalitarian partnership with the professional. However, Alison does not see it as necessarily equal, because of the vulnerability of the person who is ill. Her view of partnership is one where patients and families have as much involvement, choice and control as possible within the constraints of the ward and the hospital. But she finds that she has to undo decades of socialization which has led to acceptance that they have no active role to play in nursing care, by legitimizing this choice and control for them. She does this by checking out whether or not they want to be involved and respecting their wishes.

Alison conveyed her belief that patients had a part to play in their care by avoiding body postures and positions that are potentially intimidating to patients, such as 'towering above' them during conversations. Fieldnotes show her consistently sitting on the bed, or crouching if the patient was in a chair, so that her eyes were level with or below those of the patient. Alison shared responsibility with patients for decisions about how their clinical problems should be managed. In addition, patients were not rushed and were allowed to set the pace of care. Where patients are dependent, 'doing for' them is sometimes necessary, but Alison demonstrated that it can be done within the context of fostering as much independence as possible.

### Graceful care: 'using all aspects of self'

Graceful care has aesthetic, humanistic and spiritual dimensions. Physically, it has a beauty of form, movement and sequence and is appropriately sensuous. In the humanistic and spiritual dimensions, it is a form of moderated love given unconditionally to promote healing and growth. Graceful care is conveyed through a relationship in which there is a physical, existential and emotional closeness between the professional and patient.

It is mediated through practical caring and the practitioner's use of self by:

1 Being authentic and expressing self as person, consciously and unconsciously, through the body, comportment and touch.
2 Giving focused attention to the patient through stillness and graceful movements.
3 Helping patients to relax by using posture, movement, voice, ordering and sequencing to create a therapeutic, healing environment.
4 Being physically and emotionally present with patients and families in their suffering, through physical proximity, silence, sustained eye contact, attuned listening, reassurance.
5 Using engaged responses to patients' suffering.
6 Allowing spontaneous and intentional positive emotions to enter care and maintaining a balance between an absence and an excess of emotional engagement to sustain emotional involvement.
7 Handling negative and inappropriate emotions and keeping them out of care.
8 Using humour to facilitate closeness and connection.
9 Using all these strategies and appreciating who the patient is as a person to provide comfort.
10 Using the intimacy of practical care to foster closeness, to express a form of moderated love, and to engage and work with the physical, cognitive, affective, psychological, existential and spiritual aspects of the patient.

### *'Practical caring': being intimate and offering a form of moderated love*

Alison saw intimate personal care of patients as the very heart of nursing, and the opportunities presented by practical bedside caring as the medium through which the patient's experience of illness is transformed and personal growth and healing occurs. The unusually intimate contact associated with helping patients to wash, dress and so on, not only allowed her to make detailed observations of their physical well-being, but also gave her an immediate, privileged and close access to the patient's personal world. The closeness to the physical body and to its discomfort, its dysfunction or its deformity, soon brought her equally close to the patient's concerns, beliefs and mental, emotional and psychological states and spiritual needs.

Moments of privacy and intimacy gave Alison the opportunity to address feelings and concerns that might not be disclosed in more public or formal circumstances. Intimate space for private conversation in the middle of a busy ward appeared to be created intentionally by the use of her body. Her face was often only about nine inches away from the patient's and she spoke softly and quietly. They looked as though they were inside a bubble, as if no-one else existed.

Alison had complex goals and used a multitude of strategies during seemingly simple activities, such as bathing, which assisted the patient's recovery. She used these intimate opportunities to do psychological work, such as allaying anxiety and fear, lifting patients' moods and motivating patients. Alison's work with Tim illustrates beautifully how simple physical care can make a difference to a patient if it is approached thoughtfully and creatively. Alison used her comportment to give Tim focused attention: 'I sat on his bed with him for a few minutes, not saying very much at all, just with my hand on his hand . . . I just sat and waited for some initiative to come from him'.

Practical bedside caring was also the essential medium through which Alison expressed moderated love, in Campbell's (1984) sense, in little acts of service and compassion. This form of love embodies a skill in sustaining a balance between reason and feeling and between an absence and excess of professional engagement, and plays a symbolic role through which concern and hope are mediated for the patient. Overall, the strategies of graceful care provide ways of achieving these balances and expressing the symbolic role. In Alison's stories, we catch a glimpse of her bodily expression of attunement, tenderness and acceptance, through her stillness; a stillness created by her smooth, unhurried and gentle movements, gentle voice and facial expression, and sustained eye contact. Thus she affirmed her focus on patients' and relatives' concerns and her genuine openness and receptiveness to their experience.

This bodily expression created a feeling of safety and trust, and comforted, supported, nurtured and reached out to frightened, depressed and withdrawn patients and grieving relatives. The hand-holding, the soothing caresses, the hugs, the tears and simply 'being there' are all part of a 'closeness which is neither sexual union nor deep personal friendship' (Campbell, 1984, p. 49). It is a spontaneous physical and emotional love within limits.

Letter from Peter: Such a long journey we travel and so many meetings along the way. We touched for just a few moments, but you will remain in my heart forever . . . I shall never forget the love and tenderness that you gave one sad traveller.

## The rationality-intuitive domain

### Intentionality: 'I made a conscious decision to . . .'

Intentionality is the consciousness, self-awareness and thoughtfulness of professionals as they meet both problematic, puzzling or sensitive situations and non-problematic, very ordinary ones in their daily work. Both kinds of situation are unique in some way. The concept is realized through the adoption of deliberate strategies to facilitate the other concepts of skilled companionship and by carrying out purposeful and deliberate acts. Decisions about what purposeful action to take are informed by both intuition and rational thinking.

#### *Acting deliberately, consciously and intentionally*

Alison demonstrated intentionality as she deliberately adopted the relationship strategies in her care of Peter and Tim. It was embedded in the way she explained what she did and the rationale behind her actions. For example:

AB: I sat close enough to Peter on purpose so that I could touch him if it was appropriate and I did at one point, when he was crying, I touched him on his knee . . .

What I was trying to do here was to help him to establish, in his own mind, what support he needed, what his support networks were and how he could use them.

Intentionality imbued by both rational and intuitive decision-making is shown in Alison's rational decision to sit close enough to Peter, but deciding when to touch was probably based on intuition.

### Saliency: 'knowing what matters'

Saliency is reflected in the ability to know both consciously and intuitively what is important, what matters, what is of concern and significance, from both the practitioner's and the patient's perspectives. Saliency arising from intuition results from the professional's immersion in a meaningful world in which certain features or events, complete with nuances, stand out as more or less important than others. This kind of saliency allows the practitioner to act swiftly, appropriately and effectively. However, this framework gives special attention to the conscious form of saliency in which significance is deliberately sought. The practitioner then focuses on significant cues and clues, and plans care that will address what matters to both professional and patient.

#### *Determining saliency rationally and intuitively*

What is important stands out for Alison. For example, she could see that it was important to convey to Tim that she was 'trying to respond to his needs, as he saw them'. Her sense of saliency is also visible in the way she tells her stories: there are no extraneous, unnecessary details to cloud the important, relevant substance.

According to Alison determining what is salient is often a rational, intentional act, closely related to the collection and analysis of data in the patient-centred assessment (see Particularity: 'knowing the patient'), 'I select out from the mass of data in my head, the information I need for care planning and for communicating to others'. Alison used the strategies of **being authentic as a person, using comportment to focus and emotional** and **physical presence** to help patients to express verbally and non-verbally what was salient for them. Knowledge of what was important to her patients alerted her to how she could use all aspects of herself further and more effectively. The mutually enhancing relationship between saliency and graceful care is seen here. Knowing what is salient for the other in the professional–patient relationship increases reciprocal understanding and promotes a sense of partnership (and also shows the relationship between saliency, particularity, reciprocity and mutuality).

### Temporality: 'time, timing, anticipating, pacing'

Temporality is reflected in the nurse's understanding of the importance of attending to the particulars of past, present and future time in helping a patient to move through healing or dying processes. It is realized through the strategies of **acknowledging past, present and future time, making focused time** for this work and for developing the nurse–patient relationship, **timeliness** or acting in an opportune or timely way, **looking forward in time** or anticipating care or patients' needs, and **regulating the speed of interaction or balance of conversation** with the patient. The predominant mode of thinking appears to be rational except in the case of timeliness, where intuitive thinking is seen to play a part.

#### *Timeliness*

Timeliness is closely linked with particularity and saliency. This strategy involves taking appropriate action at an opportune time. Alison knew when the time was right to coax Tim into having a shower.

#### *Looking forward in time*

Knowing her patients helped Alison to look forward in time to anticipate patients' needs. She was able to anticipate the problems that patients might have because of her knowledge of patient populations, built up from her knowledge of individual patients. Particularity facilitated the assessment of future possibilities.

Enabling patients to work with her means that Alison often has to help patients to anticipate events, so that they can collaborate. For example, Alison tried to help Peter to anticipate his wife's death and the part he wanted to play in it.

## Therapeutic use of self domain

The therapeutic use of self domain is the dynamic, overarching domain of skilled companionship. In this domain Alison puts together any configuration of the practical strategies of the relationship and the rationality-intuitive domains and imbues them with her own unique way of knowing, being, doing and feeling, both as a person and as a nurse, as she takes herself into the nurse–patient relationship. The domain is illustrated by the stories of Alison's care of Peter and Tim. All seven concepts (see Plate 2, at the front of Section 3, p. 119) can be seen at work within the committed, involved and engaged stance of the patient-centred nurse. Both consciously and unconsciously, Alison reveals who she is as a person and how she uses herself as 'the instrument of nursing' (Titchen, 2000, p. 96).

**Table 9.1 Professional artistry**

Professional artistry may take the form of synchronicity, balance, attunement and interplay. This artistry enables the professional to do, or be, all or any of the following within any one interaction with a patient:

- Put together any configurations of the practical strategies of the relationship and rationality-intuitive domains appropriate to the individual patient and situation.
- Bring appropriate aspects of self into the practical strategies.
- Use both intuition and rational thinking.
- Use both theoretical and professional craft knowledge.
- Draw out the meaning and significance of theoretical, technical or scientific knowledge for the particular patient.
- Be aware of what is going on within self, the relationship and outside the relationship.

The skills demonstrated by Alison in these stories may seem simple and ordinary, but they are not. It is proposed that they demand professional artistry in the form of synchronicity, balance, attunement and interplay (see Table 9.1).

The artistry component of the professional craft knowledge of the expert practitioner facilitates emotional, physical, existential and sometimes spiritual **synchronicity**. Synchronicity is realized, for example, when the emotions and movements of the practitioner occur at the same time as those of the patient. Practitioners pace their physical movement through space and time to be in tune with that of their patients, and they display emotions that are congruent with the ways that both they and their patients feel. The professional and patient exist together for a period of time as a **unit**, working, growing and being together for the duration of their journey together.

Professional artistry is also embodied in practitioners' **attunement** to their patients as people and to their symptoms, responses, physical functioning and body topology. In addition, it is revealed in the complex **balancing** of the domains and managing the fine **interplay** between intuition and rational thinking and theoretical and professional craft knowledge.

## Conclusions

Patient-centred health care, characterized as skilled companionship, is founded on humanistic, spiritual and phenomenological perspectives. Skilled companionship comprises two domains of professional craft knowledge, the relationship and rationality-intuitive domains, which include process concepts and practical strategies for realizing them. The synthesis, integration, interplay and balance of these concepts with each other and with the aspects of being human in the unique situation are forms of professional artistry. This artistry occurs in the overarching domain, the therapeutic use of self, as the skilled companion takes his or her self as a person into the practitioner–patient relationship.

Within the therapeutic use of self domain, the expressive actions of the relationship domain imbue the companion's instrumental actions. Thus, acts of intimate bedside caring, such as washing patients, may permit access to the patient's inner world and concerns, as well as being a symbolic, transcendental act of caring.

Although many of the concepts and strategies contained in this conceptual framework have been identified in the empirical nursing research literature (see Titchen, 2000), they have not previously been aligned within these knowledge domains. This research has also elaborated on these ideas. The concepts of graceful care and intentionality in the context of health care and many practical strategies are newly established. The skilled companionship conceptual framework is, therefore, new, and presents a theorized account of the professional craft knowledge that practitioners use in helping relationships. The framework shows, for the first time, the theoretical (prerequisite and/or mutually enhancing) relationships between the concepts. A prerequisite concept creates the possibility and conditions for the full realization of its dependent concepts.

The largely intuitive kernel of the skilled companionship framework, namely, the relationship domain, previously considered somewhat ineffable, can now be more fully described, although it is likely that much remains unarticulated. Penetration of the kernel is, therefore, beginning to be made possible by the finding that expertise is characterized not only by intuitive judgment but also by rational, conscious thinking. The skilled companionship framework, therefore, shifts the emphasis from intuition, previously considered to be the hallmark of expertise, to a view where both intuition and rationality are seen to contribute to expertise. In this respect, the framework empirically challenges the Benner–Dreyfus model (see Benner, 1984; Dreyfus and Dreyfus, 1985; Benner and Tanner, 1987), and strengthens that aspect of the theoretical challenge mounted by Cash (1995) and Rolfe (1997). However, the later recognition by Benner and colleagues of the place of Aristotelian practical reasoning in expert clinical judgment (see Benner et al., 1996) supports my tentative proposal that professional artistry, as described in Table 9.1, is the hallmark of expertise. This proposal needs to be investigated in further research.

A possible criticism of this research could be that it is based on the study of one expert nurse. However, the large dataset produced by a series of observations, interviews and reflective conversations, over an extensive period of time, provided an adequate range of situations and ensured redundancy, clarity and confidence in the data. In addition, because the conceptual framework is supported by rigorous empirical research in a variety of nursing fields and by a rich, contextualized description (see Titchen, 2000), the potential for transferability of the findings is strengthened. There are dangers associated with an uncritical acceptance of the framework, for example, seeing the unique ways in which the expert realized the strategies as generalizable, instead of seeing the principles underlying the strategies. I also acknowledge the difficulty of seeking to reveal the complex, detailed, transparent background of everyday practice, at the same time as explicating its essence through a conceptual framework (hence the length of this chapter).

There is a possibility that the terminology used in the framework may make it difficult for practitioners to grasp or it may be designated as unnecessary, alienating jargon. It seems necessary to me, for the purposes of improved communication, to use theoretical terminology that already exists in the research literature. For, as Benner (1984) points out, it is only when nurses share a common, agreed language or discourse that they will be able to create new clinical knowledge and expose it to their own critical review and public scrutiny (see also Chapter 7).

This study has made contributions to the conceptual development of patient-centred nursing and expertise. The responses that I have received when sharing these findings with therapists, speech and language pathologists and clinical psychologists, lead me to suggest, tentatively, that the skilled companionship framework is transferable to these and possibly to other health care professions, although the strategies may differ. This research may, therefore, be useful for curriculum planners in health care education who are open to remapping professional knowledge based on investigations such as this, and for those who help practitioners to develop their expertise by reflecting upon, and learning from, their practice.

## Note

1. In this chapter, unless otherwise indicated, quotations in a different font are derived from Titchen, 2000.

## References


Benner, P. (1984) *From Novice to Expert: Excellence and Power in Clinical Nursing Practice*. London: Addison-Wesley.

Benner, P. and Tanner, C. (1987) Clinical judgment: How expert nurses use intuition. *American Journal of Nursing*, January, pp. 23–31.

Benner, P. and Wrubel, J. (1989) *The Primacy of Caring: Stress and Coping in Health and Illness*. Wokingham: Addison-Wesley.

Benner, P. A., Tanner, C. A. and Chesla, C. A. (1996) *Expertise in Nursing Practice: Caring, Clinical Judgment, and Ethics*. New York: Springer.

Binnie, A. and Titchen, A. (1999) *Freedom to Practise: The Development of Patient-Centred Nursing*. Oxford: Butterworth-Heinemann.

Campbell, A. V. (1984) *Moderated Love*. London: SPCK.

Cash, K. (1995) Benner and expertise in nursing: A critique. *International Journal of Nursing Studies*, **32**, 527–534.

Dreyfus, H. L. and Dreyfus, S. E. (1985) *Mind Over Machine: The Power of Human Intuition and Expertise in the Era of the Computer*. New York: Free Press.

Marck, P. (1990) Therapeutic reciprocity: A caring phenomenon. *Advances in Nursing Science*, **13**(1), 49–59.

Rogers, C. (1983) *Freedom to Learn for the 80's*. London: Charles E. Merrill.

Rolfe, G. (1997) Beyond expertise: Theory, practice and the reflexive practitioner. *Journal of Clinical Nursing*, **6**, 93–97.

Tanner, C. A., Benner, P., Chesla, C. and Gordon, D. R. (1993) The phenomenology of knowing the patient. *IMAGE: Journal of Nursing Scholarship*, **25**(4), 273–280.

Titchen, A. (2000) *Professional Craft Knowledge in Patient-Centred Nursing and the Facilitation of its Development*. DPhil thesis, University of Oxford; Oxford: Ashdale Press.

# 10

# Critical companionship: a conceptual framework for developing expertise

**Angie Titchen**

This chapter reports further findings of the study (Titchen, 2000) introduced in Chapter 9 (knowledge of the contents of which will assist the reader in perceiving the similarities and differences between skilled companionship and critical companionship). **Critical companionship** is a conceptual framework for developing expertise in patient-centred health care (skilled companionship) in clinical settings. While the concept was inductively derived in a study of nursing, further work is beginning to suggest that it is transferable to other health care professions. In this chapter I present the framework and illustrate, through stories and excerpts, how it can be used in two different models. The **outsider model** of critical companionship sets out the role and critical attributes of a facilitator of experiential learning, who not only helps expert practitioners to understand the nature of, and to articulate, their professional craft knowledge, but also prepares them as facilitators of others' acquisition of craft knowledge. The **insider model** describes the role and critical attributes of an insider facilitator of experiential learning, usually the expert practitioner, who helps less experienced practitioners to acquire and create the craft knowledge of skilled companionship. The parallels in the helping relationships between a practitioner and patient and between a facilitator and practitioner are revealed. The contribution of these findings to research investigating the acquisition of expertise is discussed.

## Introduction

Although a number of key characteristics of expertise are emerging in the research literature (e.g. MacLeod, 1994; Benner et al., 1996; Conway, 1996), still very little is known about how to facilitate their development in less experienced professionals. In this chapter, I am concerned with how three characteristics of expertise (being patient-centred; being able to create, use and critically review professional craft knowledge; and being self-reflective and self-evaluative) can be facilitated. These characteristics are essential dimensions of the recognition, generation, critique and ongoing review of practice knowledge which is the topic of this book.

In Chapter 9, I introduced the study and the context in which I sought to make sense of patient-centred nursing, from the perspective of expert nurses. Alison Binnie (AB), a ward sister and expert in patient-centred nursing, and I (AT) worked together with the author in a practice development project to help the ward nurses to become more patient-centred. At the outset, we found that the nurses lacked or had poor understanding of patient-centred nursing. They seemed to be more like 'passing acquaintances' than 'skilled companions' in their relationships with patients and families (Binnie and Titchen, 1999). We saw their learning needs as the development of skilled companionship and believed that Alison, as a ward sister who had her own caseload of patients, was in an ideal situation to help the nurses. However, we soon discovered that Alison needed help to shed traditional ward teaching practices (Titchen and Binnie, 1995) so that she could become a more effective facilitator of learning. The literature suggests that other experienced practitioners also need help in preparing for this role (e.g. Runciman, 1983; Fish and Twinn, 1990; Johns, 1997). Unfortunately, there is little understanding or guidance for preparing experts within the clinical area or for helping nurses become more patient-centred.

Within an overall critical social-science theoretical perspective, I used an action research approach to investigate how I, as an experienced facilitator of experiential learning, helped Alison to become a more effective facilitator of the staff nurses' acquisition of craft knowledge. My aim was to develop principles for action which could be used by others preparing expert clinicians as facilitators. Using the distinct but complementary traditions of phenomenological sociology and existential phenomenology, I conducted a parallel case study of the professional learning support Alison gave to the staff nurses in her ward. A longitudinal design allowed evaluation of the effectiveness of our strategies. Data were collected over two-and-a-half years, through participant observation, reflective conversations, in-depth interviews, story-telling and review of documentation. They were analysed using principles developed from the methodological assumptions of the action research approach and the two phenomenological traditions. From understandings gained through this work, the critical companionship conceptual framework was generated and grounded in rich, contextualizing data. It is supported by the very limited research which exists in nursing (see Titchen, 2000) and in other health care professions (Goodfellow et al., in press).

## Critical companionship as a metaphor for facilitating experiential learning

Critical companionship, for me, is a metaphor for a helping relationship in which critical companions accompany less experienced practitioners on their personal, experiential learning journeys. The metaphor implies being together for the duration of a journey and a mutual parting at the end, each party going their separate way.

The metaphor is new and reflects four theoretical perspectives. The first draws on **critical social science** and the idea of supporting critical reflection integrated with practice, using, for example, the work of Habermas (1972), Freire (1985) and Fay (1987). The second is located in **humanistic existentialism**, where I was particularly influenced by the work of Rogers (1983). The third perspective is **spiritual** in nature, elaborating on the ideas of Campbell (1984), but not within a particular religion or doctrine. It refers to the transcendental, symbolic acts of caring for others and unconditional, moderated love. The fourth perspective is **phenomenological**, in that the critical companion is concerned with addressing the learner's lived experience of practice and of learning.

## Critical companionship: a conceptual framework for developing expertise

The conceptual framework of critical companionship is laid out in a series of concentric circles (see Plate 3 at the front of Section 3, p. 119).

At the heart of the framework lies the critical companionship relationship between the critical companion and the practitioner. Radiating out is the **relationship domain** with its four process concepts which stand in a prerequisite relationship with each other, mutuality being the most dependent. The next circle represents the **rationality-intuitive domain** and its three process concepts, which comprise a set of practical tools enabling the companion to realize the relationship domain. Moving out, the next circle contains the **strategies** that realize the above concepts. In the overarching **facilitative use of self domain**, the relationship, rationality-intuitive and facilitation domains configure, interplay and are imbued by the aspects of being human, as the critical companion takes herself or himself into the relationship. (Comparison with Plate 2 shows how these domains parallel those of skilled companionship, i.e. the helping relationship between the practitioner and patient.)

In Plate 3 the **facilitation domain** and its four concepts are set out. Whilst distinct, the concepts are not mutually exclusive and they do not have prerequisite relationships with each other. Moving outwards again, the adjacent two circles show the **strategies** that realize these concepts and the broad **aspects of the situation** which are attended to. The outer circle represents the **milieu** or the opportunities for reflection which critical companionship uses. The small arrows indicate the **antennae** through which the critical companion senses what is happening within and without him/herself.

Taking the framework as a whole, the dotted lines suggest the possibility of any number of configurations and interplay between the aspects of the situation, of being human, and of the three domains occurring in the overarching domain, facilitative use of self (the large arrow).

The following definitions apply both to **outsider critical companions** (such as an educator or professional development facilitator who does not have authority in the clinical setting, but who is helping an expert practitioner working in that setting to develop experiential learning strategies) and to **insider critical companions** (who are the expert practitioners with authority in the clinical setting and who are helping less experienced colleagues to become skilled companions to their patients). For reasons of brevity, the term 'practitioner' is used to refer to the person who is being helped, whether it is the expert or less experienced professional.

## The relationship domain: concepts

### Mutuality

Mutuality is embodied in the working together of the critical companion and the practitioner in a collegiate partnership that is carefully negotiated. Critical companions are attuned to practitioners' readiness to learn, making use of opportunities for shared experiences. They build on the practitioner's starting point and tender their knowledge and experience as a resource for the practitioner to draw upon in the solution of problems and to help them learn from their practice. The critical companion enables mutuality by:

1 Helping the practitioner to understand the situation, what is happening and what is likely to happen.
2 Sharing responsibility with the practitioner for learning and decision-making about practice development.
3 Accepting and legitimizing other practitioners' involvement in critical dialogues.

### Reciprocity

Reciprocity is embodied in a mutual, collaborative, educative and empowering exchange of feelings, thoughts, knowledge, interpretations and actions between the companion and practitioner – during the development of the relationship and in the realization of particularity, mutuality and graceful care – for the purposes of mutual benefit and enhancement of the human outcomes of the relationship for all concerned. There is a recognition that both parties are recipients of gifts of care, concern, satisfaction and wisdom.

### Particularity

Particularity refers to the critical companion getting to know and understand the unique details and experience of the practitioner, within the contexts both of the specific learning situation and of the person's life (as far as the practitioner wishes to disclose). This knowing of 'where the person is at' is seen as the starting point from which the facilitation of learning is designed. Each practitioner is seen as a unique person with individual needs which need to be met in different ways. Thus, the critical companion seeks to know the practitioner as a whole person, as well as a colleague. This knowing is acquired through observing the practitioner's situation and responses and through facilitating story-telling and self-reflection. General educational knowledge is particularized in order to design, provide and evaluate learning experiences for individuals in each situation and circumstance.

### Graceful care

Graceful care is the support given to the practitioner by the critical companion through presence, comportment, use of body and touch, and through moderated love to promote personal and professional growth. The critical companion is concerned with developing cognitive, affective and psychological aspects of the practitioner. There is an existential and emotional closeness between them. Critical companions use themselves to convey:

1 Being authentic and expressing self as person, consciously and unconsciously, through the body, comportment and touch.
2 Giving focused, undistracted attention.
3 Creating a workplace culture in which practitioners feel cared for.
4 Being physically and emotionally present with the practitioner in times of stress, disappointment and frustration, through physical proximity, attuned listening and reassurance.
5 Making engaged responses to practitioners' problems and feelings.
6 Maintaining a balance between an absence or an excess of emotional engagement with the practitioner.
7 Dealing with negative or inappropriate emotions.
8 Comforting practitioners when they are distressed about either personal or professional issues.
9 Using humour to provide support.

10 Appreciating the practitioner as a person and valuing his/her unique professional contribution.

Staff nurses experienced Alison's graceful care in the following ways:

*Moira:* Alison is approachable and non-threatening because her manner is cheerful and she never seems to be down . . . She is really reliable, you know what to expect . . . She makes time for me . . . and makes me feel that I have something positive to offer . . . and I found that really encouraging.

*Harriet:* She seems to be listening to the meaning of my questions, not just for the sake of it, but really empathising with me . . . She really cares if you are having major problems with patients.

*Janice:* She gives you good feedback, always honest. It never puts you down, it's very clever.[1]

## The rationality-intuitive domain: concepts

### Intentionality

Intentionality is expressed in the consciousness, self-awareness and thoughtfulness of critical companions as they deliberately and purposefully adopt the strategies that realize the process concepts of critical companionship.

### Saliency

Saliency is embodied in the ability to know both consciously and intuitively what is important, what matters, what is of concern and significance, from both the critical companion's and the practitioner's perspectives. Saliency arising from intuition results from the companion's immersion in a meaningful world in which certain features or events, complete with nuances, stand out as more or less important than others. This kind of saliency allows the companion to act swiftly, appropriately and effectively. This framework gives special attention to the conscious form of saliency in which significance is deliberately sought. The critical companion then focuses on significant cues and clues, and plans learning strategies that will address what matters in the situation. Saliency can be seen in the following story (as can mutuality, particularity, graceful care, intentionality, temporality and the facilitation concepts which follow).

**Drawing salient information into a cluster**

*AB:* When Harriet told me the situation . . . I asked in a non-critical voice, 'How long has Daisy been in?' So I was planting or bringing to the surface information and putting it together in Harriet's mind, in a way, so the information was then in front of her. So I was making her think: Daisy has been in for a week – has she got a district nurse (yes she has) – two bits of information there. Then she's almost there herself, thinking, 'Well, I haven't actually spoken to her myself". So I didn't need to say, 'You should have phoned the district nurse' because by the time I had drawn up the relevant bits of information in a cluster, she was able to make the judgment.

*AT:* You helped her lay the significant information out and bring it together and she could then see, looking at the picture, what she should have done.

*A:* That's right. I think I try to do that quite a bit with people . . . You draw up salient points for them, out of what might be a bit of a fog, and once the salient things stand out, things suddenly make sense to them.

### Temporality

Temporality is reflected in the critical companion's understanding of the importance of attending to the particulars of past, present and future time in helping a practitioner to learn. It requires a capacity to make focused time for this work and for developing the companion-practitioner relationship, timeliness or acting in an opportune way and looking forward in time to anticipate the practitioner's needs.

## The facilitation domain: concepts

### Consciousness-raising

Consciousness-raising refers to enlightenment or the bringing to practitioners' consciousness the knowledge embedded in daily practice and a recognition of the nature of this knowledge. It includes bringing to practitioners' attention their intuitions and behaviour and its effects, whilst practising as clinicians and critical companions.

### Problematization

Problematization is making problematic some practice currently seen by the practitioner as unproblematic. The task of the critical companion is to help the practitioner bring to the surface and critique the tacit understandings that have grown up around repetitive, habituated and mindless practice experiences, to point out phenomena that are not being attended to because they do not match the practitioner's craft or theoretical knowledge and to provide the requisite knowledge to recognize a problem and/or its extent. Where practitioners do see practice as problematic, but are 'stuck', the critical companion helps them to see it from a different perspective, from which the problem becomes solvable. If practitioners are unaware of inconsistencies or contradictions in their practice, the companion points them out.

### Self-reflection

Self-reflection is a cyclical process in which practitioners critically reflect upon their experiences, rational thinking and intuitions for learning about self and for learning from and improving their practice. The critical companion helps them reconstruct their experiences and describe the salient features of their actions, behaviours, happenings in a particular situation, together with their thoughts and feelings. Positive feelings are focused upon and the companion helps the practitioner to remove obstructing feelings cathartically. Companions facilitate practitioners' analysis and evaluation of their experiences and thinking by encouraging deliberative reflection and metacognition. Assistance is given in associating new and existing knowledge and incorporating new knowledge into existing conceptual schemata. The practitioner is helped to draw conclusions about experiences and to theorize them. The implications of new practical and theoretical understandings are considered, and statements about the actions that could bring about the desired goal within these particular circumstances and context (i.e. action hypotheses) are devised. Plans are then drawn up to test the hypotheses in practice.

*AB:* Angie's skilled listening and probing, in formal interviews and in reflective conversations, help me to look very carefully and critically at my decisions, actions and experiences and to theorise about them . . . This experience has greatly strengthened my reflective and analytic abilities. I am conscious, not only in my conversations with Angie, that my everyday thinking has become much more rigorous.

### Critique

Critique entails collaborative critical reflection upon a reconstructed experience and the situation in which it took place. Through critique, personal and professional issues and meanings at work in the situation are uncovered, in addition to the influence of socio-historic factors shaping the situation. Further reflection takes place in the light of the newly gained insights, theoretical understandings and interpretations of practice. Through this confrontation with the experience, through collaborative meaning-making and a process of contestation and debate, new understandings are used to develop new knowledge about how to change the situation within the practitioner's sphere of work and within the social, cultural, historical and political contexts that shape practice.

## Facilitation of learning strategies

### Articulation of craft knowledge strategy

Critical companions use four forms of communication to make their craft knowledge accessible to others: **story-telling** (in which they analyse and interpret their own experiences); **making suggestions** (based on craft knowledge after analysis and interpretation of the practitioner's current experience); **analysing, interpreting and evaluating shared experiences** (informed by craft knowledge); and **offering non-specific maxims**. The following reflective conversation illustrates aspects of the second form.

*AT:* When I was a physiotherapist I always had two or three students working with me and I saw part of my role as facilitating their learning. I used to build in quite a lot of reflection time when I shared my knowledge with them.

*AB:* I think it's much easier when you've got two or three people to think about, but my problem is I am trying to think about the whole ward. Although when I am on the team, it should be easier in that I try to focus on the team members.

*AT:* It's the same number of people.

*AB:* Yes, which is realistic.

*AT:* I was often very deliberate in my approach. I would set things up so that we could do patient assessments together and sometimes we would arrange to observe each other . . . and then we would discuss what had been going on and reflect and evaluate ourselves . . . (That creates) a shared experience which you can then both talk about. You can debrief, you can talk about your own perspectives – the way you and the staff nurse see it. What are the differences? Why did the staff nurse see it this way and you that?

*AB:* I think that's what I need to do with the team members a little more than I do at the moment.

**Observing, listening and questioning strategy**

*AB:* My experience is that when you (AT) are around in the ward you help me to look at my own skills and my own development . . . Just talking through stories with you has helped me a lot to clarify what I am doing. You listen to a story, you help me to tell a story. But then, you make me probe and get back to the story.

The observing, listening and questioning strategy is used by critical companions to facilitate practitioners' articulation and questioning of their own craft knowledge. The companion adopts the attributes, reflexivity and skills of a qualitative researcher. The critical companion, as a participant observer, observes and listens to practitioners going about their everyday work and asks them to give a detailed account of the observed situation and the knowledge they used in it. Soon afterwards, as if conducting an in-depth interview, the critical companion stimulates recall of the situation and probes for clarification. Questions are asked about the seemingly obvious, to reveal the feelings, intentions, logic and rationale underpinning specific actions and to facilitate story-telling and the questioning of assumptions. The companion also asks questions about intuitive and rational judgments, the interplay between intuition and rational thinking and generalizations of craft knowledge being used. The strategy enables practitioners to deepen, refine, generate and test craft knowledge through verbalization, interaction and communication, and it makes this knowledge available for others to reflect upon and to debate critically.

**Feedback on performance strategy**

*AT:* The majority of your (AB) interactions with patients are short, but on a deep level. You sit on the bed and give sustained eye contact. You listen intently and are rarely distracted. You are usually holding the patient's hand or touching their arm. You give time for patients to respond and you allow long silences with contact. I observed you on a busy day, but you made time for patients when they gave you cues that they wanted to talk.

Feedback on performance is a strategy in which the companion provides the practitioner with data collected using the observing, listening and questioning strategy. The practitioner is invited to examine the data, which may be in a variety of forms such as fieldnotes, audio recordings or verbal observations. This feedback, given by the companion prior to a reflective conversation, does not include interpretations or judgments. The companion encourages practitioners in the conversation to explore the craft knowledge which may be brought to the surface through their engagement with the data. The feedback is also used to confront practitioners with their actions and their effects, to enable them to assess their progress and to guide their actions.

*AB:* My clinical role at last is having an impact which it wasn't before. People talk about it and they comment on what I do and they notice that they are learning from it. What I want to do is to be giving feedback more constructively. And this idea of making them reflect, there's not much evidence of that and that's because I don't think I have moved much further since last time we talked about it . . . I suppose I am thinking back to examples where I didn't take opportunities.

Feedback on what went well and what did not is given in detail, not only to enable practitioners to evaluate themselves, but also for naming craft knowledge and showing the interplay between rational thinking and intuition.

The companion focuses on the whole situation and gives intensive feedback about the accuracy of rational and intuitive judgments made by the practitioner. Practitioners are encouraged to check out intuitive judgments using rational thinking.

Practitioners are helped to cope with constructive criticism by being given the opportunity to evaluate their performance and self-diagnose learning needs before feedback and an objective diagnosis of learning needs is offered. Where appropriate this self-evaluation and diagnosis is validated, making any further criticism more tolerable. The critical companion draws salient information together in a non-critical way, to facilitate the practitioner's self-evaluation as in the story 'Drawing salient information into a cluster' (see p. 83).

*AB:* When people are trying something new, if you knock them down early, it is hard to pick up. People are so fragile and sensitivity is important. They are very tentative, trying so hard and they need accurate feedback, in the sense that it is important to show them where they need to develop or improve. It needs to be done quite gently, so they are not just squashed. And if they feel that they have got halfway there themselves, that just makes the rest of the criticism much more tolerable.

### High challenge/high support strategy

High challenge/high support maximizes the effect of challenge as a catalyst for learning and imbues the other facilitation strategies. Companions challenge taken-for-granted assumptions, beliefs, values, expectations, perceptions, judgments and actions in a constructive, interested and supportive way. Challenge is offered by providing opportunities for practitioners to observe critical companions' practice and make comparisons with their own. Companions also question practitioners, push them on to use new craft knowledge, to behave in new ways and to take risks.

Companions give learning support as practitioners seek new understanding of situations and problems and generate action plans. They help practitioners to rehearse new ways of working with patients. They avoid taking over from practitioners in difficult situations, providing guidance and validating practitioners' judgments (if appropriate in the situation). They also give emotional support by realizing graceful care, for example, by 'being there', using humour or supportive, connecting touch, making focused time and being attuned to the practitioners' experiences. Support is also given, for instance, by validating practitioners' self-evaluations (where felt to be accurate) and by celebrating progress and successful outcomes.

*AT:* I have seen you (*AB*) challenging the nurses as you work alongside them as a team member. There is evidence that they are watching you and learning from you which suggests that you have effectively made your intentions explicit.

### Critical dialogue strategy

Critical dialogue can involve a complex variety of configurations of all the other critical companionship strategies, facilitated by the critical companion within reflective conversations. Thus by using oral discourse, the critical companion promotes collaborative interpretations, critique and evaluation of data (provided by critical companion and practitioner). Fostering practitioners' self-awareness, reflective, critical and creative thinking prepares the way for facilitating the particularization of research-based and theoretical knowledge and creation of craft knowledge.

Particularization is attained by encouraging the practitioner's deliberative and metacognitive reflection. The companion facilitates the generation of commonsense theory (using craft knowledge) and the use of formal theory to inform further action, and assists in creating a vision for change. Further craft knowledge, acquired through the subsequent use of commonsense and formal theory in practice, is debated at a later stage.

Critical dialogue was highly effective in attuning Alison to the nature of craft knowledge and in furthering our understanding of how it is developed through experience and through the critical dialogue itself.

### Attuning Alison to the nature of craft knowledge

Before the nature of Alison's craft knowledge could be explored, she had to become attuned to it. Therefore, employing particularly the 'observing, listening and questioning' strategy, I focused her attention on the craft knowledge surfacing in her stories, for example. This was crucial because, although I had explained to Alison the nature of craft knowledge as described in the literature, and she had had no difficulty understanding that, it took her some time 'just to appreciate what level craft knowledge is functioning at' (Titchen, 2000, p. 123). Initially, she was surprised whenever I directed her attention to it.

*AT:* There have been several times when I have said to you, 'That was your craft knowledge' and you have been slightly surprised and then you have said, 'Oh, yes!' as if you hadn't thought about it before.

*AB:* That's right. But that's because of the nature of craft knowledge. You're not conscious of it at the time . . . That's the last thing you are thinking of at the time because you are so engaged in the situation.

At first, Alison saw craft knowledge in narrow terms, merely as factual knowledge. In addition, she had difficulty understanding the embeddedness of the knowledge in the skill. I helped her to see it in broader terms as we analysed one of her stories.

*AB:* You see a lot of the action was value laden; it was driven by values as much as knowledge. For example, I find if somebody starts a conversation that's not related to the patient, over the patient, I tend to drop the conversation because I don't like doing that, and that's a values thing rather than knowledge. I just think of this poor guy dying and bleeding to death and I don't want to talk about the off-duty over him, even if he can't hear. I'm sure that's nothing I know really, but I believe that it's a sign of disrespect or insensitivity.

*AT:* But isn't that knowledge – ethical knowledge? And it requires knowledge to know how to realise those values in practice . . .

*AB:* Ethical knowledge is something we draw on quite a lot; it's part of our craft knowledge . . . It is quite an interesting thing. I shall be thinking all the time now, 'What knowledge is this?'

### *Identifying how craft knowledge is developed*

Alison believed that she had developed her craft knowledge of patient-centred nursing in three ways. First, she used theoretical principles in her practice:

*AB:* I think an awful lot of it has really grown out of the Rogerian theories. I think that is what got me started. Now the kind of detail I've shared with you isn't published in his work, but once you start to just use the basic principles – acceptance, being open, being empathetic and genuinely there in the situation – then you've got a whole new world that opens up really. And I think that these are things that I have learned to fine-tune. It's a whole approach that I've learned the principles of. I really understand them, have internalised them and am committed to the principles. But the fine-tuning detail . . . is just how you learned yourself, that you can best realise these principles in daily practice.

The second way of developing professional craft knowledge was merely being there, immersed in the situation and encountering a puzzling or confusing situation, or feeling irritated by something and then working things out for herself. The third way combines the first two, in which a problem is met in the use of theoretical principles and the problem solution occurs through a process of trial and error as the 'nitty-gritty' practicalities are worked out. Alison believed that she learned not only through close involvement of heart and head in the situation, but also being able to stand back and reflect upon it.

I found two other ways in which Alison acquired craft knowledge. First, our critical companionship helped her to refine her craft knowledge of nursing patients and to acquire knowledge about facilitating nurses' learning. Second, the unconscious transfer of her craft knowledge of working with patients to her facilitation work with nurses led to the creation of new craft knowledge. 'There's so much craft knowledge in this; it's about helping people. It's all the same stuff really' (Titchen, 200, p. 125). When the craft knowledge of skilled companionship was used in her role as a facilitator of learning, that knowledge required modification and fine-tuning in the new context; thus new craft knowledge was developed.

### *Facilitating theorization of practice*

Theories were used to inform our understanding of what was happening. For instance, I introduced socialization theory to help us to understand how the pervasive influence of a traditional ward learning culture was influencing the nurses' experience of Alison's facilitation. This understanding gave us ideas about how to change things, giving rise to decisions about appropriate action hypotheses to test. I also introduced educational theories as a resource to help Alison to improve her facilitation of learning skills. Building on my own commonsense theorization of a situation, I used theories to make suggestions for action.

*AT:* My impression is that the nurses don't see practical bedside care as having the same opportunities that you do, which makes the situation interesting for you. They feel bored and don't see the possibilities because they haven't really internalized patient-centred care. And, of course, Martha MacLeod's work shows that expert nurses attempt to meet multiple goals in basic care, so perhaps we need to think about how you could help them to use the opportunities provided by so-called basic care to address psychosocial issues as well as meet physical needs.

Alison experienced my theorization in these contexts as helpful.

*AB:* You make the process explicit at a theoretical level, so I can use that theoretical image to guide my actions next time.

Then she began to join in the process, but it took some nine months before she initiated it spontaneously.

*AT:* Today, you said, for the first time, 'I am now theorising', and you have never said that before . . .

*AB:* (laughs) Yes, well, I think that's because I'm conscious that that's what we're doing. I've been conscious that I've moved on from merely thinking, 'What's going on here?' to theorising, that is, asking, 'Why?', 'What are the principles here?', 'What's the relationship?', 'Where are the connections?'.

### Role-modelling strategy

Role-modelling is a strategy used to help a practitioner to become a facilitator of experiential learning, in which the companion demonstrates how the process concepts of consciousness-raising, problematization, self-reflection and critique can be realized in all the strategies above. The practitioner has a direct experience of the strategies and thus knows what it is like to be on the receiving end. Within the critical dialogue strategy, the companion helps the practitioner to transfer this experience to facilitating the experiential learning of others. Practitioners as critical companions for their junior colleagues consciously use this strategy as they go about their everyday work of looking after patients, to demonstrate their tacit knowledge and the strategies that realize the concepts of skilled companionship. Role-modelling is much enhanced by combining it with the articulation of craft knowledge shortly after the role-modelling has occurred.

*AB:* I am thinking of the way you help me to look at my work with the nurses on an individual basis. You know, how I am trying to get to grips with helping them to reflect on their practice and that comes from you and the way you help me to tell the story, to reflect and to theorise.

*AT:* You're having the experience with me of how it feels to have one's reflection and evaluation facilitated.

*AB:* That's right. Then I try to help them to do that. That is a role-modelling.

## Facilitative use of self domain

The facilitative use of self is the 'pathway' or overarching domain of critical companionship. It is complex and dynamic, involving multiple configurations of the facilitation, rationality-intuitive and relationship domains and their interplay. It also involves interplay with the **human aspects** (i.e. knowing, being, doing and feeling) and with the **situational aspects** which are determined by the particular. For example, to help an expert practitioner to become a critical companion, the aspects on which to focus might be fostering self-awareness, understanding of the nature of professional craft knowledge, and skill in facilitating its acquisition and creation. To help less experienced practitioners to become more patient-centred, the focus might be on articulating the craft knowledge of skilled companionship and promoting self-awareness, critical thinking and professional craft knowledge acquisition and use.

In the facilitative use of self domain, critical companions use 'antennae' to sense what is going on within themselves, the practitioner and their interactions and what is going on in the clinical setting. There is also an interpretive and associative interplay between theoretical and craft knowledge (see Eraut, 1994), as well as between intuition and rational thinking.

This use of self occurs when the facilitation, rationality-intuitive and relationship domains of critical companionship are shaped by the critical companion as a person. Self-aware and self-knowing engagement with the practitioner and use of these domains demands professional artistry, in the form of synchronicity, balance, attunement, interplay and perspective trans- formation.

The following story illustrates this domain. The context is a reflective conversation, during which Alison and I analysed a supervision session that I had observed five days previously between Alison and Dave. In their session, they had discussed Annie, Dave's patient, who had had a stroke and had been left with a communication problem. Dave recounted how he had discovered that if he gave Annie time, she could make herself understood. He had observed that her relatives did not give her time and always spoke for her. Although he had felt that this situation was not in Annie's best interests and that he would have liked to intervene with her relatives, he did not see it as his place to do so. I had observed Dave with Annie the morning before and had questioned him about her, so in the story, I am using my understanding of the situation in the conversation.

**Using the body to facilitate self-evaluation**

*AT:* When you got to the bit about the daughters speaking for Annie, can you remember what your intentions were then?

*AB:* My intention was to try to help him to rethink his own approach, rather than telling him that I thought that it was wrong. But I didn't particularly want to tell him that, certainly at the beginning. I wanted him to think again.

*AT:* He told you about deciding not to approach the daughters and then he very quickly introduced a question mark into his voice.

*AB:* Yeah.

*AT:* He said, in effect, that he didn't think that it was his place to intervene with the daughters. Then in the next sentence he said, but that's what I've been thinking about – that maybe I should.

*AB:* What I was trying to do – just in my facial expression, really – instead of responding (verbally), you just are silent and you look a question mark really, don't you?

*AT:* Mmh. Just the raise of an eyebrow.

*AB:* Mmh. It's not a judgment, just 'Well, is that really the only way of looking at it?' Just a way of making them pause, isn't it?

*AT:* Mmh.

*AB:* So they do go back and question themselves. It's much more satisfying.

*AT:* It's through your body language that you are demonstrating that there is a salient feature here.

*AB:* Yeah.

*AT:* And you're asking them to analyse this particular aspect again in the light of your questioning expression and they think, 'Oh, I have to look at this again, maybe I'm not right'.

*AB:* Once he had started to question it – he had taken the lead on that – I think I remember following up with a few more probing questions, 'Do you think that's your role?', 'Could you intervene there?' He was saying that it wasn't his role to intervene with the family or whatever and I asked something to the effect of 'How does Jessie react when they speak for her?'

*AT:* And he said she just seems to accept it.

*AB:* So he's brought the subject up now. He's initiated it and now I'm helping him, so I can move into slightly more active, more focusing mode now.

*AT:* Presenting new perspectives.

*AB:* Yeah. But on material that he has brought to me which is so much more comfortable than me saying, 'Well, there is a situation here that you are not handling very well' (laughs) which would just terrify them.

*AT:* And he knows what Jessie's reaction is, because he immediately uses his own body to show you (Dave had indicated Jessie's resignation to the situation by shrugging his shoulders).

*AB:* So that brings out another salient feature for him to reconsider, 'Well, if that is her reaction, perhaps I should be doing something.'

**The milieu**

The milieu in which critical companionship takes place is determined by whether or not the critical companion has a clinical caseload in the practitioner's clinical setting. If not, the milieu encompasses **reflective conversations** away from the clinical area and of **focused conversations** within it. The latter usually follow from the observing, listening and questioning strategy. If the critical companion has a caseload and is thus able to work alongside the practitioner in the clinical setting, the milieu consists of **clinical supervision integrated with practice**. This requires building reflection time into caring for patients. For example, in the story above, Alison and Dave negotiated time together to discuss his patient Annie in the staffroom during a tea break. In addition, the milieu may include **in the midst of practice**, where the companion uses whatever is happening, for instance, bedside shift handovers and clinical team meetings.

## Conclusions

Underpinned by critical social science, humanistic, spiritual and phenomenological perspectives, critical companionship is a new framework for facilitating the development of three characteristics of expertise: skilled companionship (or being patient-centred); being able to create, use and critically review professional craft knowledge; and being self-reflective and self-evaluative. Two models of critical companionship have been presented, an outsider model for preparing an expert practitioner as a facilitator of experiential learning, and an insider model that is used by the expert to help others develop expertise within the clinical setting. Whilst some evidence of the effectiveness of the models has been set out here, more detailed evidence is reported elsewhere (Titchen, 2000).

Supported by the very little empirical research already available in nursing, the framework makes a conceptual contribution to this neglected area. Experience in disseminating this framework to other health care professions suggests that the critical companionship framework is transferable. I propose that the framework should be tested in different contexts and professions.

Overall, three strong messages emerge from this study. First, the recognized parallel relationship between patient-centred health care and the facilitation of experiential learning is confirmed and attention is paid to distinctions and modifications. Second, professional artistry is essential not only to patient-centred health care, but also to being an effective facilitator of learning. Third, story-telling, dialogue and journeying together on physical, emotional, psychological and metaphysical levels play a significant role in helping patients to move forward and in facilitating practitioners' development of expertise. The foundation of each of these areas is professional craft knowledge, which plays a fundamental role in the effectiveness, artistry and humanity of quality professional practice.

## Note

1. In this chapter quotations in a different font are derived from Titchen (2000).

## References


Benner, P. A., Tanner, C. A. and Chesla, C. A. (1996) *Expertise in Nursing Practice: Caring, Clinical Judgment, and Ethics*. New York: Springer.

Binnie, A. and Titchen, A. (1999) *Freedom to Practise: The Development of Patient-Centred Nursing*. Oxford: Butterworth-Heinemann.

Campbell, A. V. (1984) *Moderated Love*. London: SPCK.

Conway, J. (1996) *Nursing Expertise and Advanced Practice*. Dinton: Quay Books.

Eraut, M. (1994) *Developing Professional Knowledge and Competence*. London: The Falmer Press.

Fay, B. (1987) The basic scheme of critical social science. In *Critical Social Science: Liberation and Its Limits* (B. Fay, ed.), pp. 28–41, 219–220. Cambridge: Polity Press.

Fish, D. and Twinn, S. (1990) *How to Enable Learning Through Professional Practice: A Cross-Profession Investigation of the Supervision of Pre-Service Practice*. Twickenham: West London Institute of Higher Education.

Freire, P. (1985) *The Politics of Education: Culture, Power, and Liberation*. Basingstoke: Macmillan.

Goodfellow, J., McAllister, L., Best, D., Webb, G. and Fredericks, D. (2001) Students and educators learning within relationships. In *Professional Practice: in Health, Education and the Creative Arts* (J. Higgs and A. Titchen, eds). Oxford: Blackwell Science.

Habermas, J. (1972) *Knowledge and Human Interests*. London: Heinemann.

Johns, C. (1997) Becoming an effective practitioner through guided reflection. PhD thesis, University of Luton.

MacLeod, M. (1994) It's the little things that count: The hidden complexity of everyday clinical nursing practice. *Journal of Clinical Nursing*, **3**, 361–368.

Rogers, C. (1983) *Freedom to Learn for the 80's*. London: Charles E. Merrill.

Runciman, P. J. (1983) *Ward Sister at Work*. London: Churchill Livingstone.

Titchen, A. and Binnie, A. (1995) The art of clinical supervision. *Journal of Clinical Nursing*, **4**, 327–334.

Titchen, A. (2000) *Professional Craft Knowledge in Patient-Centred Nursing and the Facilitation of Its Development*. DPhil thesis, University of Oxford; Oxford: Ashdale Press.

# 11

# Personal frames of reference in professional practice

**Anne Cusick**

The focus in most professional education, training and development is the acquisition and mastery of specialized knowledge and skill. This knowledge and skill can be technical or reflective in nature (Harris, 1993). By achieving appropriate standards in their understanding and application of specialized knowledge and skill, practitioners demonstrate competence in their fields (McGaghie, 1993) and earn their place as 'professionals'. They are recognized as colleagues and peers by those who already have the status and privileges of the specialty. They are also recognized as 'experts' by the community they serve. Specialized knowledge and skill is therefore important in the way professionals define themselves and the way the community views those who call themselves professional (Friedson, 1986).

The importance of specialized professional knowledge and skill in practice is indisputable. It is the special knowledge and the unique services which make particular professions needed and valued by the community; and it is the specialization which differentiates one profession from another. Consequently, it is not surprising to find that those groups seeking to attain or retain professional status emphasize the need for specialist knowledge. They do this through calls for research or scholarship to demonstrate the uniqueness of their practice and through suggestions for supervision and mentorship to promote practice quality. But specialist knowledge, be it scholarship or craft knowledge, is only part of the picture of professional practice. Professionals are people long before they become professionals. This chapter explores the way in which being a person affects and is affected by professional practice.

## Becoming a professional

Professionals are not born. At some point in life, a person decides to become a professional. Although each person is unique, the process of becoming a professional has common features for everyone. In essence, individuals must take on a new role and make the professional role theirs. Theoretically speaking, they engage in the processes of **role-taking** (Mead, 1934; Turner, 1962; Miller, 1981; Hurley-Wilson, 1988) and **role-making** (Turner, 1962, 1980; Conway, 1988).

These processes are proposed to be quite conscious (Cohen, 1989). Once the decision has been made to become a professional, an individual's energy and actions are directed towards developing the professional role. This is usually done through long periods of socialization structured as educational programmes where the novice learns the specialized knowledge and skill that constitute shared meanings of the professional group. In addition to learning and practising the use of knowledge and skills, novice professionals have opportunities to reflect on their progressive attainment of the professional role through events and interactions which verify their new status; for example, through milestones like their first unsupervised field placement, first public exhibition, or the awarding of certificates of achievement. Once the individual is accepted as a member of the professional group, role-taking and role-making do not finish. The person continues to change and modify the professional role as a result of further professional interaction. Things that were considered important early in a career may change and the professional role may be adjusted accordingly.

Role-taking and role-making are processes which assume that individuals take actions based on the meaning they have about a given situation or thing (Rose, 1962; Collins, 1985; Hoover, 1986; Jacob, 1987). These meanings arise through social interaction with other people (Stryker, 1981) and are actively handled or modified through reflection (Blumer, 1969; Vidich and Lyman, 1994). This is why meanings can change over time, as people experience new social encounters and have opportunities to reflect on their significance. Consequently, the process of becoming a professional does not stop with entry as a new graduate or practitioner. Rather, it is an ongoing process of development as new encounters bring new meanings and opportunities for reflection.

## Person as professional

Role-taking and role-making are important constructs which explain the way in which people become professionals. Both constructs demonstrate that the person with his/her unique views, actions and reflections is the focal point of professional development. In discussions of professional knowledge where specialist expertise is often the focus, this important centrality of the person can sometimes be overlooked. Specialist professional knowledge and practice is not a 'stand alone' thing which the individual learns and implements. Rather, it is something which the individual will encounter, make sense of, derive personal meaning from, determine what to do about, engage in and reflect on within the context of being a person. The processes of professional action and development in interaction with self are facilitated by personal reflection and interpersonal interactions.

Given the importance of role-taking and role-making in the development of professionals, there is a need to further consider the individual view, or personal frame of reference, and the way in which it contributes to professional practice and knowledge. The part played by the views or meanings held by the person who becomes a professional is highly significant. Individual frames of reference are starting points for a person who is to make sense of the professional experience. I propose that three aspects of personal frames of reference illuminate the importance of these frames of reference to professional practice. They are personal world views, professional development, and personal morality in professional behaviour. These are now explored.

## Personal world views

Personal frames of reference are significant components of the knowledge used in practice, because unique meanings held by individual professionals will play a role in the actions they take in any given situation. So although professionals will share some common understanding about practice, it will inevitably be mediated by an individual's values and beliefs (Fleming and Mattingly, 1994) or personal paradigm (Schell and Cervero, 1993). These personal frames of reference may well go beyond parameters of the profession's area of interest. A person's **world view** may thus be the framework through which professional situations, knowledge and skill are interpreted to determine their meaning and significance for action as a professional.

A world view is described as 'a total vision of life' (Griffioen, 1989, p. 84). Holmes (1983, cited in Hooper, 1997, p. 328) describes world view as 'personal or communal, pretheoretical commitments about the relationship of self to others, and the relation of humans to the nonhuman world'. World views are deeply held beliefs about reality and the nature of the self and other human beings. These beliefs are influenced by the unique combination of personal, cultural and historical contexts experienced by each person. World views are thus personal frames of reference that describe and explain our vision of the world, give meaning to things we encounter and underpin the actions we take in the world.

Professionals' personal world views have been suggested to directly influence practice actions. Hooper (1997), for example, studied the case of a therapist whose world view was based on the principles, visions and practices of Hinduism. This case study described the way in which the therapist's world view directly influenced the way she understood disability, her approaches for intervention and her practice actions. In particular, pre-theoretical commitments about reality, life and death, human nature and knowledge were central to the way in which she delivered service as a professional. Pre-theoretical commitments based on Hinduism influenced the way in which she encountered, reflected and acted on the specialist theoretical and craft knowledge and skills of her profession. This influence was not immediately observable in therapy sessions. She used a reductionist biomechanical approach in intervention, where exercise was prescribed and facilitated during activities. But in explaining her view of the intervention experience, she referred to constructs such as destiny and the need for the patient to develop inner strength. These, she explained, were important dimensions of her Hindu belief, which guided and encouraged her in her interactions with patients.

As professionals take on roles and make them their own, world views they hold will inevitably influence their practice. According to Fleming and Mattingly (1994, p. 340) professional practice is supposed to be 'value free', or at least underpinned only by the values of the profession: 'no prior assumptions, values or preferences of the clinician should intervene between the problem and the scientific mind of the practitioner'. If 'world view' is a framework of assumptions about reality, human beings and the self, which is deeply held and influences the way in which individual meaning is constructed, then such value-free approaches are unlikely to occur in professional practice. Indeed, Fleming and Mattingly (1994, p. 341), in studying the practice of therapists, found that professionals used personal values to 'guide, promote, and defend care and quality of life for their patients'.

Professions have acknowledged the role of beliefs and values in practice by encouraging students and practitioners to reflect on their personal assumptions and the way they might influence their practice. Reflective journals, supervision meetings, use of fieldnotes or creation of artefacts based on experience are examples of strategies used in professions to encourage such reflection. By encouraging such reflection, professions seek to make tacit pre-theoretical assumptions explicit, so that practitioners can apply theoretical knowledge with a view less coloured by hidden assumptions about the world and people. Recognizing pre-theoretical world views and then working with the theoretical and craft knowledge of a specialty is a key task facing the professional. It is a major task in professional development, which will now be explored.

## Professional development

The processes of role-taking and role-making suggest that becoming and being a professional are dynamic states. The role itself brings opportunities for new social interaction, novel situations and resulting new points of view, or 'standpoints' (Strauss, 1959). This is particularly the case in professions where the base of knowledge is inherently incomplete and practice actions are therefore often autonomously decided within uncertainty (Hardy and Hardy, 1988). Professional development is thus inextricably linked to personal development as individuals move through their life course and encounter new situations and reflect on them. One example of professional role development is the transition from novice to expert practitioner with resultant development in performance and competence (Benner, 1984; Dreyfus and Dreyfus, 1986; Mattingly and Fleming, 1994; Robertson, 1996; Schell, 1998). Professional development, such as the change from novice to expert, is something that happens for the whole person, not just for the part called 'service provider'.

Professionals need to be able to relate well to other people and to have an understanding of themselves, in particular of those attributes that might affect their ability to communicate and to perform specialist functions. Bernstein (1999) suggests that service professionals should therefore consider their personal motives, strengths and limitations to relate this self knowledge to the service task and context. She suggests that, in the first instance, professional development means understanding oneself and engaging in reflection and action to change oneself in ways that will help make the professional role more effective.

Consider this example: 'If one of your values is empowerment, you may need to learn to teach decision-making skills to the people you serve... Also, you need to be able to monitor yourself and look for ways in which you can help people make their own decisions as well as ways in which you hinder their independent decision-making' (Bernstein, 1999, p. 49). The conscious focus on taking and modifying or making roles is clear in this example. Here the emphasis in professional development is clearly on recognizing personal values, learning specialist skills which can support those values, and actively reflecting to decide on new actions or behaviours in relation to the personal value of empowerment. The personal frame of reference here influences what behaviours are considered important in professional practice. Likewise, professional practice experiences influence the way in which personal values are considered. The two operate in dynamic synergy. Professional development thus requires personal development for real change to occur, and personal development will inevitably develop the professional. It is therefore essential to recognize the significant part which personal frames of reference play in development of the professional.

## Personal morality in professional behaviour

In addition to world view and professional development, the processes of role-taking and role-making suggest that individual professionals have ownership of actions taken. Role-taking in particular is proposed to be a conscious process for adults, where the meanings of objects and events are considered, decisions are made and actions taken in the light of the person's views. If exposure to and interaction with the professional role has been adequate, the actions taken by an individual professional in this process should be in line with expectations and norms of the professional group (given the constraints of the situation). There will be things that are 'right' and 'proper' for the professional to do, and things that are not.

In many practice professions, there is a separation between moral judgment and practice judgment (Fleming and Mattingly, 1994). The assumption is that a reliance on theoretical knowledge for decision-making in practice will minimize the risk of social prejudice affecting service delivered (Fleming and Mattingly, 1994). This separation is, however, artificial, as personal values and beliefs, in particular world views, can influence practice.

It would seem more important, therefore, to recognize the significant role in practice of personal views about how human beings should live and what constitutes a 'good' life. These are essentially moral issues. They are of particular importance because professionals often work with vulnerable groups who have their trust. These groups trust that not only will professionals do the 'right thing' for them, but also that the advice and expert assistance given by professionals will enhance their quality of life in a 'good' way. Professionals, because they work with people, must come face to face with the complex issue of the way in which their moral principles and their consequent moral conduct affect the quality of life of others for good or ill.

This issue of morality in practice is commonly termed 'professional ethics', and in many professions it is represented by a list of rules or principles that must be adhered to for 'good' practice. This is an absolutist approach, where certain things will be either right or wrong, and the professional who 'crosses the line' will be considered unacceptable to the group. But in day-to-day practice, moral problems are rarely absolute. There are many variables that can make a problem unclear and an ethical solution relative. As a result in professional practice, it is often the individual who determines whether or not professional rules of practice have meaning, and whether or not those particular ethics will guide day-to-day decisions. Personal moral principles are likely to frame views about professional ethics, the presenting problem and the actions ultimately taken by autonomous professionals.

Morals are concerned with the distinction between right and wrong, good and bad, acceptable and unacceptable, in relation to human behaviour. Professionals use specialist knowledge to contribute some service to the community, and as a consequence of dealing with other human beings, they face on a daily basis moral problems where decisions need to be made and actions taken. These will be practical decisions, as moral problems are essentially practical ones where the question is about what one ought to do in a given situation (Hare, 1952, 1963, 1972). To come to an ethical decision, the person must consider issues of good and bad, in addition to factual questions which relate to the consequences of alternative actions (Hare, 1952). Statements of professional ethics can help guide a practitioner about 'what one ought to do'; however, the individual will have the ultimate responsibility of considering whether or not that principle or rule will and should apply in a given situation. Professionals who aim to practise in an ethical manner need to reconcile personal morals with professional codes of conduct.

## Conclusions

This chapter has explored the way in which being a person affects and is affected by professional practice. It has been argued that becoming a professional means taking on the role of 'professional' and making it one's own. Through the processes of role-taking and role-making, specialist professional knowledge is encountered, made sense of, personal meaning is derived, action is taken and reflection on the experience and new meanings occur. Through these processes, which necessarily involve social interaction, the person develops as a professional.

The key feature of using the constructs of role-taking and role-making to explain the way people become professionals is that it clearly places the person with his/her unique views, actions and reflections, at centre stage. Personal world views and personal frames of reference for moral conduct become critical starting points for understanding and developing professional behaviour. The challenge for professions is to work out how best to acknowledge the important role personal frames of reference play in the lives and practice of their professionals, at the same time as supporting and advancing the development of specialist theoretical and professional craft knowledge which underpins their existence.

## References


Benner, P. (1984) *From Novice to Expert*. Menlo Park, CA: Addison-Wesley.

Bernstein, G. S. (1999) *Human Services? That Must Be So Rewarding*. Philadelphia: MacLennan & Petty.

Blumer, H. (1969) *Symbolic Interactionism: Perspective and Method*. Englewood Cliffs, NJ: Prentice-Hall.

Cohen, J. (1989) About steaks liking to be eaten: The conflicting views of symbolic interaction and Talcott Parsons concerning the nature of relations between humans and non-human subjects. *Symbolic Interaction*, **12**, 191–213.

Collins, R. (1985) *Three Sociological Traditions*. New York: Oxford University Press.

Conway, M. E. (1988) Theoretical approaches to the study of roles. In *Role Theory: Perspectives for Health Professionals*, 2nd edn (E. Hardy and M. E. Conway, eds), pp. 63–72. Norfolk, CA: Appleton & Lange.

Dreyfus, H. L. and Dreyfus, S. E. (1986) *Mind Over Machine: The Power of Human Intuition and Expertise in the Era of the Computer*. New York: Free Press.

Fleming, M. and Mattingly, C. (1994) Action and inquiry: Reasoned action and active reasoning. In *Clinical Reasoning: Forms of Inquiry in a Therapeutic Practice* (C. Mattingly and M. H. Fleming, eds), pp. 316–342. Philadelphia: F. A. Davis.

Friedson, E. (1986) *Professional Powers: A Study of the Institutionalization of Formal Knowledge*. Chicago: University of Chicago Press.

Griffioen, S. (1989) The world view approach to social theory. In *Stained Glass: World Views and Social Science* (P. A. Marshall, S. Griffioen and R. Mouw, eds), pp. 81–119. New York: University Press of America.

Hardy, M. E. and Hardy, W. L. (1988) Role stress and role strain. In *Role Theory Perspectives for Health Professionals* (M. E. Hardy and M. E. Conway, eds), pp. 159–240. Norwalk, CT: Appleton & Lange.

Hare, R. M. (1952) *The Language of Morals*. Oxford: Oxford University Press,.

Hare, R. M. (1963) *Freedom and Reason*. Oxford: Oxford University Press.

Hare, R. M. (1972) *Applications of Moral Philosophy*. London: MacMillan.

Harris, I. B. (1993) New expectations for professional competence. In *Educating Professionals: Responding to New Expectations for Competence and Accountability* (L. Curry and J. F. Wergin, eds), pp. 17–52. San Francisco: Jossey-Bass.

Holmes, A. F. (1983) *Contours of a World View*. Grand Rapids, MI: Eerdman.

Hooper, B. (1997) The relationship between pretheoretical reasoning assumptions and clinical reasoning. *American Journal of Occupational Therapy*, **51**, 328–338.

Hoover, M. C. (1986) Adorno and Mead: Toward an interactionist critique of negative dialects. *Sociological Focus*, **19**, 189–205.

Hurley-Wilson, B. A. (1988) Socialisation for roles. In *Role Theory: Perspectives for Health Professionals*, 2nd edn (E. Hardy and M. E. Conway, eds), pp. 73–110. Norfolk, CA: Appleton & Lange.

Jacob, E. (1987) Qualitative research traditions: A review. *Review of Educational Research*, **57**, 1–50.

Mattingly, C. and Fleming, M. H. (1994) *Clinical Reasoning: Forms of Inquiry in a Therapeutic Practice*. Philadelphia: F. A. Davis Co.

McGaghie, W. C. (1993) Evaluating competence for professional practice. In *Educating Professionals: Responding to New Expectations for Competence and Accountability* (L. Curry and J. F. Wergin, eds), pp. 229–261. San Francisco: Jossey-Bass.

Mead, G. H. (1934) *Mind, Self, and Society*. Chicago: University of Chicago Press.

Miller, D. I. (1981) The meaning of role taking. *Symbolic Interaction*, **4**, 167.

Robertson, L. J. (1996) Clinical reasoning, Part 2: Novice/expert differences. *British Journal of Occupational Therapy*, **59**, 212–216.

Rose, A. M. (1962) A systematic summary of symbolic interaction theory. In *Human Behaviour and Social Processes* (A. M. Rose, ed.), pp. 3–19. Boston: Houghton Mifflin.

Schell, B. (1998) Clinical reasoning: The basis of practice. In *Willard and Spackman's Occupational Therapy*, 9th edn (M. E. Neistadt and E. B. Crepeau, eds), pp. 90–100. Philadelphia: J. B. Lippincott.

Schell, B. and Cervero, R. (1993) Clinical reasoning in occupational therapy: An integrative review. *American Journal of Occupational Therapy*, **47**, 605–610.

Strauss, A. (1959) Language and identity. In *Symbolic Interaction: A Reader in Social Psychology* (J. G. Maris and B. N. Meltzer, eds), pp. 379–385 (2nd edn, 1972). Boston: Allyn & Bacon.

Stryker, S. (1981) Symbolic interactionism: Themes and variations. In *Social Psychology: Sociological Perspectives* (M. Rosenberg and R. H. Turner, eds), pp. 3–29. New York: Basic Books.

Turner, R. H. (1962) Role taking: Process versus conformity. In *Human Behaviour and Social Processes* (A. Rose, ed.), pp. 20–40. Boston: Mifflin.

Turner, R. H. (1980) *Family Interaction*. New York: Wiley.

Vidich, A. J. and Lyman, S. M. (1994) Qualitative methods: Their history in sociology and anthropology. In *Handbook of Qualitative Research* (W. K. Denzin and Y. Lincoln, eds), pp. 23–59. Thousand Oaks, CA: Sage.

# 12

# Patient-centred practice: an emerging focus for nursing expertise

**Brendan McCormack and Angie Titchen**

This chapter explores the relationship between professional craft knowledge and nursing expertise. It demonstrates that one of the characteristics of expertise is being patient-centred. It argues that being patient-centred requires an engagement with the professional craft knowledge of developing, sustaining and closing person-centred relationships. Common features of this kind of professional craft knowledge have been identified by numerous research studies despite their different methodologies. McCormack's (1998) conceptual analysis of autonomy of older people in hospital is an exemplar study that shows these commonalities. Findings from that study are presented and are supported by evidence from Titchen's (1998, 2000) study of patient-centred nursing and its development. (See Chapter 9 for a fuller description.) We conclude that person-centredness is a key characteristic of expert nursing practice, and that it can be facilitated through critical companionship strategies. Early evidence in our ongoing research suggests that this is also the case in other health care professions.

## Expert practice

The key attributes of an expert nurse as defined by Manley and McCormack (1997), derived from the work of Benner (1984) and Benner et al. (1996), are as follows:

- **Holistic practice and holistic knowledge**. Synthesizing different types of knowledge about a patient and different ways of knowing in order to work holistically.
- **Saliency**. Seeing the most pertinent issues in the situation and the most appropriate ways of responding to them.
- **Knowing the patient**. Knowing the patient as a person and knowing his/her typical patterns of response in order to make a skilled judgment about the most appropriate nursing response.
- **Moral agency**. Having concern for responding to the patient as a person, respecting his/her dignity, protecting personhood in times of vulnerability, helping him/her feel safe, providing comfort and maintaining integrity in the relationship.
- **Skilled know-how**. Demonstrating performance that is fluid and seamless and highly proficient. Actions reflect attunement to the situation, which is shaped by the patient's responses, and does not rely on conscious deliberation.

The factors that enable this expert practice to be sustained are (Manley and McCormack, 1997):

- the ability to reflect on the effectiveness of practice;
- authority in and accountability for practice;
- therapeutic interpersonal relationships with team members and patients;
- a practice environment that enables a person-centred approach to the organization of care services.

In her study of expert nurses, Titchen (2000) identified patient-centredness as key to expertise. Her findings support Manley and McCormack's (1997) assertions and provide a new conceptualization of patient-centred nursing and its place in expertise. She found that to put the ideas and values of humanism, holism, partnership, empowerment, existentialism and the methods of phenomenology into action required the creation and use of professional craft knowledge. Distinct domains of professional craft knowledge (see Chapter 9) enable nurses to take themselves as persons into healing relationships with patients and families.

Benner and Tanner (1987), from their study of expert nurses, claim that intuitive judgment rather than rational thinking is the hallmark of expertise. However, Titchen (2000) concludes that expertise is hallmarked by professional artistry which involves rapid interplay and a balance of intuition and rationality whilst engaged in action-oriented work, and in deliberative reflection and metacognition (thinking about thinking) when bringing this interplay under critical control and scrutiny by oneself and others. Expertise also involves the therapeutic use of self and the complex harmonization of the domains of professional craft knowledge and theoretical knowledge.

Nurses clearly have difficulties in describing their 'everyday practice' and it has been argued that this is because they do not think as they have been taught, in terms of systems and structures, and do not address the issue of problem-solving through a mechanistic, linear approach (Benner, 1984; Benner and Tanner, 1987). Rather, they think holistically. Expert practitioners 'always know more than they can tell' and by acknowledging intuitive thought can act on 'hunches', draw on tacit knowledge and engage in holistic problem-solving (McCormack, 1992). The problem with this kind of knowledge is that it is difficult to quantify, and it is rare to find a chief executive who responds well to statements like 'I know this intuitively!' As a result, the need for expert registered nurses is often challenged, and they are replaced with care assistants whose role definitions reflect task-based reactive care rather than holistic anticipatory care, which is central to patient-centred practice.

## Patient-centred care

The traditional style of practice 'emphasized the service of medicine as a means of serving patients and was essentially concerned with the dutiful completion of a hierarchy of practical tasks' (Binnie and Titchen, 1998, p. 7). The most appropriate and efficient work design for this style was influenced by the industrial production-line model in which tasks were completed in the least possible time by the appropriately qualified nurse. It has been widely recognized that the lack of continuity of care, however, denied patients the comfort and support of sustained, caring relationships (e.g. Meleis, 1991).

Humanistic caring (e.g. Watson, 1988; Benner and Wrubel, 1989; Johns, 1994; Binnie and Titchen, 1999; Titchen, 2000) through a 'person-centred' philosophy is one such way of attending to the human experience in care. This style of practice demonstrates a deep respect for the autonomy of the patient as a person. Acknowledgement and valuing of each patient's biography and his or her individual perception and health care experience is fundamental to this way of nursing. This valuing of individuals aims to transform the patient's experience of illness and to be therapeutic in its own right. The role of the person-centred nurse is to be there, offering personal support and practical expertise, while enabling patients to follow the path of their own choosing in their own way. This style of nursing reflects an existentialist philosophy and the resultant humanistic psychology which has influenced many contemporary nurse theorists (e.g. Benner, 1984; Watson, 1988; Boykin and Schoenhofer, 1993; Johns, 1994). At the heart of this style of nursing is the therapeutic nurse–patient relationship, which requires continuity of care and the acceptance of responsibility for the outcomes of care. Such a philosophy is also recognized by other professional groups (Fulford et al., 1996; Hope, 1996; Kitwood, 1997; Williams and Grant, 1998). McCormack's (1998) study of the autonomy of older people in hospital demonstrates how the conceptualization of autonomy as 'authentic consciousness', underpinned by a shared understanding of nurses' and patients' values, enabled the articulation of a patient-centred practice framework. To illustrate the shared understandings that exist between McCormack's (1998) and Titchen's (2000) studies, data extracts from Titchen's work are used to illustrate the framework of person-centredness developed from McCormack's research.

## Conceptualizing patient-centredness

### Developing a conceptual understanding of 'autonomy' among older people in hospital

(McCormack, 1998)

The literature about professions and professionals emphasizes the conflict that exists in professions between loyalty to the organization or professional group and the profession's drive to do good for the people they serve. The literature dealing with professional autonomy further emphasizes the conflict that exists between the exercise of individual professional autonomy and a changed societal attitude that demands partnership in decision-making through a focus on consumerism (Dingwall and Lewis, 1983; Dingwall et al., 1988).

From a review of the literature, two opposing decision-making positions are possible for nurses. Firstly, as in Rawls' (1992) 'veil of ignorance', the nurse could be expected to act impartially and separate her moral deliberations from her knowledge of the situation. She would be obliged to evaluate the merits of particular actions solely on the basis of general considerations and the law of universality. In contrast, the nurse could adopt a contextualized position and believe that there is no objective reality on which to base decisions, and that each situation is unique, thus requiring a unique set of principles.

McCormack set out to develop a 'compromise' position, a position that recognized both the importance of the universal principles of care underpinning accountable nursing practice, and the value of the individual's biography (see Benner and Wrubel, 1989) underpinning the uniqueness of each caring experience. McCormack's research aims were to:

- create greater conceptual clarity about the concept of autonomy in relation to the notions of professional and personal autonomy;
- describe and explore the necessary and sufficient conditions for autonomy to exist in the relationship between nurses and older patients.

McCormack considered two questions to be of particular importance to this research:

- What is the meaning of autonomy in a relationship between a nurse and an older patient?
- When working with older people, can the nurse promote the principle of patient autonomy while functioning as an autonomous practitioner?

The research approach was guided by the hermeneutic philosophy of Gadamer (1993); conversational analysis (see Drew and Heritage, 1992) was utilized as the theoretical framework within which the initial analysis of data was framed. To be able to extrapolate actual practice for scrutiny, an approach to data collection was adopted that captured the interactions of nurses and patients. The recording of 'naturally occurring' conversations between nurses and patients was used as the primary source of data collection. The data were transcribed, coded and interpreted using techniques of conversation analysis (Drew and Heritage, 1992), reflective conversations (Bergum, 1991) and focused group discussions with expert nurses and older people.

### Achieving patient-centredness through an understanding of autonomy as authentic consciousness

From the research data, the key issue appeared to be the ability of the nurse to move between differing modes of being in the relationship with a patient, in order to reach the best patient outcome. The data suggested that nurses need to be able to take into account the particular person that the patient is, the particular relationship that exists between themselves and the patient, and the particular understandings and expectations implicit in the relationship (as argued by Blum, 1982). Such an understanding is achieved through an understanding of the person's authentic values:

> By authentic is meant a way of reaching decisions which are truly one's own – decisions that express all that one believes important about oneself and the world, the entire complexity of one's values. (Gadow, 1980, p. 85)

Nurses' knowing about another's authentic values requires caring about the other in a way which appreciates each patient as an individual human being, in a particular relationship with themselves. Such a particular caring knowledge of patients is necessary to determine the particular course of action to take from a variety of potential options.

Authentic consciousness is understood as a consideration of the whole of one's life in order to sustain meaning in life. Authentic consciousness is not a hierarchical ordering of possible desires, but instead is the clarification of one's values in order to maximize one's potential for growth and development. It is based on the clarification of values and the recognition of the importance of these values in decision-making. The role of the other in a caring relationship is to enable the clarification of values in order to maximize opportunities for growth and the making of authentic decisions, decisions that are representative of one's life as a whole. For older people, when autonomy is understood as authentic consciousness, the potential for the reduction of the person to a 'thing' is eroded and personhood is maintained.

The recognition of people's history acknowledges their social, psychological and cultural biographies, and this acknowledgement in turn recognizes that development continues throughout life, forming the tapestry of life (Selder, 1989). Such lives are imbued with personal meanings, beliefs and values which are essential to the way people see themselves and the way their world is constructed. While many aspects of an individual's reality may be shared with others so that common understandings can exist in order to form a sense of community, it is the individuality of our personal meanings that determines 'who we are'. It is this tapestry of meaning that creates the foundation on which the structures of our lives are built. When the threads of such a tapestry are severed and torn, as occurs through major life events (such as illness), then a once-stable foundation becomes unstable and the structures of people's lives fall.

In Chapter 9, the story 'Establishing some sense of Peter and Mary's life together' shows how an expert nurse came to know, through the process of particularity, the details of her unconscious patient's life. It also illustrates how she sought to understand the authentic values of the patient's husband, so that she could help him to clarify them and to cope with the severed tapestry of his life.

McCormack (1998) suggests that it is not enough just to take note of another's beliefs, values, views and experiences (their signs). These signs must be integrated into the being in the world for that individual. Being conscious of another's beliefs and values does not tell the nurse what to do, but rather it orients the nurse to a particular way of being. McCormack interprets this as meaning that the recognition of beliefs and values does not provide a prescription for action, but rather guides the nurse towards the most appropriate approach for action based on the individual's life experience. As Gadow (1980) argues, the recognition of the other's beliefs and values allows the patient and the nurse to have the kind of caring relationship that they want to have, appropriate to the context of care. Taking note of 'signs' enables the nurse to place actions in context, or as MacIntyre (1992, p. 210) suggests, 'the act of utterance becomes intelligible by finding its place in a narrative'.

Being person-centred relies on getting closer to the person; it goes beyond traditional notions of respecting individuality and individualized care, such as choices about food and drink, hygiene and waking and sleeping patterns. McCormack developed a framework for patient-centred practice utilizing the concepts of:

- **Informed flexibility**. The facilitation of decision-making through information sharing and the integration of new information into established perspectives and care practices. Titchen (2000) demonstrates such informed flexibility in the following account of an expert nurse's (Alison) interaction with a patient (Gertie):

  Alison: Fieldnote: I established that Gertie attributed her illness to the tragic death of her husband and son some eighteen years ago. If we are going to help Gertie to understand her heart condition, it will be no good us going straight in and saying to her, 'Your heart problem is due to a blocked artery' when for her it is related to her tragedy.

- **Mutuality**. The recognition of the other's values as being of equal importance in decision-making. Titchen (2000) illustrates this as follows:

  Alison demonstrated this recognition by accepting (a husband's) Peter's decision not to participate in (his wife's) Mary's care without question. Knowing patients' and family members' backgrounds and values, she was in a position to explore sensitively the options facing them, where appropriate, and to acknowledge and share the burden of responsibility with them.

  Letter: ... We also really valued the honesty and patience with which you discussed available possibilities of medical interventions with us. You showed great skill in approaching these issues in a way that neither interfered with our choices or left us feeling alone in the decisions we took.

- **Transparency**. The making explicit of intentions and motivations for action and the boundaries within which care decisions are set. Transparency is shown in a conversation between Alison and a staff nurse:

  Fieldnote: (*Alison*) I often think it's worth offering the spouse some time on their own because they may be worried about things that they don't want to say in front of their husband because they think they may worry him more. But you've got to do that in such a way that you've got permission from the patient. What's quite a good idea is to ask him, 'How's your wife coping?', 'Does she seem anxious about all this?' and then, if he says, 'She does seem a bit worried' or whatever, then try to get round to saying, 'Would it be helpful if I had some time with her by herself, so she can ask me questions on her own?', so that you've got the patient's permission.

(Transparency is shown in this exchange between Alison and Barbara, a staff nurse.)

*Barbara*: Mmh. And they know that you're not going behind their backs.

*Alison*: And they know you're doing it to help the wife, rather than to go behind his back and tell him things he's not allowed to know.

(Titchen, 2000)

- **Negotiation**. Patient participation through a culture of care that values the views of the patient as a legitimate basis for decision-making while recognizing that being the final arbiter of decisions is of secondary importance.

  Titchen found that Alison engaged with her patients as a partner and not as an expert who would offer solutions. Rather she offered her expertise to help patients to find their own solutions. This stance reflects her commitment to freedom, choice, personal responsibility and psychological growth. By working creatively with patients and families and by making a commitment to see problems through with them, she was able to fine-tune her practical and emotional support to match their special, personal needs and to achieve the best possible outcomes with them. Thus, she was able to maximize patients' control of their own recovery. Within the process of mutuality, Alison worked with her patients by responding to their needs as they saw them, rather than imposing on them what she felt was best. Professional knowledge in patient-centred nursing is, therefore, a negotiable resource for patients, rather than a source of power and control.

  (Titchen, 2000)

- **Sympathetic presence**. An engagement that recognizes the uniqueness and value of the individual, by appropriately responding to cues that maximize coping resources through the recognition of important agendas in daily life.

  A sympathetic presence was communicated, not only by Alison's attitude and attentiveness but also through the conscious use of physical closeness, silence, attuned listening and touch. During interactions, Alison intentionally placed herself in close proximity to the patient or relative. The attuned way that she listened to patients' stories appeared to mobilise patients' coping resources, as we have seen with Peter in the story in Chapter 9.

  (Titchen, 2000)

## Two studies – one shared understanding

Both McCormack's (1998) and Titchen's (2000) work articulate the complexity of patient-centred practice. Through the study of the participating nurses' world views of their practice worlds, the contextual, attitudinal and moral dimensions of humanistic caring practices are exposed. These dimensions have not been presented as disengaged concepts, driven by a desire to recreate the boundaries of nursing practice. Instead, the discourse of practice and the dialogue created between nurses, researchers and practice have been used to locate and illustrate the potentials of patient-centred practice and to further articulate the dimensions of expert practice. The reader who engages with both studies begins to 'live' the realities of patient-centred practice and explore approaches to developing expert patient-centred practices. Both studies require nurses to move beyond a focus on technical competence and to conceptualize the essence of the caring relationship within the concept of authenticity. For Titchen, being authentic transcends the relationship between nurse and patient and is one of the central values in being a critical companion developing others' professional craft knowledge of patient-centredness (Titchen, 1998). Both studies extend the current body of knowledge in this area (e.g. Watson, 1988; Boykin and Schoenhofer, 1993; MacLeod, 1994).

## Conclusions

From our experience in nursing, we conclude that if person-centred practice is to be made a reality, there is a need for large-scale organizational change that can enable growth through the acquisition of the kind of professional craft knowledge exhibited by Alison, and a need for 'critical companions' to accompany learners on their professional journeys. (See Chapter 10.) In discussion with colleagues working in other health and social disciplines, it is evident that person-centred practice is perhaps more advanced as a movement in nursing than elsewhere. Nonetheless, practitioners in these disciplines are consistently experiencing consumers who are expecting improved practices from their professions (Higgs, Radovich, Ryan, Irwin, personal communications). The form of these improved practices extends beyond the quality of technical performance to include a greater role for the patient/client in the decision-making process and a greater demonstration of person-centred caring in interpersonal interactions within health care and health promotion processes.

## References


Benner, P. (1984) *From Novice to Expert: Excellence and Power in Clinical Nursing Practice*. Menlo Park, CA: Addison-Wesley.

Benner, P. and Tanner, C. (1987) Clinical judgement: How expert nurses use intuition. *American Journal of Nursing*, **87**(1), 23–31.

Benner, P. and Wrubel, J. (1989) *The Primacy of Caring: Stress and Coping in Health and Illness*. Wokingham: Addison-Wesley Publishing.

Benner, P., Tanner, C. and Chesla, C. (1996) *Expertise in Nursing Practice. Caring, Clinical Judgement and Ethics*. New York: Springer Publishing Co.

Bergum, V. (1991) Being a phenomenological researcher. In *Qualitative Nursing Research: A Contemporary Dialogue* (J. Morse, ed.), pp. 55–72. London: Sage Publications.

Binnie, A. and Titchen, A. (1998) *Patient-Centred Nursing: An Action Research Study of Practice Development in an Acute Medical Unit*. Oxford: Royal College of Nursing Institute, Report No. 18.

Binnie, A. and Titchen, A. (1999) *Freedom to Practise: The Development of Patient-Centred Nursing*. Oxford: Butterworth-Heinemann.

Blum, L. A. (1982) *Friendship, Altruism and Morality*. London: Routledge and Kegan Paul.

Boykin, A. and Schoenhofer, S. (1993) *Nursing as Caring: A Model for Transforming Practice*. New York: National League for Nursing Press.

Dingwall, R. and Lewis, P. (1983) *The Sociology of the Professions – Lawyers, Doctors and Others*. Oxford: The Centre for Socio-Legal Studies, Wolfson College, University of Oxford.

Dingwall, R., Rafferty, A. M. and Webster, C. (1988) *An Introduction to the Social History of Nursing*. London: Routledge.

Drew, P. and Heritage, J. (1992) *Talk at Work: Interaction in Institutional Settings*. Cambridge: Cambridge University Press.

Fulford, K. W. M., Ersser, S. and Hope, T. (1996) *Essential Practice in Patient-Centred Care*. Oxford: Blackwell Science.

Gadamer, H. G. (1993) *Truth and Method*. London: Sheed & Ward.

Gadow, S. (1980) Existential advocacy: Philosophical foundations of nursing. In *Nursing: Images and Ideals – Opening Dialogue with the Humanities* (S. F. Spicker and S. Gadow, eds), pp. 79–107. New York: Springer.

Hope, T. (1996) *Evidence-Based Patient Choice*. London: Kings Fund.

Johns, C. C. (1994) *The Burford NDU Model: Caring in Practice*. Oxford: Blackwell Science.

Kitwood, T. (1997) *Dementia Reconsidered: The Person Comes First*. Milton Keynes: Open University Press.

MacIntyre, A. (1992) *After Virtue – a Study in Moral Theory*. London: Duckworth.

MacLeod, M. (1994) 'It's the little things that count': The hidden complexity of everyday clinical nursing practice. *Journal of Clinical Nursing*, **3**(6), 361–368.

Manley, K. and McCormack, B. (1997) *Exploring Expert Practice. Masters in Nursing Distance Learning Module*. London: Royal College of Nursing Institute.

Meleis, A. I. (1991) *Theoretical Nursing: Development and Progress*. Philadelphia: J. B. Lippincott.

McCormack, B. (1998) An exploration of the theoretical framework underpinning the autonomy of older people in hospital and its relationship to professional nursing practice. Doctoral thesis, University of Oxford.

McCormack, B. (1992) Intuition: Concept analysis and application to curriculum development. Part 1: Concept analysis. *Journal of Clinical Nursing*, **1**, 339–344.

Rawls, J. (1992) *A Theory of Justice*. Oxford: Oxford University Press.

Selder, F. (1989) Life transition theory: The resolution of uncertainty. *Nursing and Health Care*, **10**(8), 437–451.

Titchen, A. (1998) *A Conceptual Framework for Facilitating Learning in Clinical Practice*. Occasional Paper 2. Lidcombe, Australia: Centre for Professional Education Advancement, The University of Sydney.

Titchen A. (2000) *Professional Craft Knowledge in Patient-Centred Nursing and the Facilitation of its Development*. DPhil thesis, University of Oxford; Oxford:Ashdale Press.

Watson, J. (1988) *Nursing: Human Science and Human Care. A Theory of Nursing*. New York: National League for Nursing.

Williams, B. and Grant, G. (1998) Defining people centredness: Making the implicit explicit. *Health and Social Care in the Community*, **6**(2), 84–94.

13

# Acting and the limits of professional craft knowledge[1]

**Ian Maxwell**

> The enlightened Lesbonax of Mytilene called pantomimes 'manual philosophers' ... The term 'pantomime' ... scarcely exaggerates [that] artist's versatility ... It is his profession to show forth human character and passion in all their variety ... Wondrous art! ... Other arts call out only one half of a man's powers – the bodily or the mental: the pantomime combines the two
>
> Lucian of Samosata (c. 125–180 AD)[2]

## The wondrous art

In 1970, director Peter Brook revolutionized the Royal Shakespeare Company, requiring the cast for his production of *A Midsummer Night's Dream* to attend daily classes. Each morning, the actors juggled, tumbled and swung on trapezes, developing new performance skills and routines (Selbourne, 1982). Here is the very paradigm of professional craft knowledge (PCK) (Higgs and Titchen, 1995): highly skilled practitioners collectively developing and exchanging new skills, new practices.

The ensemble, in which a group of actors can accumulate, over time, a shared rehearsal and performance vocabulary, style and skill base – in other words, in which PCK can be consciously, productively structured – is perhaps the ideal, even necessary, condition for the development of a healthy theatrical culture.[3] Funded generously by the British Council, Brook enjoyed this luxury: a core of actors rehearsing and working together over an extended period. By contrast, professional theatre (both subsidized and commercial) in Australia is characterized by short rehearsal periods and contract-based employment – actors employed for 4–5 weeks of rehearsal and the season of the play, rather than on a continuing basis.

In such conditions, theatrical practice tends towards orthodoxy; PCKs circulate as shorthands, facilitating the verbal, textual, physical and spatial negotiations constituting the work of rehearsal. To make the most of short rehearsal times, directors tend to cast actors with whom they have worked before, and stylistic and practical innovation and experimentation tend to take second place to the expediencies of simply getting shows on. Further, to earn a reasonable living, actors must diversify their range, away from the stage-centred training offered by training institutions, into television, film, commercial and voice-over work (plus other, para-performative, jobs actors take to pay the rent, such as amusement park characters, clowning and so on; many actors, additionally, find themselves teaching classes to each other, further contracting the circle of pedagogic reinforcement). Actors learn 'on the job'; for example, watch a relatively inexperienced actor in a soap opera (the actor's bread and butter). Newcomers talk about being taken under the wing of more experienced campaigners, being shown the tricks of the trade: how to make the most of key lights, how to work to the camera, and so on (Flaus, 1992). Given that there is always an oversupply of 'talent', actors quickly learn to accumulate experience and skills, simply to avoid unemployment.

This chapter explores the place of PCK in contemporary theatre practice; that field in which, as Lucian of Samosata wrote two millennia ago, the actor (pantomime), as 'manual philosopher', calls out both halves of a man's [sic] power: the mental – the realm of theoretical, propositional knowledge – and the bodily – where knowledge arrives by other means.

## An actor prepares

In 1937, the Russian director Constantin Stanislavsky published *An Actor Prepares*, recounting, in the form of a series of diary entries, the journey of a young actor through training under the guidance of an all-seeing, all-knowing master, Tortsov ('the Director'; Stanislavsky, 1937). The reader shares the student's experiences, stumbling through a series of mysterious, reality-warping exercises, wrestling with common preconceptions about acting, falling flat on his face, witnessing the humiliations and failings of his classmates. Throughout, he is hostage to the apparent omniscience of the Director: a charismatic figure who, at the end of each session, explains all, reveals what has been happening, making sense of everybody's experience. As the students move through training, and the pieces fall into place, Tortsov's intentions become apparent: the shape of what we now know as the 'Stanislavsky System' emerges.

Here, the process of actor-training involves a series of trials and errors: baited traps, set to lead the student astray, the better to correct him. At its best, this process is what the Polish director/teacher Jerzy Grotowski (following in the footsteps of Stanislavsky) would, 25 years later, call the *via negativa*, a process involving the stripping away of what one already knows in order to 'access' or 'uncover' (metaphors pervading acting training) an **essence** (Grotowski) or a **spirit** (Stanislavsky), hidden beneath, or occluded by, the obfuscations set up by the process of living (Grotowski, 1968). More sinisterly, it involves the construction of an absolute dependence, an almost explicitly oedipalized relationship between the actor (*qua* analysed) and teacher/director (*qua* analysand): the naïve, starry-eyed student learns, first and foremost, that they know nothing, must 'free' themselves of what they thought that they knew, and give themselves over to the teacher, who knows. Who, most importantly, knows this: what it is to be human; the secrets of those aspects of being human which we all hold as most preciously ours, defining of ourselves as selves: our memories and our emotions. And because this figure knows these things, he apparently knows the student better than the student knows him or herself. For the student actor in Tortsov's studio, the pedagogic contract is this: 'trust me, because I know'.

Stanislavsky's quasi-phenomenology of the actor-in-training is itself a literary (perhaps, better, a dramaturgical) device, a trope for his own career as a reformer of the theatre. A handsome young man, born into a show business family in the late nineteenth century, Stanislavsky was appalled at the lack of any systematicity in acting work. Companies produced repertoires of melodramas, with standardized characters played as caricatures or as types rather than as discrete personages. The task of the actor involved signalling, as much as experiencing, emotional states, through the display of a system of conventional gestures and the declaiming of speeches out, towards the audience. Actors learned their craft on the job. Companies were constructed around patrifamilial lines; the central figure was the actor-manager, who secured engagements, taking lead roles, organizing other players on the stage, slotting new members of the company into established staging and characterizations. As in the itinerant commedia dell-arte of Renaissance Italy, the pre-revolutionary stages of France and the English Restoration, actors specialized as comics, lovers, tragic heroes and so on.

In place of this artisan, master–apprentice model of acting training, Stanislavsky claimed to be creating a rational **system** of acting, using a combination of 'psycho-technique' and rigorous textual analysis to develop a role. The system was grounded in a complex of implicit propositions – assumptions about human behaviour drawn from the fledgling science of psychology; in particular the work of Théodule Ribot (1839–1916) and Ivan Pavlov (1849–1936) (see Counsell, 1996, pp. 28–30).

Stanislavsky's research did not, however, proceed propositionally, but as **practice**. The theoretical grounds of his work were neither rigorous nor explicit, but articulated as quasi-scientifically informed common sense. His books (written as afterthoughts to subsidize his later work) have recourse to homey, anecdotal examples to support his assertions. The unfinished, work-in-progress nature of theatre practice, and, indeed, the very contingent nature of the work itself (if it works, it works, and damn the theory), accounts for the reluctance of theatre practitioners to commit their work to paper. Nonetheless, the implicit theorization (uncharitably, perhaps, the 'folk-psychology') grounding Stanislavsky's work has been massively influential. As an orthodoxy, his system (and its subsequent evolution in the USA into the Strasberg 'Method'), has become the model for acting training throughout the Western world: a 'default' setting, and the naturalized background against which alternative models are predicated. However, notwithstanding Stanislavsky's attempt to systematize (indeed, rationalize) the process of training actors, and the flourishing of written theorizations of acting throughout the past century, in practice, actor training (and the ongoing development and maintenance of skills and knowledge) might best be seen as an institutionalization of an artisan tradition, shoehorned uncomfortably into the field of tertiary education.

While it is a relative commonplace to speak of theatre as being grounded in an oral rather than literate tradition, this is only part of the story. Acting is an **embodied** tradition: knowledge is constituted in and through bodies in space. PCK is explicitly prioritized over propositional, theoretical knowledge, to the extent that the latter, understood as being predicated non-experientially, is discredited and often dismissed as not being real knowledge at all.

That is not to say that propositional or theoretical knowledge does not inform this field: it certainly does, but in disguise, verified by its demonstrable effectiveness in a practical context (stagecraft, for example: those craft knowledges predicated upon 'what works' on stage, in front of the camera), its phenomenological resonance ('that feels right'), and authorized through the body of the teacher. The identification of particular forms of knowledge with 'naturalness', 'instinct', and the prioritizing of certain phenomenological, experiential knowledge, however, construes other forms of knowledge as being inauthentic, as distorting, identifying them with a figuring of 'culture' as that which stands in the way of real knowing.

## Contemporary acting training in Australia

Actor training in contemporary Australian institutions broadly follows the Stanislavskian/Grotowskian model, varying with the backgrounds of specific teachers. At the heart of this model is the studio: a protected space, abstracted from everyday life, within which the (carefully selected) actors-in-training are encouraged, under intensive tutelage, to 'explore' themselves, psychologically and physically. Isolated within the institution, and often discouraged from taking up outside activities (particularly acting jobs, and, to an extent, part-time jobs, leading to what becomes an explicit valorization of the struggling artist), students are given heavy workloads of physically exhausting classes, and set tasks outside class (e.g. visits to zoos). Many students relocate interstate to attend higher-status institutions, creating isolation and sense of sacrifice, contributing to a sense of knowledge as being won through hardship.

Here, my brief exploration of these knowledges, based upon my experience as an actor-in-training, takes the form of a critique.[4] The prioritizing of particular forms of experiential knowledge brings with it a complex of interrelated problems: a failure to produce critical, reflective thought, instead reifying technique as fact; not 'this is one model of acting' but simply 'this is how to act'. Additionally, as part of this same complex, this construction of knowledge tends towards creating learning subjects dependent upon authoritative figures – teachers, gurus, masters, directors – who claim knowledge not only of the craft of acting, but of the learning subjects themselves; suggesting to the learner, as mentioned earlier, that 'I know you better than you know yourself: trust me, and I will show you yourself'.

## A hidden world

Susan Letzer Cole (1992) has written of theatrical rehearsal as a 'hidden world', shrouded in mystery and secrecy. Acting training creates around itself an even more marked air of secrecy. Actors talking about their training are reminiscent of old soldiers recounting boot camp stories that outsiders simply cannot understand. Further, within the theatre industry there are disincentives to 'owning up' to a university background. A prominent Sydney director, for example, completed a Masters thesis analysing the centrality of gossip and anecdote to rehearsal, but avoided furnishing the university department that bestowed the degree with a copy of the dissertation for fear that she would somehow be exposed as a thinker rather than as a doer. Similarly, having enquired about university graduates with successful careers in the performing arts, a journalist called me back: the agents of the actors I had named had claimed that their clients had 'not gone to Sydney University' but were, in fact, graduates of the National Institute of Dramatic Art (NIDA), as if the two were mutually exclusive. Here is another actor's account:

As an actor both at N.I.D.A. and out in the industry, I survived by pretending to be . . . insane or neurotic or stupid . . . the most threatening thing I could do was to engage in intelligent debate with the director . . . An intelligent actor in the mainstream is regarded with a raised eyebrow, as a strange and possibly inconvenient aberration . . . I watched myself and other actors avoid public dialogue on theatre, in order to land the next job . . . in such a fear-driven environment, how can the true beauty of theatre . . . ever flourish?

(Broinowski, 1997, p. 125)

## Knowledge of self: scenes from training

Within the Stanislavskian rubric, knowledge is constituted in the first instance as knowledge of self. To create roles, actors draw upon their experiences. Training involves developing techniques which allow actors to access their experiences and memories which, in the course of everyday life, perhaps because of their unpleasant nature, are hidden. Everyday life is construed as creating obstacles within the individual; training involves processes of unblocking, in order to arrive at pure emotional states. During our first week, we were introduced to the axiomatic ground of our training: a radical, embodied deconstruction of a cultural bias towards rational, propositional knowledge. 'Outside', we were told, 'in the world, you are encouraged to think, to be rational, to analyse, at the expense of developing other ways of knowing. Here, in the safety of this place, we will privilege other ways of knowing: the emotional, the knowledges of the body.' Hence, the pervasive injunction: 'Don't think; do'. Inverting the Cartesian devaluing of emotional, subjective knowledges as idiosyncratic and contingent, here, to think was to allow doubt to creep in, to 'block' one's impulse, to lock out, or censor authentic responses, the truth. With vulgar-psychoanalytic methods we were lulled into reveries of 'chaotic thinking', halfway between asleep and awake, and told that there we would start to find our uncensored states of being, to 'release creativity' from 'the mind's habitual dulling of the world' (see Johnstone, 1979, pp. 26–32).

Daily 'voicework' sessions encouraged us to relax, to get back in touch with our 'natural' bodies – the broad consensus of contemporary voice theory being that the experience of living, with all its vicissitudes, creates tensions which physiologically impede the flow of sound through the body's structures, inhibiting the production of an expressive, resonant, intimate voice (see Berry, 1973, 1987; Linklater, 1976, 1992; Rodenburg, 1992, 1993). Naturalness was equated with emotion and intuition, coded as desirable but lost, in contrast to culture, which was equated with thought and rationality, a problem to be dealt with and removed en route to re-establishing contact with one's ('hidden', 'lost') centre. Thought, and the kind of knowledge gleaned from thought, was taken as misleading, and not to be trusted.

In the charged context of the studio, effective technique can be mistaken for fact, craft knowledge taken as propositional knowledge. Understanding such slippages as what philosophers call 'category errors' can avoid the pitfalls of debates between practitioners and theorists, such as one recently played out in a prominent theatre journal; an academic writer interpreted PCK discourses of voice teachers as statements of propositional knowledge, and offered academic, philosophically compelling critiques of the metaphysical assumptions she saw underlying those discourses. Responding, the practitioners replied that the academic, as someone who hadn't herself experienced the techniques in question, was not justified in making her critique (see Werner, 1996; Berry et al., 1997).

The problem is that different modes of knowing produce different knowledges. More importantly, however, this pedagogical context furnishes PCKs with a rhetorical force and authority which shifts them into a different, more problematic set of claims. The heavily metaphoric (and, importantly, highly effective) nature language of breath control ('breathe through your groin', e.g., or the discourse of 'centredness', with its implicit metaphysics of a pre-cultural, essential self) is effaced; a complex metaphorical language is taken to be a simple descriptive language, producing particular horizons of (self-)knowledge.

## Emotional recall

Perhaps the most striking aspect of actor training, however, drawing most directly upon the Stanislavskian/Strasbergian tradition, involved emotional recall. Members of the class were asked to select from memory their most 'X' moment. We were to fill in the X (revealingly, a vast majority of the class selected traumatic moments) and to recall this moment in minute detail: where it took place, who was there, where they were in relation to each other, what was done and said, by whom and in what order, with particular attention to what our bodies did throughout. With a group of other students we presented these moments, not as drama but as re-enactment, recreating the material and psychic conditions of the original experience. We were told that our bodies usually avoid configurations in which we experienced trauma or discomfort, but that in this exercise we were to risk placing ourselves in those positions.

The exercise was extraordinarily powerful. As each student performed/enacted these moments, we witnessed massive outpourings of emotion. My own experience of the exercise was no exception: I chose a happy moment, and even then was shaken by the intensity of the experience. At the most practical level, we were learning the potential of the human body to recall emotional states, and the necessity of involving our bodies (as well as our memories) in the process of producing our stock in trade: emotions. The lesson here was that, notwithstanding our greatest fears, the emotions released from the Pandora's boxes of our embodied memories would not destroy us, that we could journey to these emotional extremes and come back intact, stronger. Having overcome the fear (of something like potential psychological dissolution) once, we were told ('trust me'), next time we would find it easier: soon we would be able to conjure real emotional states, drawn from our experience, on cue, as roles demanded. These were unforgettable lessons, their 'truthfulness' sustained by the evidence of our own experience.

Subsequently, I read Stanislavsky, where this process is described in step-by-step detail; prior to this, I had attributed the exercise to my teacher: he had known what would happen – we had trusted him, and he had shown us shakingly extraordinary things about ourselves. I cannot overemphasize the power of this knowledge, of our apprehension of his knowledge. Even now, ten years later, 'professional craft knowledge' seems too neat, too clinical a term to describe the experience; even now I feel inclined (and what a giveaway this is: my knowing is here subordinated to a 'feelingness') to claim what I learnt in that class (and a number of classes like it) is the most real knowledge I have ever known.

This knowledge was construed as being, first and foremost, **embodied**: we could not, we were told, learn this in books. We had to **do** it; only after we had actually experienced the work would we be able to claim knowledge. Simultaneously, however, we were also learning a dependency. Throughout the exercise, the teacher reassured each student, exhorted us to trust him; he literally held distraught students in his arms at the end of their re-creations, reassuring them – us – that they were 'safe', 'all right', 'whole'.[5]

Stanislavsky was never named as the origin of these exercises; others were, but only when teachers claimed embodied lineage to the figure in question. While Rudolph Laban and Moshe Feldenkrais, for example, both figured as (lower case) labels for approaches to work, we were never invited to read their writings, or to approach their work as theoretical or propositional knowledge. So 'laban work' was authorized through one teacher's attendance at a Laban institute in Canada, 'feldenkrais work' through another teacher's training with someone taught by Feldenkrais himself. 'No-one', we were told, 'is allowed to teach the technique unless they learnt it through Feldenkrais or one of his disciples [sic].' As I write now, I have in front of me the mimeographed notes distributed by my laban teacher, bearing this admonition on the title page:

**Notes to Supplement ACTIVE Class Participation**

Contained in these notes are extracts from some of Laban's work . . .

An intellectual understanding only is useless.

The only way to understand is to DO it . . .

. . . this work deals with sensation so words are inadequate.

My point here, as throughout, is not that our teachers were involved in some kind of misrepresentation or epistemological fraud; it is absolutely the case that I could not have learned these lessons in the same way through reading. I may have learned them as a set of theoretical propositions, but that would have constituted knowledge of a completely different order, arguably of an order that would be of little if any use to me on stage. It is emphatically the case that one must actively experience the exercise in order to arrive at the requisite craft knowledge. This learning is explicitly phenomenological: knowledge of one's self, gained through an exploration of one's own embodied experience and memory. The knowledge is a **technos**: a practical skill. In this context of learning, however, given the intensely personal nature of the learning process, its being steeped in discourses of 'self-discovery', 'journey', and so on, and the power of the teacher, professional craft knowledge comes at the expense of critical reflective knowledge.[6]

## Notes

1 Editors' note: Readers may be surprised to see this chapter about acting in a book focusing on the health professions. We have included it, based on an assumption that we learn effectively from contrasting and critiquing cases. Presenting an intriguing opposition to the predominant epistemological values in the health professions, Ian Maxwell shows how, in the preparation of actors, professional craft knowledge is valued and taught almost exclusively. Through a critique of subsequent effects on students' learning, Maxwell builds an argument for the development of students' critical reflective knowledge. This argument mirrors others put forward in this book, in terms of the critique, integration and harmonization of all kinds of knowledge, albeit from a very different starting point.

2 In Nagler (1959, p. 29).

3 Despite recent attempts (notably The Bell Shakespeare Company and Company B at Belvoir St, both based in Sydney) there are currently no ensemble theatre companies working in Australia.

4 I trained at the Victorian College of the Arts School of Drama, 1987–89.

5 Dean Carey, a Sydney acting teacher, recently called for a 'code of conduct' to protect acting students from 'scars, not just of physical intimidation, but also emotional and sexual violation' (*Sydney Morning Herald*, 29 May, 1998, p. 13).

6 Editors' note: This chapter, perhaps, serves as a timely reminder to us about the importance of valuing all kinds of knowledge equally and of helping students and less experienced professionals to develop expertise in using them in critical, integrative and balanced ways. We might also reflect on whether some of us prioritize particular forms of experiential knowledge to the detriment of developing students', less experienced colleagues' and our own critical, reflective thinking. Is there evidence in our own practices, of creating dependency in those we help to learn – vestiges of the omniscient teacher as the 'one who knows' and 'who knows the student better than the student knows him or herself'. Do we contribute to a culture in which 'doers' are more valued than 'thinkers' or vice versa?

## References


Berry, C. (1973) *Voice and the Actor*. New York: Collier.

Berry, C. (1987) *The Actor and His Text*. London: Harrap.

Berry, C., Rodenburg, P. and Linklater, K. (1997) Shakespeare, feminism, and voice: Responses to Sarah Werner. *New Theatre Quarterly*, **13**(49), 48–52.

Brcinowski, A. (1997) Why did the actor cross the road? In *About Performance 3: Theatre as Performance* (J. L. Lewis and I. Maxwell, eds), pp. 121–128. Sydney: Centre for Performance Studies, University of Sydney.

Cole, S. L. (1992) *Directors in Rehearsal: A Hidden World*. New York: Routledge.

Counsell, C. (1996) *Signs of Performance: An Introduction to Twentieth-Century Theatre*. New York: Routledge.

Flaus, J. (1992) Thanks for your heart, Bart. *Continuum: Film – Matters of Style*, **5**(2), 179–224.

Grotowski, J. (1968) *Towards a Poor Theatre*. London: Methuen (republished 1976).

Higgs, J. and Titchen, A. (1995) The nature, generation and verification of knowledge. *Physiotherapy*, **81**(9), 521–530.

Johnstone, K. (1979) *Impro: Improvisation and the Theatre*. London: Methuen.

Linklater, K. (1976) *Freeing the Natural Voice*. New York: Drama Book Publishers.

Linklater, K. (1992) *Freeing Shakespeare's Voice: The Actor's Guide to Talking the Text*. New York: Theatre Communications Group.

Nagler, A. M. (1959) *A Source Book in Theatrical History*. New York: Dover Publications.

Rodenburg, P. (1992) *The Right to Speak: Working With the Voice*. New York: Routledge.

Rodenburg, P. (1993) *The Need for Words: Voice and the Text*. New York: Routledge.

Selbourne, D. (1982) *The Making of 'A Midsummer Night's Dream': An Eye-Witness Account of Peter Brook's Production from First Rehearsal to First Night*. London: Methuen.

Stanislavsky, C. (1937) *An Actor Prepares*. London: Eyre Methuen (republished 1980).

Werner, S. (1996) Performing Shakespeare: Voice training and the feminist actor. *New Theatre Quarterly*, **12**(47), 249–258.

# 14

# Professional practice: artistry and connoisseurship

**Sarah Beeston and Joy Higgs**

Inherent in the practice of the professionals we recognise as unusually competent is a core of artistry.

(Schön, 1987)

This chapter propounds the notion that there is an element of artistry at the heart of the kind of professional practice that is acknowledged to be outstanding and to which we all aspire. This artistry encompasses, but goes beyond, competence and what we might describe as technical expertise. It is owned by an individual who possesses a blend of qualities built up through extensive and reflective personal knowledge and experience. It is difficult to describe and impossible to commodify (i.e. to reduce to a commodity, or a definable, saleable item). However, this professional artistry is recognized and greatly desired by others in the field, and is worthy of consideration and exploration in order to make it accessible to a greater number of people.

Having come into being under the umbrella of the medical profession, many of the allied health care professions have had to struggle to discover and articulate an identity of their own. They have attempted to delineate the core knowledge of their profession; they have built models of practice (Reed, 1984; Aggleton and Chalmers, 1986); they have undertaken professionally relevant research. For the most part these ways of understanding and describing practice have been pursued by researchers who are also engaged in the education of practitioners within universities. More recently, and as a result of greater collaboration between researcher and practitioner, there has been an increasing interest in identifying the growth of practitioners from novice to expert (Benner, 1984; Jensen et al., 1999). Such research is rooted in the world of practice and begins to throw light on what is meant by the term professional artistry (Schön, 1983).

Donald Schön (1983, 1987) was the first of a number of professional educators who came to think of professional practice as an artistic endeavour which needed to be explored. He called this kind of practice 'professional artistry'. He suggested that we should be questioning 'what we can learn from careful examination of artistry', which he saw not as 'inherently mysterious', but as 'an exercise of intelligence, a kind of knowing, though different in crucial respects from our standard model of professional knowledge' and as 'rigorous in its own terms' (Schön, 1987, p. 13).

Another proponent of artistry within professional practice was art educator Elliot Eisner, who described artistry as comprising the two elements of **connoisseurship** and **criticism** (Eisner, 1985). These terms had specific meanings which mirrored but went beyond everyday language. In art, these terms denote a way of knowing and seeing which demonstrates an expert critical appreciation and an ability to disclose or express what has been seen and known. In Eisner's view both elements are essential to artists if they are to contribute to their art in ways which have impact and produce change.

This chapter is concerned with the notions of artistry and connoisseurship and with the assumption that professional artistry is worth examining in exploration of the nature of professional practice.

We begin by identifying some characteristics of professional practice which are pertinent to the discussion of artistry and connoisseurship which follow. We then consider what kinds of knowing might be embedded in artistry: what kinds of expression are associated with it and what kind of rigour is inherent within it. We conclude by considering the implications for education and research in the health professions.

## Characteristics of professional practice

Professional practice is not a clearly bounded entity or a given phenomenon. It is a dynamic, developing process which builds upon the specific origins and traditions of a particular profession, which give it character and make it recognizable. The notions of professional artistry and connoisseurship need to be understood within the context of professional practice. Otherwise they are likely to become abstract constructs with little value for the practitioner.

### Professional practice lies within a tradition

The term **professional practice** can be used in two ways. Practice can refer to the activity of a single practitioner, and also to what has been described as a 'whole tradition in which particular activities are related together as part of a social project or mission' (Golby, 1993, p. 4). The two are part of the whole; the practice of the individual sits within and is influenced by the broader tradition of the particular profession within which it is located. Thus individual practitioners practise within their profession in ways similar to the way in which artists carry out their art: within a tradition and displaying certain characteristics which are understood within a genre. Within some practice professions these traditions are implicit rather than explicit; in all professions they are challenged and changed as knowledge is developed. Nevertheless, professional practice and artistry are located within a tradition.

### Professional practice is dynamic

Practice is not a fixed, taken-for-granted phenomenon. It is not the case that practice presents itself as a series of well-defined instrumental problems that lend themselves well to one of a number of predetermined solutions. This would limit the practitioner to the role of an applied scientist whose practice is constrained by knowledge available from existing research in application to identified problems (Schein, 1973). This may once have been the expectation of professionals, but with increasing levels of technology and new knowledge it is acknowledged increasingly that the problems that present themselves to practitioners are predominantly 'uncertain practical problems' which do not lend themselves to procedural solutions (Reid, 1978). In contrast to the traditional view of professional practice, which assumes that theory is applied to practice in a technical-rational way (Schön, 1983), those who perceive advanced practice as being characterized by artistry view practice and the practice environment as complex and unpredictable, requiring 'wise judgement under conditions of considerable uncertainty' (Eraut, 1994, p. 17). This view requires of professionals that they use their skills and knowledge as an extension of themselves, in a manner similar to the way in which an artist may use a brush or a conductor may use a baton.

Moreover, practice is not a solitary pursuit. Increasingly, practice shares power and decision-making. Like artists, practitioners involve others in what they are doing. Practice is created through interaction and participation within a specific situation. Thus artistic practice is a dynamic process which is embedded in practice in specific contexts and with particular clients, requiring imagination and creativity to cope with the ambiguity and uncertainty of practice situations.

### Professional practice presupposes technical competence

Professional practice is constructed upon the foundation of technical competence. By virtue of self-regulation within the health professions the starting point for all practitioners is that the novice practitioner has a basic level of knowledge of different kinds: **propositional knowledge** associated with practice that is based on theory and research; **professional craft knowledge** derived from professional experience which provides the essential skills for practice; and **personal experiential knowledge**, which each individual brings to whatever he or she does (Higgs and Titchen, 1995). This is the starting point, not the end goal. Becoming a complete professional requires more than technical competence: it calls for professional artistry.

Technical competence comprises the set of professional tools, skills and knowledge which practitioners bring to their practice and which they continue to hone throughout their professional lives. The development of artistry requires attention to the dimensions of practice, which are often invisible, the values, beliefs, attitudes, assumptions, expectations, feelings and knowledge that lie below the surface and behind the actions of the practitioner (Fish, 1998). For professional artistry to develop within the practitioner there must be a growth in personal knowledge as well as in propositional and professional craft knowledge, because personal knowledge, including the practitioner's beliefs and values, provides a frame of reference for the individual to act and to engage with others. It is likely to be through an exploration of those aspects of practice which are hidden to the observer that the unique growth of the individual happens. So technical competence is both the starting point of professional practice and the essential foundation for the development of professional artistry, while experiential knowledge supplements and enhances this technical knowledge base in the refinement of professional artistry.

### Professional practice is pluralistic

In common with other professions, the recent development and growth within the health professions has led to a new pluralism within individual professions. Where there may once have been a broad consensus as to what constituted the core skills and knowledge of the profession, the role of the professional, and the values inherent in practice, this has long since ceased to be the case (Schön, 1983). Today it is more realistic to talk of best practices (plural), each being found to be credible as well as situationally relevant. This pluralism challenges previous cultures and traditions within specific practice professions. These traditions have their roots in the underlying philosophies of a profession and are demonstrated in the modalities which lie within its accepted scope of practice.

Within professions, for instance, differences are now exhibited in relation to the management of different client groups, the use of different modalities, and the work undertaken in different contexts of care. These differences are demonstrated by the increasing number of specialisms and special interest groups within the individual health professions, each promoting a different perspective. If one looks at practice as comprising actions, knowledge and values (Handal and Lauvas, 1987), it can be seen that for practitioners to engage effectively within professional practice they need to understand the complexities and underlying assumptions of these differing approaches and to be able to adopt a number of different theoretical stances and practice frameworks. Thus, along with increasing complexity in the types of problem brought to the practitioner there is also increasing complexity in the responses available to the practitioner. This requires professionals to exercise the art of problem-setting as opposed to problem-solving, whereby they reframe the situation encountered, examining it from a number of perspectives before negotiating with the client the 'best fit' response (Schön, 1983).

A positive effect of pluralism is that it encourages practice which is creative and innovative. A negative effect is that it becomes more difficult to establish and maintain professional expectations and traditions. Pluralism militates against shared values, language and norms, and against the capacity to articulate one's practice to others and to agree about its role. Since pluralism on the one hand engenders professional artistry and on the other challenges professional traditions, there is a heightened need for the traditions[1] of practice to be made explicit rather than implicit. A greater degree of transparency would provide a form or mode of operation which would help to set the boundaries of practice and articulate the values, knowledge and actions of the profession, thus encouraging creativity and innovation within a tradition or culture that makes debate possible and valuable.

## Connoisseurship and criticism

The existence of the characteristics of the health professions discussed above challenges us to examine further the notions of artistry and connoisseurship. This section considers the concepts of artistry and connoisseurship and seeks to understand them in terms of the kinds of knowing, kinds of expression and kinds of rigour to be found within them.

### What kinds of knowing?

The kind of knowing associated with professional artistry is an individual[2] knowing. It is a knowing whereby the individual practitioner develops awareness of various types of knowledge through experience in the field and blends experiential with other types of knowledge. It requires the practitioner to place personal experience within a framework of propositional and professional knowledge in a way which gives this experience meaning and ultimately allows expression of that meaning to others. Eisner conceived of knowing as connoisseurship. He described it as a way of paying attention, and the accompanying notion of criticism as a way of disclosing or expressing what had been seen (Eisner, 1985). It is important to note that both concepts are essential to his view of artistry. Perhaps this is because without personal meaning there can be no clear expression of knowledge.

Eisner compared the process of becoming a connoisseur of practice with that of becoming a connoisseur of wine (Eisner, 1985). Both are intentional activities. Both involve paying attention to something in which the use of the senses and the emotions as well as the mind is important. In appreciating wine we rely on a well-developed sense of smell and of taste. These senses must be educated if we are to be connoisseurs. Wine-tasting classes offer experience of differing wines, encouraging comparisons and providing information which allows the taster to develop his or her understanding of the production and properties of the wine. One can know a lot about wine from a book, but without the personal knowledge gained from tasting and smelling the wine, one can never become a connoisseur.

In this illustration of connoisseurship one can see the individual's knowledge lying within and incorporating within itself the kinds of knowing associated with propositional knowledge and professional craft knowledge of the profession (Higgs and Titchen, 1995). In addition, connoisseurship encompasses a great depth of individual, personal knowing that comes from a high level of reflective awareness of self and others as people and professionals. The personal knowledge of the connoisseur of wine is a knowing that allows fine discrimination between wines and an appreciation of the differences between them. It involves the whole person, senses, intellect and emotions. This knowing has been gained through a procedure of wine-tasting shaped by those in the trade, those with the appropriate craft knowledge. The capacity to discuss and justify one's personal judgment in relation to wine is dependent in turn upon having a framework of knowledge with a conceptual or theoretical basis that is shared by others within a tradition. This framework offers alternative perspectives on the experience of the connoisseur, allowing his or her judgment to be refined. It does not predetermine or prescribe the experience or its interpretation but provides frameworks for reflection upon the experience which enable the individual to make sense of the experience.

Similarly, within health and educational practices there is the development of individual knowledge or a way of knowing that emerges from within a context provided by professional craft knowledge and propositional knowledge. Lawrence Stenhouse spoke of such knowing within teaching. He likened the role of teacher to that of orchestral conductor. He wanted teachers to probe the meaning of educational ideas within a curriculum, just as a conductor develops understanding of the meanings of the composer within a score. In the same way that the conductor, steeped in the music of the composer, involves the orchestra in discovering meaning within form, so the teacher steeped in the meaning of the curriculum develops ideas and through educational action involves learners in knowledge discovery. Thus the teacher sees the curriculum as 'the medium for learning the art of teaching' (Stenhouse, 1980, p. 43). Within this context one sees again that propositional and professional craft knowledge have a distinct role to play. They provide a form and a tradition, within which the artist aspires to discover 'new teaching moves – moves that were not a part of one's existing repertoire' (Eisner, 1983, p. 11), while at the same time acknowledging that 'there is no mastery, always aspiration' (Stenhouse, 1980, p. 42).

In the health professions, skilled practitioners learn the knowledge and craft of their profession and gain competence. For the expert this is not enough, and for the professional artist there is much more to be learnt. Through experience, reflection, critical self-appraisal and ongoing self-directed learning, skilled practitioners learn many additional dimensions to their skills, such as the subtlety of touch, the heightened awareness of the intangibles and nuances of interpersonal relationships, the complex skills of professional judgment and practice wisdom. None of these attributes are easily learnt and many would argue that beyond the basics they cannot be taught, and they are out of reach or even eschewed by some. Yet they constitute the same fineness or finesse that characterizes the quintessential artist, critic or connoisseur in many realms of endeavour.

Within the context of professional practice, different professions will develop their own styles of connoisseurship. This may require a highly developed use of specific senses in order to recognize such cues as 'the tone of a voice or musical instrument, the feel of a muscle or a piece of sculpture' (Eraut, 1994, p. 42). The traditions of different professions will provide different theories and professional knowledge which will shape novice practitioners as they develop meaning through such engagement.

Thus the kind of knowing associated with artistic practice is individual knowing. It is gained through participation within the particular field of practice but must be framed and shaped by theories and traditions found within the propositional and professional craft knowledge unique to that field of practice. Individual knowledge is characterized by creative thinking that goes beyond procedures and protocols and results in professional judgments which may prove to be innovative in nature.

## What kinds of expression of knowledge?

The ways in which a practitioner comes to know and test ideas may be a private affair but there comes a point when this knowledge must be given public expression if it is to be acknowledged as professional artistry in Eisner's terms. If connoisseurship is characterized by individual knowledge that exhibits meaning, then the mediation of that meaning requires appropriate expression, an expression that makes the meaning accessible to others and which invites their response and criticism.

The current climate in which health professionals work lays great emphasis on the presentation or expression of practice in ways which demonstrate the evidence base of their practice. This has created a demand for an expression of practice that is formal and research-based, and that focuses on the outcomes of practice as opposed to the processes or contexts of practice. It results in research papers which are valuable to those who seek publicly verifiable evidence, since it demands adherence to 'publicly codified rules' (Eisner, 1981). These papers may also inform the individual practitioner but they are not readily conducive to the expression of personal meaning.

In contrast, artistic practice is embodied often unconsciously within the practice of an individual as he or she works with a patient or client. Others who recognize the artistry may watch and intuitively grasp the meaning as a result of their own experience, but the artist is not fulfilling the requirement of disclosure. More public communication of professional practice can be achieved by means of master classes where artistry is enacted in a more conscious way and where meanings are made explicit, and via publications and research reports which seek to explore the value of professional artistry (see, e.g., Binnie and Titchen, 1999).

However, there are significant barriers to be overcome if practitioners are to find ways of communicating meaning which allow for criticism from their peers. Before artistry can be expressed publicly it must be articulated privately, and this is often a barrier. The work of Mattingly and Fleming (1994) within occupational therapy suggests that the lack of a shared language through which to express ideas is a major impediment to expression. Another hindrance is the fact that the majority of the health professions do not have a long tradition or clear identity within which practitioners can locate their conceptions and experiences of practice. Explicit frameworks for practice are at an early stage of evolution in many health professions; such frameworks are often not addressed during the initial education of health professionals. Underpinning these barriers is the likelihood that the demand for evidence in a form with which practitioners are unfamiliar, and the stipulation to practise only what has proven effectiveness of outcome, result in practitioners being slow to value and reluctant to express their artistry. Instead they are vulnerable to responding to the demands of external agencies rather than taking the initiative to express their practice in their own terms.

The challenge remains to discern the kinds of expression which would give voice to artistry within the health professions. Consider the following example of how such artistry could be expressed:

> (*Nurse*) That was when I sat on the bed, facing her with my back to the rest of the room, and I held her hand. I wanted to be able to make eye contact with her and keep us together as a unit, if you like. I felt that if I sat the other way that I would be like the team, which was not what I wanted. And she held my hand really tightly . . . and she stroked it with her thumb. It was a very close gesture. We talked in quiet whispers while they were there.
> (Binnie and Titchen, 1999, p. 170)

We have identified the need for explicit expression of the traditions of individual professions within which practitioners can locate their ideas (Golby, 1993). Other ideas in relation to the expression of artistry are considered in the closing section of the chapter.

## What kind of rigour?

Schön (1987, p. 13) described professional artistry as being 'rigorous in its own terms'. We turn now to look at the kind of rigour associated with professional artistry, in relation to both connoisseurship and criticism. Rigour can be considered as the application of sound, defensible strategies for ensuring that the knowledge and skills, indeed the attitudes, that the professional employs meet high standards. In the absence of certainty in practice (which can be both a desirable as well as problematic factor) the standards set by a professional will often be individual rather than peer-referenced or externally set. It is, in fact, the essence of professionalism to act in the best interests of the person(s) being served, with a conviction and commitment to providing quality and accountable service. Similarly, it is the professional who must determine what methods to use to ensure this rigour, this quality service. Strategies which can be used to achieve rigour include:

- immediate strategies – such as metacognition and reflection-in-action, which provide ongoing monitoring and instantaneous feedback or control of performance and cognition;
- strategic or longer-term strategies – such as reflection-on-action, performance appraisal, critical review or research, to provide a mechanism for constant revision, updating and refining of knowledge, skills and attitudes.

At the stage of developing connoisseurship, practitioners develop their artistry privately within their practice. They test their ideas in action within a form provided by different theoretical frameworks. In so doing they are reviewing and developing the meanings associated with their individual knowledge base within the context of the professional craft knowledge and propositional knowledge of their profession.

We can look to education for an illustration of knowledge framing and testing. Within education the traditions of teaching are communicated in part within the curriculum, which provides the form or structure for the teacher's practice. However, the rigour of the artistic professional lies not in strict adherence to these forms but in a testing of different ways of working within them. Work in progress evidences rigour in ways similar to 'the sketchbook of a good artist, a play in rehearsal, a jazz quartet working together' (Stenhouse, 1980, p. 42). Thus, the professional artist becomes a practitioner-researcher in his or her own ward, clinic or classroom, able to conduct investigations based on ideas emerging from practice and testing those ideas in the laboratory of practice (Stenhouse, 1975). For health professionals, the form of this professional artistry may lie within a shared model of practice or a set of guidelines or protocols derived from theory and research.

Practitioner-researchers will not work within just one form or frame of reference when dealing with the complexity of practice. They will be concerned with the process of problem-setting as well as problem-solving. This requires the practitioner to consider a variety of frames of reference when considering a situation. Problem-setting is central to the processes of reflection-on-action and reflection-in-action which Schön (1983) puts at the heart of professional artistry. Reflection requires rigour in thinking within different disciplines or knowledge bases, or the capacity to respond to new and complex situations and to use one's knowledge in newly formulated ways. This level of creative thinking requires an internalization of the traditions and ways of working of a profession or subset of a profession.

The rigour associated with connoisseurship has little in common with the rigour associated with research in the positivist tradition. The requirement for rigour within the positivist tradition is necessitated by the goal of the research, i.e. the desire to generalize from its findings. The aim of the professional artist is not to develop propositional knowledge but to generate meaning. This meaning will begin at a level personal to the individual but will then be tested by the professional community. In keeping with this aim, the major instrument of data collection in the connoisseurship model is the practitioner through whom the meaning is developed and expressed (Eisner, 1981).

The rigour associated with the expert skill of criticism or expression comes within the context of a community. In the context of professional practice, Schön (1983, p. 33) wrote of knowledge being 'embedded within the socially and institutionally constructed context shared by a community of practitioners'. This is the professional knowledge by which practitioners 'make sense of practice situations, formulate goals and directions for action, and determine what constitutes acceptable professional conduct' (Schön, 1983). This knowledge will vary between different health professions and within individual professions as they work with specific client groups or within specific contexts of care. We see here how traditions are social entities which emerge from practice and are shared by communities of practitioners. Beyond individual critique and metacognitive scrutiny, rigour is achieved by testing knowledge through exposure to the professional community. Rigour is dependent on criticism from within the community and is exercised by those who are actively involved in practice.

The rigour used within these communities has certain characteristics. It is concerned with credibility and transferability rather than with validity (Krefting, 1991). The type of rigour associated with the expression of professional artistry requires that others in the community of practice find the meaning that is expressed to be credible in terms of the traditions of practice, and that they find it can be transferred to their own practice and applied in other contexts. It is also accepted that within individual interpretations there will be some inventiveness, or artistic licence (Eisner, 1981). Professional artistry interpretations can be expressed through role-modelling and articulation of professional craft knowledge (see, e.g., Titchen, 2000). Other strategies could include videotapes of practice, photographs, poems, stories or critical dialogue.[3] (Exploring ways of communicating professional artistry is an important direction for future research and education.)

It can be seen that the rigour associated with professional artistry must include rigour within both the development and the expression of artistry if the relevant professional community is to adopt the artistic evidence before them. Rigour to achieve artistry is not only a planned cognitive activity as a component of systematic reflection-on-action for instance, but also requires the application of a high level of awareness or attention to thinking within practice.

Mezirow, for instance, uses the term 'transformation learning' to mean 'the process of learning through critical self-reflection, which results in the reformulation of a meaning perspective to allow a more inclusive, discriminating, and integrative understanding of one's experience' and a greater capacity to act on these insights (Mezirow, 1990, p. xvi), i.e. to employ rigour or critical appraisal in practice. He describes the continuous development of the individual as 'perspective transformation' (Mezirow, 1981).

William Torbert (1978) contends that increased consciousness is the key to liberating education. It involves 'a higher quality of attention than we ordinarily bring to bear on our affairs' (Torbert, 1978, p.109). Such attention, he says, is necessary for the search for shared purpose, self-direction and quality work which 'create the possibility for adult relatedness, integrity, and generativity and therefore represent the essence of genuinely liberating higher education' (Torbert, 1978, p.110).

By bringing the higher level of attention (as per Torbert, 1978) to our professional reasoning and decision-making we are able to enhance our understanding of the clinical problem, to become more aware of, and more able to deal effectively with the many complex factors influencing reasoning and decision-making, to enhance communication, and to decrease the level of potential bias and error in our reasoning (Higgs and Jones, 1995). This ability is an important reasoning dimension of professional artistry.

## Implications for research and education within the health professions

Professional artistry could be described as the meaningful expression of a uniquely individual view within a shared tradition. If such artistry is to make a contribution within the health professions, then approaches to research and education need to foster and develop the capacity for connoisseurship and criticism among its members. We will turn now to a consideration of how this might be done.

To begin to appreciate professional artistry and connoisseurship there first needs to be a greater understanding of the variety of and need for different ways of knowing. (This is explored in Chapters 1 and 2.) In addition, the professions and the scientific community need a greater understanding and appreciation of the variety of ways in which research can be conducted, recognizing the roles particularly of the interpretive and critical research paradigms in the exploration of human phenomena, as well as the importance of empirico-analytical research methods. In the end, the research approach adopted needs to be able to illuminate the phenomenon being investigated, not destroy it. There is a need for greater use of research approaches which are applicable to the goal of practice development (as well as practice measurement and testing), amenable to practice settings and achievable by and attractive to practitioners as well as academic researchers.

More value needs to be placed on the practitioner as researcher and on different types of collaborative research. There will need to be training in relevant research methods. Education at both the initial and continuing stages will need to enhance the artistic aspects of practice as well as provide a theoretical basis on which to draw and build. The need is for a model of continuing professional development or lifelong learning that will involve practitioners in knowing and expressing the artistic core of their practice.

### Implications for research

There are implications for the way in which research is conceived, conducted and expressed. For example, practitioner research can be viewed as a pursuit of truth within a single case study design undertaken to test the efficacy of a particular intervention which has been isolated through the design of the case (Ottenbacher, 1986). Alternatively, practitioner research can be a reflective process used to test and refine new combinations of ideas and actions. Rather than the research method being the sole key to development of professional artistry, we need to consider first the aim and purpose behind practice-based research.

The felt need to provide more evidence for practice interventions in many of the health professions has led to an increase in the number of collaborative research projects being undertaken. Commonly, such projects are managed by means of partnerships between clinical and academic staff and are designed to advance research in clinical practice (Glen and Smith, 1999). This model contrasts sharply with that described by Titchen (2000). Her collaborative research was conceived as an exploration of the nature of professional craft knowledge within nursing and was conducted in a strongly collaborative way which resulted in the personal and professional development of her collaborator and herself as researcher, as the two worked alongside one another, both demonstrating the attributes of professional artistry (Titchen, 2000).

For artistry to be fostered within the health professions, the appropriate types of research need to be encouraged as part of clinical practice and continuing professional development. Health professionals have written about the value of the deliberative process as a means of personal and professional development (Fish and Coles, 1998). This approach goes beyond reflection and demands an engagement with the more contentious issues underlying practice. Fish and Coles (1998) compared the processes of reflection and deliberation with reference to the work of Schön and Schwab. Schön's work encouraged critical thinking associated with practice and promoted the reframing of ideas through the use of alternative frames of reference. Schwab (1969) advocated 'the language of the practical', which entailed 'the exercise of the art of the practical with its associated method of deliberation'. This method 'is complex and arduous. It treats both ends and means and must treat them as mutually determining one another. It must try to identify with respect to both, what facts might be relevant' (Schwab, 1969, pp. 318–319).

Clearly, this is a time-consuming and demanding approach in attempting to express professional artistry. Nonetheless it would enable practitioners to identify what it is they have come to know through their experience as they made sense of it through the language, concepts and frameworks of others. This process would go beyond the identification of cause-and-effect relationships, to explore values and attitudes and other invisible aspects of practice. Practitioners might use the framework used by Handal and Lauvas (1987) as they encouraged novice teachers to explore their practice by means of identifying the actions, knowledge and values embedded within it. Alternatively, they might use the more detailed framework of Fish and Coles (1998), which involves identifying that part of their professional 'doing' and 'saying' that is the visible portion of the iceberg, and the knowledge, feelings, expectations, assumptions, attitudes, beliefs and values that lie hidden below the water line (Fish and Coles, 1998, pp. 305–306). To explore practice in such a way is to acknowledge the primacy of practice as the starting point for research.

## Implications for education

Artistry grows out of a way of knowing and seeing that is informed by theory, enabled by competence in action, and shaped by personal experience.

At an individual level professionals must be equipped with the theory and technical competence essential for practice and must know how to test their ideas through evaluation and research. They will need the capacity for lifelong learning, which includes the continuing development of the senses that are particularly relevant to their field of practice and the capacity for metacognition, critical self-appraisal and reflective transformation. The growth, recognition and refinement of artistry in a profession will require an explicit articulation of the traditions of practice specific to their area – traditions which emanate from that practice and which have not been separated from the practice base through the traditions of the universities within which they are educated. Education will need to play a continuing and vital role in the continuing development of such professionals.

In terms of preparation for practice, the world-wide expansion in technical and theoretical knowledge challenges the notion that students can be taught all that they need to know prior to entering professional life. Careful selection of material from a range of knowledge bases needs to be made by curriculum developers. This makes it essential that curriculum developers choose between competing fields of knowledge in preparing undergraduate curricula. Otherwise there will be little time and opportunity for the development of the non-propositional aspects of learning which are essential to the continuing development of the novice. The development of the capacity of students to learn from experience must continue to be fostered within the initial education of health professionals.

The inevitable consequence of a crowded curriculum within initial education is that much remains to be learnt after graduation. It is often at this stage that practitioners begin to develop connoisseurship in terms of the use of senses, the refinement of reasoning and the metacognitive skills which are central to their practice, and which are often associated with particular specialisms within their ever-expanding scope of practice. The use of mentors and clinical supervisors in the workplace and of practice-based courses can do much to provide the continuing professional development (CPD) which is essential to artistry.

In terms of the development of professional knowledge, the growth of the CPD movement brings with it the requirement for decisions about what constitutes professional knowledge. It raises the question as to whether CPD should be conceived of in terms of 'topping-up' theoretical knowledge gained prior to entering a profession or in terms of building upon the knowledge gained through experience of practising within the profession. The development of professional artistry requires the latter.

## Conclusions

The focus of this chapter has been on the notion of artistry within professional practice. In an age when the unquestioned supremacy of science and the scientific method is being challenged, we support a dynamic approach to practice expertise which embodies professional artistry and which develops both the practitioner and the practice. We propose that connoisseurship and criticism are appropriate to an understanding of professional artistry. We suggest that connoisseurship moves beyond technical competence and scientific knowledge and that it deepens the professional's understanding of the nuances, subtleties, wordless being and interactions which comprise excellent professional practice. Further, we call for greater exploration of professional artistry and for the development of new forms of expression, so that practice wisdom and graceful care can be made more accessible to others.

## Notes

1 In using the term 'traditions' we are speaking of the culture of a profession, with its associated values and norms, rather than implying traditional practice, which could refer to outdated and superseded practices.

2 The use of the term 'individual' does not imply that the knowing/knowledge is kept private or hidden from public scrutiny, rather that it is personal and unique in its configuration and derivation.

3 Refer to Chapter 7 for a discussion of the role of a critical companion in facilitating development and awareness of professional artistry.

## References

Aggleton, P. and Chalmers, H. (1986) *Nursing Models and the Nursing Process*. London: Macmillan.

Benner, P. (1984) *From Novice to Expert: Excellence and Power in Clinical Nursing Practice*. Menlo Park, CA: Addison-Wesley.

Binnie, A. and Titchen, A. (1999) *Freedom to Practice: The Development of Patient-Centred Nursing*. Oxford: Butterworth-Heinemann.

Eisner, E. (1981) On the differences between scientific and artistic approaches to qualitative research. *Educational Reader*, April, pp. 5–9.

Eisner, E. (1983) The art and craft of teaching. *Educational Leadership*, **40**, 4–13.

Eisner, E. (1985) *The Art of Educational Evaluation: A Personal View*. London: The Falmer Press.

Eraut, M. (1994) *Developing Professional Knowledge and Competence*. London: The Falmer Press.

Fish, D. (1998) *Appreciating Practice in the Caring Professions: Refocusing Professional Development and Practitioner Research*. Oxford: Butterworth-Heinemann.

Fish, D. and Coles, C. (1998) *Developing Professional Judgement in Health Care*, Oxford: Butterworth-Heinemann.

Glen, S. and Smith, K. (1999) Towards new models of teaching and researching nursing: The research practitioner. *Nurse Education Today*, **19**(8), 628–632.

Golby, M. (1993) *Case Study as Educational Research*. Oxford: Butterworth-Heinemann.

Handal, G. and Lauvas, P. (1987) *Promoting Reflective Teaching: Supervision in Action*. Milton Keynes: Society for Research into Higher Education and Open University.

Higgs, J. and Jones, M. (1995) Clinical reasoning. In *Clinical Reasoning in the Health Professions* (J. Higgs and M. Jones, eds), pp. 3–23. Oxford: Butterworth-Heinemann.

Higgs, J. and Titchen, A. (1995) Propositional, professional and personal knowledge in clinical reasoning. In *Clinical Reasoning in the Health Professions* (J. Higgs and M. Jones, eds), pp. 129–146. Oxford: Butterworth-Heinemann.

Jensen, G. M., Gwyer, J., Hack, L. M. and Shepard, K. F. (1999) *Expertise in Physical Therapy Practice*. Newton, MA: Butterworth-Heinemann.

Krefting, L. (1991) Rigor in qualitative research: The assessment of trustworthiness. *American Journal of Occupational Therapy*, **45**(3), 214–222.

Mattingly, C. and Fleming, M. (1994) *Clinical Reasoning: Forms of Inquiry in a Therapeutic Practice*. Philadelphia: F. A. Davis.

Mezirow, J. (1981) A critical theory of adult learning and education. *Adult Education*, **32**, 3–24.

Mezirow, J. (1990) Preface. In *Fostering Critical Reflection in Adulthood: A Guide to Transformative and Emancipatory Learning* (J. Mezirow and Associates, eds), pp. xiii–xxi. San Francisco: Jossey-Bass.

Ottenbacher, K. J. (1986) *Evaluating Clinical Change: Strategies for Occupational and Physical Therapists*. Baltimore: Williams & Wilkins.

Reed, K. (1984) *Models of Practice in Occupational Therapy*. Baltimore: Williams and Wilkins.

Reid, W. (1978) *Thinking About the Curriculum*. London: Routledge & Kegan Paul.

Schein, E. (1973) *Professional Education*. New York: McGraw-Hill.

Schön, D. A. (1983) *The Reflective Practitioner: How Professionals Think in Action*. New York: Basic Books.

Schön, D. A. (1987) *Educating the Reflective Practitioner*. San Francisco: Jossey-Bass.

Schwab, J. J. (1969) The practical: A language for the curriculum. *School Review*, **78**(1), 1–24.

Stenhouse, L. (1975) *An Introduction to Curriculum Research and Development*. London: Heinemann Educational Books.

Stenhouse, L. (1980) Curriculum research and the art of the teacher. *Curriculum*, **1**(1), 40–44.

Titchen, A. (2000) *Professional Craft Knowledge in Patient-Centred Nursing and the Facilitation of its Development*. DPhil thesis, University of Oxford; Oxford: Ashdale Press.

Torbert, W. R. (1978) Educating toward shared purpose, self-direction and quality work – the theory and practice of liberating structure. *Journal of Higher Education*, **49**, 109–135.

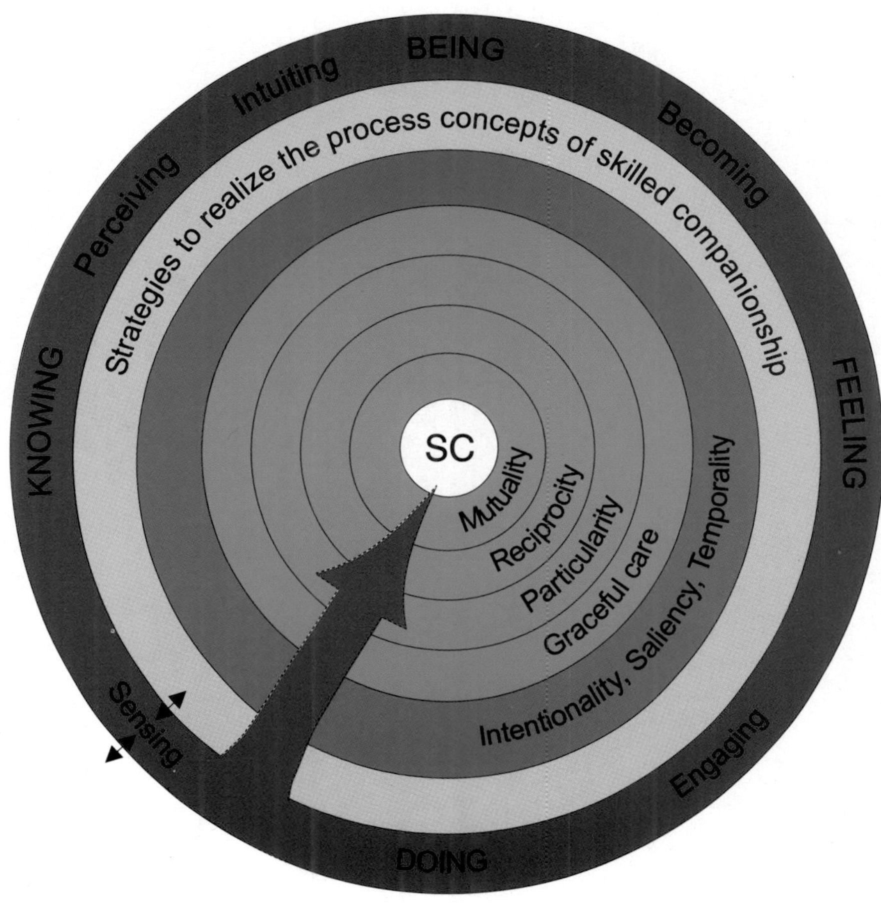


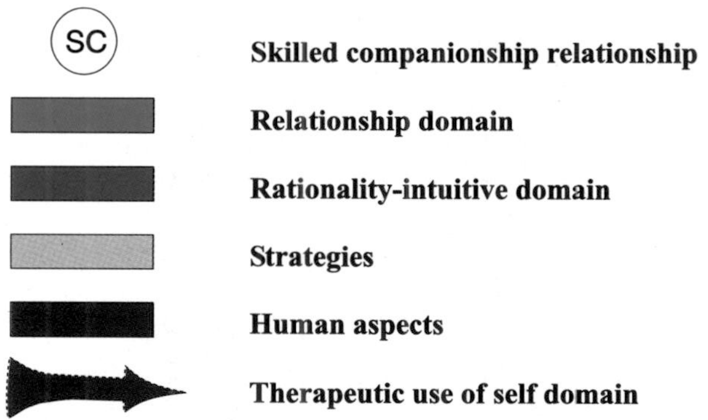


**Plate 2** Skilled companionship: a conceptual framework for patient-centred health care

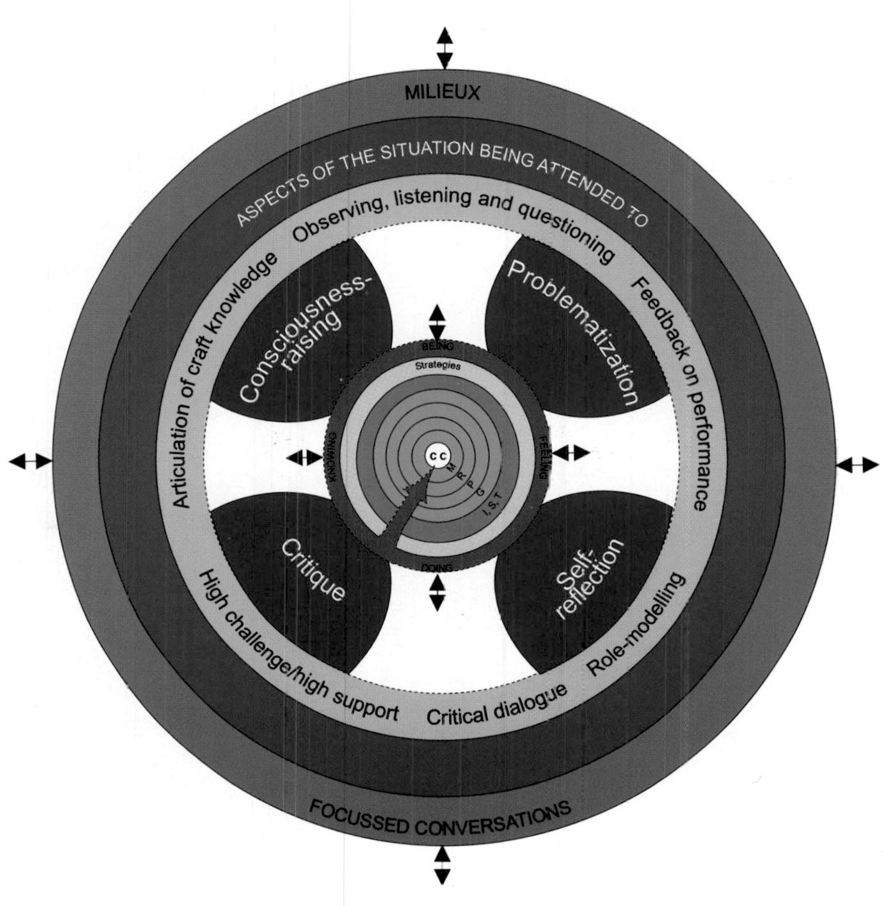


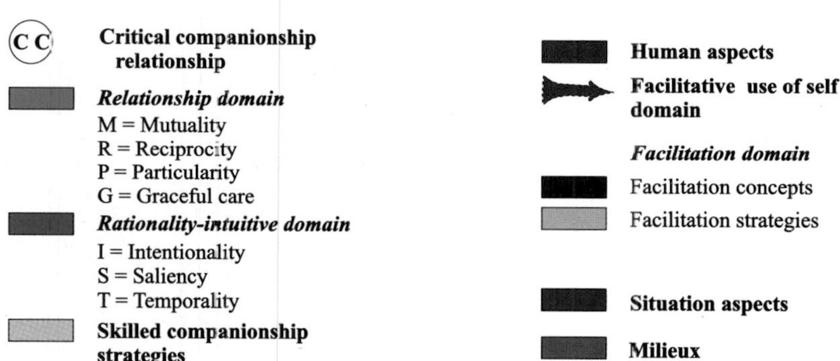


**Plate 3** Critical companionship: a conceptual framework for developing expertise

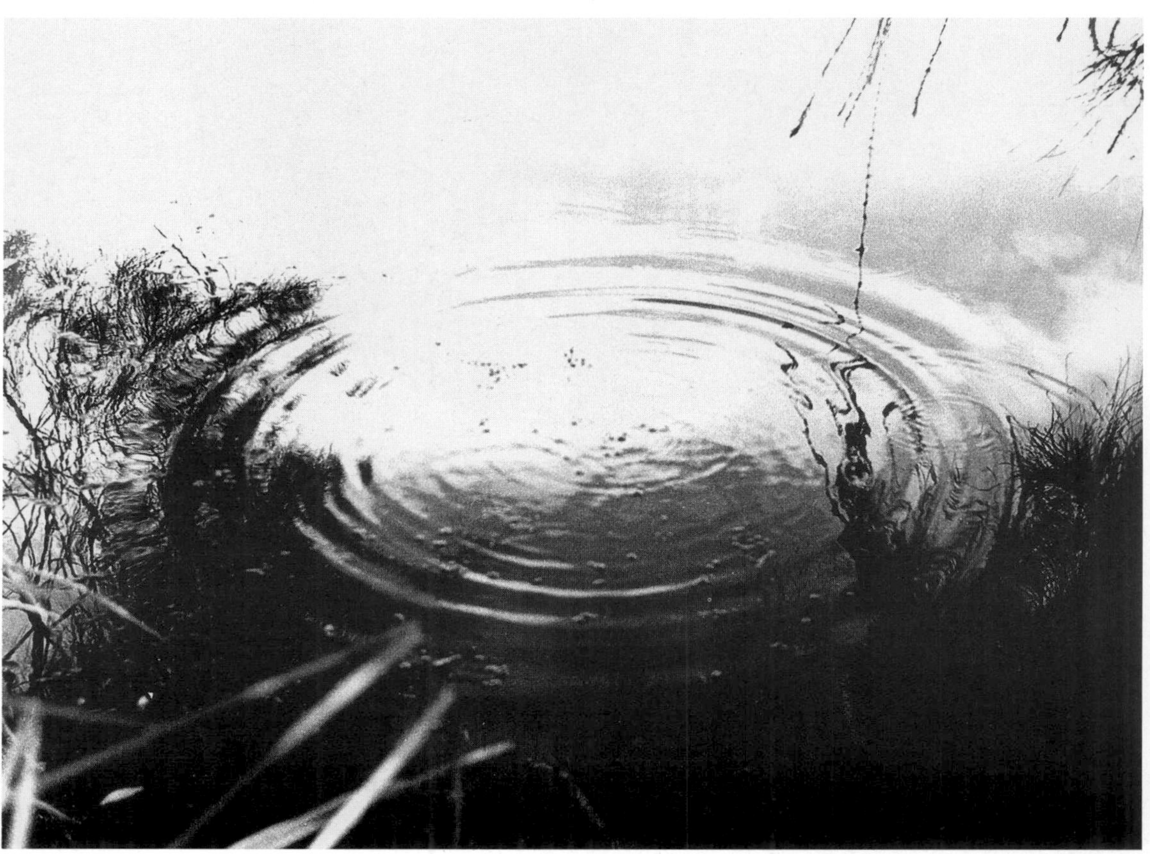

**Plate 4** Quiet pool and ripples

# Section Three

# Practice knowledge in action

# 15

# Reflection as a tool for developing professional practice knowledge and expertise

**Jane Gamble, Philip Chan and Hal Davey**

As a newly graduated occupational therapist, I (J.G.) recall asking my supervisor to explain her actions in relation to a particular clinical case. She had just conducted an occupational therapy work assessment where there were multiple and complex problems which she had dealt with easily, with creativity and to the satisfaction of the client, the employer and the rehabilitation provider. She truly demonstrated wisdom, expertise and professional craft knowledge. What she did find extremely difficult, however, was to explain to me how she had achieved this, the steps she took and why, and the critical things she had noticed about the situation as it occurred. My challenge was to understand this complex situation, the therapist's action and to learn how to attain some of her abilities.

How do therapists use their everyday professional experience, and what role does reflection play in the development of professional practice expertise? We explore this question in this chapter. We also explore some important related topics, to illustrate how they influence the use of reflection to develop professional practice knowledge and expertise.

## Defining reflection

Firstly, we should explain our conception of reflection, as there are many differing definitions, both in the literature (e.g. Boud and Walker, 1990; Schön, 1991), and also in the use of the term 'reflection' in everyday language. This often leads to ambiguity as people try to discuss 'reflection' without having clarified what they really mean.

In this chapter, we define reflection as firstly, the process by which an experience is brought into consideration, while it is happening or subsequently; and secondly, the creation of meaning and conceptualization from experience (Brockbank and McGill, 1998). Critical reflection, which occurs as a result of critical debate within oneself and possibly with others, may develop one's potential to look at things as other than they are. This type of reflection is important in the development of new ways of being a professional, and in creating transformative learning consistent with the critical paradigm (Mezirow, 1981) as it relates to knowledge generation. Such transformative learning is essential in the way it empowers learners to face the challenges of future learning and professional life enriched with a broader, more insightful knowledge base.

## Experience as a basis for learning

Central to understanding the use of reflection to develop professional knowledge and expertise is recognition of the importance of experience as a basis for learning (Boud, 1993). With experience, individuals engage in transactions with the world of professional practice, using their existing knowledge, skills and attitudes within the context of professional service delivery. The following propositions from Boud (1993) provide a foundation for our understanding about the use of experience in learning:

- Experience is the foundation of and stimulus for learning.

- Prior experiences will influence all learning.
- Learners construct their own experience.
- Learning is socially and culturally constructed and occurs in a socio-emotional context.
- Learning is not purely a cognitive process. It also has affective and conative features and as such is a holistic process in which feelings, emotions and action are as necessary as the cognitive processes which occur during and after the experience.

These propositions can be applied equally well to higher education students and to professionals who, in the development of a repertoire of approaches to practice, draw on professional practice experiences and interact with consumers, clients or patients and with other professionals. Professional practice experience, used as a foundation for learning, provides the opportunity for professionals to rethink their practices and to develop their professional knowledge and expertise or professional craft knowledge.

## Defining professional craft knowledge

Professional craft knowledge consists of practical knowledge, procedural knowledge, and theory-in-use (Higgs and Titchen, 1995). Practical knowledge (Heron, 1981; Benner, 1984) or procedural knowledge (Biggs and Telfer, 1987) encompasses practical expertise and skills. The term, professional craft knowledge, gives a sense of the intuitive, aesthetic and of knowing what, when and how (Higgs and Titchen, 1995).

Professional craft knowledge guides the expert practitioner to react to the whole situation and to make highly skilled judgments without being conscious of a deliberate way of acting. Professional craft knowledge is frequently tacit in nature because it is generally taken-for-granted and is perceived as so obvious and ordinary that it is rarely articulated. For example, when expert occupational therapists are asked about the finely tuned observation skills they have used in observing an injured worker, they are likely not to mention the taken-for-granted knowledge that they use every day. This could include the sophisticated task analysis they perform almost automatically, which will include all aspects of the worker's physical performance, the social-emotional and contextual aspects of the task as well as the layers of meaning ascribed to the task by the worker. We suggest that it is through the use of reflection about experience that such practitioners can enhance the development of their professional craft knowledge and expertise.

Higgs and Titchen (1995) suggest that the expert practitioner's depth of clinical judgment is born of a wealth of personal experience of practice in combination with the processing of prior learning. In processing prior learning, the expert practitioner is developing mastery of the knowledge base underpinning practice. The expert develops competency and confidence in selecting critical steps to formulate and test hypotheses. When processing learning in the practice context, the expert may have subconsciously observed significant variations and patterns, attending to them all at the same time (Bowden and Marton, 1998). The more this expert practitioner observes these variations and patterns, the more proficient the performance will be, to the extent that the expert can do it intuitively, as part of professional craft knowledge. The 'intuitive' ability to discern fine individual variations in the task analysis example above, and the ability to use short cuts to arrive at reasonable conclusions, both illustrate the development of this therapist's professional expertise and professional craft knowledge.

We suggest that it is through the use of reflection on experience that expert practitioners can enhance the development and awareness of their professional craft knowledge and expertise; furthermore, they have the potential to contribute towards collective professional knowledge by making their insights public.

## Learning from experience using reflection

The model that we have used to explain the use of reflection in the development of professional expertise is based on the model developed by Boud and co-workers (Boud et al., 1985; Boud and Walker, 1990). Their model of learning from experience consists of three key phases. The first phase is preparation before the event. In this phase, consideration is given to what the learner or practitioner brings to the event that may enhance or inhibit professional learning; consideration of what the event or milieu has to offer; and of the learning strategies that the practitioner may employ. The second phase is the occurrence of the experience itself. In this phase, the practitioner/learner engages with the milieu. Learning occurs by noticing, by intervening and through reflection-in-action.

The third phase is reflection on the experience after the event. In the third phase, the practitioner/learner returns to the experience to recapture it in as much detail as possible, attending to positive and negative feelings, re-evaluating the experience in order to link new learning to old and to consolidate the learning from experience. It is this reflective learning process that occurs when using experience as a foundation for the development of new practice knowledge and expertise, or professional craft knowledge.

The literature (Boud and Walker, 1998) and our work with graduate health science students[1] (Gamble et al., 1999) show that the ability to learn from experience and to use a reflective approach are influenced by certain conditions related to the practice context and to the practitioner or learner.

Reflection requires conscious effort and recognition of the value of reflection as a tool for learning from experience, as well as a sense of confidence in one's ability to effectively use reflection as a tool for learning. Actively using reflection to deal with professional experiences, particularly those experiences that are complex and which create uncertainty, as one graduate student observed:

> allows you to step outside of yourself, so you can actually try and imagine yourself in that situation and think, OK, I can learn from this and will change it next time.

This reflective process is sometimes difficult, particularly when the situation that one is reflecting on arouses ambivalent or negative emotions. Confidence that returning to the experience and reflecting on the experience will result in a useful outcome helps the professional to persist with what may initially seem like a process of going round in circles or being stuck in a rut of ideas and feelings.

To quote one of our graduate students:

> so if it *[the case study]* is meaningful, then you reflect on that, and what you would do in the real life situation. And at the time you think, this is a really hard case. And then you go back and think, gee, I really learnt so much from that particular case study.

Thus we are finding that graduate professional entry students incorporate reflection into their learning, becoming more sophisticated in their ability to use this strategy as they develop as learners.

Reflection is a skill that can be developed through practice and with time spent on the development and use of the skill.

> In the initial stages of using reflection, it wasn't very helpful for me. I would just go around in circles. But I think that over the two years I have gained more experience and have developed a more structured way of using the reflective process. Now I reflect better, and can take myself out of the situation and look at it more objectively. It has also become a more automatic process.

## Time for reflection

Another significant factor in the effective use of reflection is the availability of time to reflect.

> I think it *[reflection]* is enjoyable and I think you do get benefit, but I don't think it is a highly valued thing because if it was more valued then we would get more time to incorporate it into our lives. It is kind of, like . . . it is a luxury.

However, by allowing the luxury of time, one can use reflection to enhance professional understanding and the resultant professional expertise developed through learning from the experiences of service delivery. In contrast, the structure of many professions seems to preclude reflection in practice. Sinclair (1998, p. 73) suggests 'there is a definite need to teach managers and practitioners the efficacy of reflection in the long term' to the benefit of clients and of the service. Additionally, using reflection as a conscious process also provides an awareness of one's professional development; it can in itself be a source of satisfaction and intrinsic reward.

## Using reflection to develop professional knowledge and expertise

Professionals and students have reported utilizing different strategies as tools for reflection. Strategies often mentioned are contemplation, professional writing (Morrison, 1996), journalling (Walker, 1985), discussion with peers or experts about one's experience (Candy et al., 1985), reflective listening, and reflection as part of action research cycles (Carr and Kemmis, 1986).

Preferred strategies for reflection are individually determined, as illustrated by the following quotes from our graduate students:

I need some time to reflect on my own before I can talk to others about what happened and how I felt, as I couldn't really express what I am thinking and feeling.

I prefer to start reflecting alone, especially if there is a difficult situation.

*[it was]* . . . where you sat down and talked about what we had really learned and what we are good at and if we have covered all areas. I thought that was really useful reflection to me.

It would be easier to express in my own language. If I have to write it in English I find it more difficult to reflect. I would rather write in Chinese . . . Reflection might be just going on in your head and you don't necessarily express it in language form and sometimes you have got that feeling and it is so difficult to put into words, not even to write it down on paper.

The above quotes, taken from our research on reflection in learning (Gamble et al., 1999), illustrate the variety of meanings that this group of graduate professional entry students ascribe to using reflection in their development as occupational therapist health care practitioners.

Using an example from professional practice, we now illustrate how experienced professionals use professional craft knowledge and how it can be enhanced through the use of reflection. An occupational therapist is conducting a detailed observation and task analysis during a work visit for an injured factory worker. During the work visit, the therapist considers the dimensions of work likely to be affected by the worker's hand injury. These dimensions include the tool usage and related hand function, the sequential organization of task steps, including the use of tools for some steps, and the social relationships between workers sharing tools. The experienced therapist can focus on the key and critical areas. In the observation of the worker, the expert will identify that, as well as difficulty using scissors through the effects of the injury, the worker has the added task dimension of sharing scissors with two other co-workers. One co-worker is overly possessive about keeping control of the scissors and is impatient about the extra time the injured worker is taking to use the shared scissors.

Using the sophisticated, internalized, expert professional craft knowledge, this therapist is making recommendations about the rehabilitation, work task modifications, and return to work, linking in to her previous experience with similar situations and the professional expertise or craft knowledge that she has developed over time. In this example, her recommendations may include a request for purchase of additional tools, the repositioning of tools and recommendations for restructuring work tasks.

Often, this therapist has difficulty in explaining the links between the comprehensive observations and the recommendations she has made. However, with the use of reflection, this therapist can make explicit the reasoning and professional knowledge about her activity analysis and this complex work observation. The process of reflection will assist the therapist in understanding her reasoning better, in learning from her experience, and in informing other therapists about her expert practice.

Reflection helps professionals unpack their experience and the different layers of meaning within it, allowing them to explain the experience to themselves or to another. In the above case example the therapist is assisted by the use of reflection on the work visit experience in her preparation for writing a medico-legal report to the insurance company about the injured worker and his work. She can also add new hypotheses to her professional craft knowledge or modify existing hypotheses about her practice, particularly related to her use of skilled observation and task analysis. This growth in knowledge is valuable for use in similar situations in the future.

## Exploring reflections with an expert or a peer

We now consider a novice therapist who is conducting the same work visit as the therapist in the previous example. In contrast to the expert practitioner, the novice may not be able to observe as quickly, may miss some parts of the activity analysis, may not analyse as quickly, and may not be able to synthesize observations as quickly across task dimensions in order to identify the central issues for the injured worker. There may also be difficulty in clearly identifying critical elements or subtle variations within the situation. This novice practitioner does not have the same extensive professional craft knowledge as the expert, and is using practice knowledge in a check-list approach to observation and activity analysis. In retrospect, the novice practitioner may realize that she or he had not identified some of the areas of difficulty experienced by the worker, for example, overlooking some of the social factors in the work environment. As a result, the novice therapist may experience some frustration and need reassurance about her or his performance.

By describing the experience in detail to a peer or an expert, the novice can use reflection to revisit the situation and to consider the experience, observations and actions across the broader layers or dimensions of the task analysis – as well as in other aspects of the work visit. The novice can also describe the resulting therapy recommendations as well as recalling and discussing previous similar work situations. Through discussion with expert colleagues, the novice's reflections can lead to new insights. For example, novices can learn that they need to consider and attend simultaneously to the effect of the social context and its influence on sharing of tools (scissors, in the above example) as well as the many other dimensions of the work tasks.

Our research has shown that trust is an important condition whilst reflecting on experience with a peer or colleague. Comments about reflecting with others highlight the importance of this collegial relationship:

> [Reflection works well] as long as it's the right relationship and you have been listened to . . . [and] . . . you are not, I guess overbearing them with what you are reflecting on.

When commenting about using reflection to learn during fieldwork education, students also highlighted the related importance of the organizational environment. Students value

> an open and flexible organisation, so you can show your weaknesses and vulnerabilities.

The ability to work effectively as part of a team is important for service delivery. Graduate students have commented on the value of reflection in developing their teamwork:

> Reflecting has helped us define our relationships as well as our learning . . . when you know where someone is coming from you can actually learn from them rather than being offended by them, you know.

In developing relationships, reflection can assist practitioners to accept individual differences and gain understanding about the effect they have on professional practice. This understanding about working with and learning from colleagues also becomes part of the professional's repertoire of professional craft knowledge.

By reflecting with others, be they peers or experts, in a relationship conducive to supportively identifying inadequacies and difficulties as well as proficiency, professionals gain a broader perspective on their experience. Sharing reflections about professional practice can develop understanding and craft knowledge as professionals, thus fostering the development of expertise.

## Difficulties in the creation, recognition and testing of professional craft knowledge through reflection

Using reflection to develop professional craft knowledge is not always a straightforward process; it can at times be problematic. In returning to the experience, the literature (Boud et al., 1985), our research with graduate students (Gamble et al., 1999), and our personal experience indicate that there may be feelings of discomfort associated with reflection, particularly if there are negative emotions or conflict associated with the experience. This can lead to avoidance of reflective processes as well as a failure to recognize the potential for new learning within the experience. The continuing development of professional craft knowledge and expertise may be limited by this avoidance.

Another common pitfall in using reflection in developing professional craft knowledge is that the experience and resultant insights and knowledge may be devalued, because of the commonsense and everyday nature of the experience and the resultant knowledge generated. For example, in the case situation mentioned earlier, the occupational therapist has developed fine-tuned activity analysis abilities and extensive professional craft knowledge about alternative and complementary approaches in the analysis of work-related activity. However, when reflecting on or being asked about this area of her knowledge, she may consider that activity analysis is a foundation occupational therapy skill that many possess, without any awareness of her highly sophisticated professional expertise in the area.

A third potential problem in using reflection to develop expertise and knowledge relates to the difficulties that professionals have in converting their craft knowledge into propositional knowledge. Because of the intangible nature of the reflective process and the apparently random and circuitous nature of reflection, it is often difficult to identify patterns emerging in the development of the insights gained. It can be helpful for the professional to use a journal to record the reflections and to review the journal entries from time to time, to analyse emerging themes and concepts. This is one of a number of strategies which can be used to access the tacit, taken-for-granted knowledge and insights which typify professional craft knowledge.

The analysis of reflection on professional experience and the insights gained about professional practice can be approached more formally, by incorporating reflective practices into professional review and development. One such strategy is to use qualitative research methodologies such as action research (Carr and Kemmis, 1986). Other less formal strategies for critical analysis include journal writing (Walker, 1985; Morrison, 1996), reflective discussions and reflective listening.

Importantly, reflection in the development of professional craft knowledge needs to be recognized as a mechanism for the development of inquiring minds, used to foster the development of empirical truth rather than used as a gimmick, a strategy to control, or a universal solution to practice knowledge generation. We cannot stress enough the importance of trust and of ethical practice when professionals agree to share their reflections about practice experience. We refer to both qualified and student professionals. Frank, honest sharing is the motivation which underlies the use of reflection to learn from one's own and others' experiences, whether novice or expert.

## Summary

In this chapter we have presented reflection on experience as a basis for learning for professionals. We have explored the place of reflection in the development of professional craft knowledge and expertise, using a model of learning from experience through reflection, informed by our research with graduate students. We have stressed the need for time for reflection to develop professional expertise. We have also attempted to describe the use of reflection in professional practice, using experience as a tool for developing professional craft knowledge. We contend that reflection is a legitimate tool that can be used in a number of forms by expert or novice, alone and with others. There are difficulties that can be barriers to reflection, and we have highlighted them and suggested strategies, especially the use of ethical behaviour, to attempt to overcome them.

We acknowledge and are grateful for the shared wisdom of the graduate students who agreed to participate in our research on reflection in learning, and who entrusted us with their insights. The power of their quotations in this chapter illustrates the value placed by these students on reflection as a learning tool for use in professional practice as they move from novice to expert.

To return to the opening scene, my (J.G.'s) supervisor took the time to explain her practice, exploring what she had just done. We both gained a greater understanding of the situation, using reflective conversations to access her professional craft knowledge, thereby enhancing knowledge for us both. Reflection played a key role in making explicit the expert therapist's tacit professional craft knowledge.

## Note

1 From this point onwards the quotations in a different font represent the voices of students from our Master of Occupational Therapy professional entry programme.

## References

Benner, P. (1984) *From Novice to Expert: Excellence and Power in Clinical Nursing Practice*. London: Addison-Wesley.

Biggs, J. and Telfer, R. (1987) *The Process of Learning*. Sydney: Prentice-Hall.

Boud, D. J. (1993) Experience as the base for learning. *Higher Education Research and Development*, **12**, 33–44.

Boud, D. J. and Walker, D. (1990) Making the most of experience. *Studies in Continuing Education*, **12**, 61–80.

Boud, D. J. and Walker, D. (1998) Promoting reflection in professional courses: The challenge of context. *Studies in Higher Education*, **23**, 191–206.

Boud, D. J., Keogh, R. and Walker, D. (1985) Promoting reflection in learning: A model. In *Reflection: Turning Experience into Learning* (D. J. Boud, R. Keogh and D. Walker, eds), pp. 18–40. London: Kogan Page.

Bowden, J. and Marton, F. (1998) *The University of Learning: Beyond Quality and Competence in Higher Education*. London: Kogan Page.

Brockbank, A. and McGill, I. (1998) *Facilitating Reflective Learning in Higher Education*. Buckingham: SRHE and Open University Press.

Carr, W. and Kemmis, S. (1986) *Becoming Critical: Knowing Through Action Research*. Geelong, Victoria: Deakin University Press.

Candy, P., Harri-Augstein, S. and Thomas, L. (1985) Reflection and the self-organized learner: A model of learning conversations. In *Reflection: Turning Experience into Learning* (D. J. Boud, R. Keogh and D. Walker, eds), pp. 100–116. London: Kogan Page.

Gamble, J., Davey, H. and Chan, P. (1999) Student experiences of reflection in learning in graduate professional education. Paper presented at HERDSA Annual International Conference, Melbourne.

Heron, J. (1981) Philosophical basis for a new paradigm. In *Human Inquiry: A Sourcebook of New Paradigm Research* (P. Reason and J. Rowan, eds), pp. 19–35. Chichester: Wiley.

Higgs, J. and Titchen, A. (1995) The nature, generation and verification of knowledge. *Physiotherapy*, **81**, 521–530.

Mezirow, J. (1981) A critical theory of adult learning and education. *Adult Education*, **32**, 3–24.

Morrison, K. (1996) Developing reflective practice in higher degree students through a learning journal. *Studies in Higher Education*, **21**, 317–332.

Schön, D. A. (1991) *The Reflective Practitioner: How Professionals Think in Action*. Aldershot: Avebury

Sinclair, K. (1998) Reflective practice in health care. In *Occupational Therapy: New Perspectives* (J. Creek, ed.), pp. 66–76. London: Whurr.

Walker, D. (1985) Writing and reflection. In *Reflection: Turning Experience into Learning* (D. J. Boud, R. Keogh and D. Walker, eds), pp. 52–68. London: Kogan Page.

# 16

# Facilitating the acquisition of craft knowledge through supported reflection

**Jan Dewing with contributions by Andy Woodrow**

This chapter focuses on supported reflection carried out through a system known in the UK as clinical supervision. In particular it describes how I, as an experienced practitioner and clinical leader, made use of a range of theoretical principles to guide and facilitate another, less experienced, practitioner to become more effective in her work with patients, relatives and colleagues.

In the context of the practice setting and the practitioner described in this chapter, **becoming more effective** means:

- being open to the experiences of being available to others and developing appropriate ways in dealing with the consequences of being open, available and authentic;
- becoming more person-centred; moving from patient- to person-centredness (holistic to humanistic);
- practising in ways that live out an expressed philosophy and model of care on a day-to-day basis that others can see;
- becoming sensitively skilled in the ways of using craft knowledge in day-to-day practice.

## Clinical supervision: guided structured reflection

Clinical supervision is a system in which practitioners meet with another more experienced practitioner and discuss issues related to their practice. The particular features of clinical supervision are:

- There is a contract that includes confidentiality within professional boundaries.
- Supervisees bring to the session practice encounters or critical incidents that they have begun reflecting on.
- It makes use of reflection, preferably through a model of guided reflection such as that of Johns (1993).
- The supervisee works at being open to challenge and support from the supervisor.
- The supervisor uses a variety of models and methods to challenge and support supervisees to learn and increase their ways of knowing about specific incidents and also to generalize their learning for the future.
- Written notes are kept of each session.
- Supervision is formally evaluated by both supervisee and supervisor at specified intervals.

Obviously, there is much more to clinical supervision than what has just been described here, and I return to this subject later in the chapter. There is a healthy debate current in the UK, for example, around the expected benefits of clinical supervision and the ways in which it can or does influence the development of practice. There is also a debate about whether or not a manager can be a practitioner's supervisor, as happened in Andy's case.

## The practitioner

Andy qualified as a Registered General Nurse in 1985. Within one year she gave up nursing because of family commitments. In 1995 Andy decided to return to nursing, and successfully completed a formal **return to nursing** programme. As part of her clinical placements, she worked at Burford Community Hospital (see below). Andy then went on to work at Burford and other places through nurse agencies. In 1996 Andy applied for, and was appointed to, a staff nurse post, working part-time. Andy says that not long after this appointment she recalls becoming aware of clinical supervision. She heard a range of comments, from those who were 'suspicious' of supervision and its purpose and those who made much more favourable remarks. In particular,

> a much trusted colleague whose opinion I listened to and respected described the benefits of supervision and advocated it as being positive

Andy made the decision to approach me (in my role as hospital manager and clinical leader) about entering into clinical supervision.

## The context

Burford Community Hospital consists of a small hospital of 11 beds, a multi-agency day unit, a nurse-led minor injuries unit, and outpatient clinics. There are no resident medical staff, with medical care being provided by the patients' general practitioners. Burford provides a nursing-led service, where nurses coordinate admissions and discharges on behalf of the health care team. The hospital provides multidisciplinary rehabilitation, as well as respite and palliative care and care for older people with dementia. Burford had a well-established history of being a Nursing Development Unit (NDU) (see, e.g., Pearson, 1988; Johns, 1994). The hospital, through the work of Johns (1994), developed the Burford Nursing Development Unit Model (see Table 16.1) on which practice was based.

The model of leadership used by me, as the clinical leader, was most closely related to **transformational leadership** (Bennis and Nanus, 1985, p. 3). I also valued Kouzes and Posner's (1988) leadership characteristics, such as inspiring a shared vision, enabling others to act, and modelling the way. Supervision using guided reflection and a counselling approach was an ideal method for living out my style of leadership, developing the professional craft knowledge of the practitioners and supporting the hospital philosophy. The hospital philosophy and model inevitably meant there were implications for the sort of learning and education that the team needed in order to develop themselves and their nursing skills.

The National Health Service Trust of which the hospital is part offered a wide range of formal education opportunities that could be found in any good organization. Formal education opportunities provided the practitioners at Burford with technical and rational knowledge (Schön, 1983). But there comes a point in the development of most nurses, especially those who are moving towards humanistic or person-centred nursing, where something else is needed. This could perhaps be described as the missing link in Carper's (1978) ways of knowing or Kikuchi's (1992) private ways of knowing. Professional craft knowledge usually holds within it tacit and intuitive knowledge (Carr, 1989; Titchen, 1998, 2000). The key to practitioners being able to assimilate the required knowledge and attitudes underpinning humanistic nursing is accessing their personal knowledge. This combination is essential for working with people to facilitate re-enablement and healing, and for coping with the consequences of working in this way.

Clinical supervision was seen as a way of helping nurses to develop the missing link. It was,

**Table 16.1 The Burford Nursing Development Unit Model (from Johns, 1994, p. 41)**

- Who is this person?
- What health event brings this person into hospital/here?
- How must this person be feeling?
- How has this event affected this person's usual life patterns and roles?
- How does this person make me feel?
- How can I help this person?
- What is important for this person to make their stay [in hospital] comfortable?
- What support does this person have in life?
- How does this person view the future for him or herself and for others?

therefore, offered to all nurses in the hospital and more latterly to therapists, because of the following reasons:

- It was essential that the mutuality, intersubjectivity and heightened state of connectedness characterized by caring was nurtured (Montgomery, 1993, p. 101).
- It was a method for living out transformational leadership.
- It was a method to facilitate skilled companionship (Titchen, 1998, 2000) or the development of nurses in ways that seemed to bring out person-centred or humanistic caring skills to a greater degree.[1]
- It was both a learning and support system complementary to the practice philosophy and model that ensured nurses engaged with patients as far as they were able. In addition, it was a system that helped nurses to cope with the stress that person-centred caring can induce. It must be noted, however, that full engagement in caring does not necessarily lead to burnout. There are many accounts of successful caring experiences being self-reinforcing and energizing for nurses (e.g. Binnie and Titchen, 1999). In this case, structured guided reflection or clinical supervision builds on this energizing process.

## Clinical supervision: the theory

There are various definitions and descriptions of clinical supervision, usually with more commonalities than differences (e.g. Hawkins and Shohet, 1989; Butterworth and Faugier, 1992; Kohner, 1994). The term 'clinical supervision' is, in my experience, looked upon unfavourably by some nurses. 'Clinical' makes it seem cold or aloof, and 'supervision' has, for many nurses still emerging from hierarchical organizational cultures, distinct reminders of being checked on by a manager or of fault finding.

Platt-Koch (1986) describes clinical supervision as a process for expanding knowledge, and developing clinical expertise and proficiency, self-esteem and autonomy. I would not disagree with this view, but suggest that all definitions of supervision are incomplete without a clear description of what is meant by developing clinical expertise. For example, does it mean developing knowledge about technical aspects of nursing? Does it mean reducing length of stay, or ensuring that all patients comply with a rehabilitation programme? Does it mean developing the graceful care of skilled companionship (Titchen, 1998, 2000; see also Chapter 9)? Perhaps it means developing the professional artistry which Titchen concluded is the hallmark of expertise. Clinical practitioners do not all agree about what good nursing care is or what patients' needs are. Nurses have different visions about what nursing is and how far it should extend into the domains of healing and spirituality. Visions of what nursing can potentially be are also influenced by the nurse's personal and often private values and beliefs.

Bond and Holland (1998, p. 12) describe the process of clinical supervision as being a:

> regular, protected time for facilitated, in depth reflection on clinical practice. It aims to enable the supervisee to achieve, sustain and creatively develop a high quality of practice through the means of focused support and development.

I would suggest that the means by which creativity develops is through focused support and challenge, rather than the more loosely structured idea of development. Sometimes, very technically skilled and efficient nurses have had difficulties with developing professional artistry. Clinical supervision enables nurses to look into the heart of nursing practice and come to understand better both themselves and the essence of their practice.

According to Johns (1995), clinical supervision offers:

> an 'ideal milieu' for the guidance of reflective practice just as reflective practice offers an ideal method to structure what takes place in clinical practice.

In other words, clinical supervision becomes a structure for guided reflection on practice. I would argue that many nurses struggle with reflection, if trying to do it on their own, in private. Lauder (1994) suggests that reflection fails to link theory and practice because it separates thought and action. Quite often nurses who reflect on their own make no progress beyond the descriptive level of reflection as described by Mezirow (cited in Burns, 1994).

## Clinical supervision: the practice

Clinical supervision or structured guided reflection takes time to establish within most clinical areas, and is best introduced in an organized and collaborative way.[2] The supervisee makes appointments for the session, usually 1 hour every 4–6 weeks. The session takes place in a private and quiet room where the supervisee and supervisor will not be disturbed. The supervisee has prepared for the session by using a reflective model to work through an encounter from practice that has meaning, perhaps because it was challenging, very positive or puzzling. This is also referred to as a critical incident or significant experience. Such experiences from practice can be complex and many key issues can be identified. For example, take Andy's incident during one of her sessions:

I wanted to talk about Monday . . . I went home feeling totally guilty. Well, not guilty but dissatisfied. I hadn't done everything that I needed to do, but I didn't have a minute to myself all day. I remember feeling I was flitting about all over the place and not doing anything particularly well. I don't know if it's my ability to prioritise my work. I did not perceive any complaints from patients. Perhaps its just my own feelings and that I'm not feeling positive about what I did that day. I wonder if it's common for others to feel like this – going home feeling dissatisfied?
*(fourth supervision session)*

It is possible to identify several key issues from what Andy told me by using observation, listening and questioning as Titchen (1998, 2000) suggests in her model of critical companionship. However, the point of supervision is not for me to identify the issues, but for Andy to sort out the wood from the trees and do it for herself. Sometimes the supervisor, like the critical companion, brings together material gathered by the supervisee for critical reflection and self-evaluation. The supervisor and critical companion may point out salient features in the situation, but only after helping practitioners to do this for themselves. Andy was only into her fourth session and wasn't always clear about what the key issues were. She continued:

Perhaps I think too much about whether or not I'm doing the right thing with my time.

Following this, we explored what the day was like in much more detail. We discussed, for example, how she felt when she came to work (returning from two days away and not knowing the patients). Andy was able to talk about what she hadn't done, in considerable detail.

There was a dressing that I hadn't done. I hadn't managed to spend any time with Doreen because she had her family with her all morning. I know it's important for her to have visitors, but she hadn't had a wash at all. I do know it's not life threatening for her not to have had a wash, but I think it would have been nice for her visitors if she had. I just didn't seem to be involved that morning.

*JD* (supervisor): If you weren't having an input in that area, let's have a look at what you were doing. Tell me about what you did achieve that day?

*AW:* I worked with EG and spent quite a bit of time with her. I attended to her leg and gave it a massage – really well. I also spent some time with FT and helped him to soak his feet. He did say it was really good and he looked pleased. I spent a lot of time with ME (a patient being admitted) when he came in and helped him to settle in to the ward, by orientating him with the building and what was happening around him. The patients all seemed happy, it was just me that wasn't.

In an earlier part of the session, Andy had described how she had read all the notes and care plans and was aware of other patients and their ability to self care. She said that she knew what the care assistant was doing and how she regularly went in to see how Doreen and her family were.

Perhaps Andy felt frustrated because she could not see, and therefore appreciate, the level of skill she was applying to her work and just what work she had achieved. At one point she described how she 'popped in and out of Doreen's room'. I challenged Andy about what she meant by this expression. She replied:

I suppose I was giving snippets of care, but it could be that I was facilitating the care to be given by her husband and other family members . . . I knew what had and hadn't been done and I was able to hand this over to the next nurse taking over from me.

We spoke of the benefits of this approach for Doreen and her family. Over the following sessions Andy returned to the theme of how she was spending her time and how effective she was being. She began to develop a sense that collaboration between the nurse and patient, at a deeper level, is more likely to occur when:

- the doubts of the practitioner are explored;
- the practitioner has an opportunity to devise and test out alternative hypotheses;
- the practitioner can scan these hypotheses for their consequences;
- the practitioner has a sense of control over her or his possible biases.

Andy became more comfortable with not knowing everything and accepted that there will always be things that remain unknown. She also was able to articulate that in her actual practice, even if the nurse–patient interaction and subsequent action was not textbook perfect, the reflective process was leading her to an increased understanding of what was happening and of the interrelationship between theory and practice and the private and public domains of herself, the nurse. Indeed, Benner and Wrubel (1989, p. 395) suggest that nurses try to reconcile the ideal with the realities of practice. These authors suggest that nurses who are experts at caring can view reality as a source of possibilities, rather than as a deficit in relation to fixed theoretical ideals. Once Andy had identified what she was doing, I was able to help her to acknowledge, and then accept, that what she was doing was valuable and therapeutic work that kept the patient as a person at the core.

In an hour-long session of supervision or structured guided reflection, there is usually time to reflect deeply on only one or two of the key issues raised through the critical incident. I use a range of supportive and challenging interventions to encourage supervisees to develop their appreciation of an incident and to learn from it. I generally utilize Heron's Six Category Intervention Analysis (Heron, 1975), but not exclusively. However, using Heron's model to achieve high challenge and support complements the critical companionship model (Titchen, 1998, 2000). Adding depth to the critical discussion enables the supervisee to consider the 'micro' world of the nurse–patient relationship. Supervisees will sometimes come to a session and say to me:

I asked myself what you would have asked me to think about.

This is evidence that the supervisee is beginning to develop self-supervision and is moving supervision into daily practice, especially if there is evidence of reflection or attempting to answer the question. The supervisee usually gradually develops greater levels of confidence in challenging and supporting colleagues and becoming more questioning and creative in practice. Therefore, she will begin to model or live out and explicate it to others in day-to-day practice (and in relationships with colleagues). This can be seen in Andy's comments later in this chapter.

## Helping strategies

Framing a dilemma or problematizing it in supervision, to make it more comprehensible, can be a good strategy for a supervisor. In her eighth session, Andy described to me her work and relationship with a woman who was dying. The woman's only visitor had been a female friend who now seemed unable to visit and had been approaching Andy outside the hospital to find out how the patient was. When I asked her what options she could identify for managing the friend's enquiries in ways that were respectful and confidential, Andy was able to identify and give a rationale for one way of working through this situation. This indicated to me that Andy had not deeply reflected on the problem, since otherwise she would have been able to talk about a range of options and their likely consequences. I was able to suggest that this 'problem' was not going to stop, and to ask how Andy would prepare the patient's friend for the impending death. I also asked Andy to consider the needs of this patient's friend to be involved in the dying process, in a way that she could cope with and that was acceptable for her:

How can you effectively work with this person when they do not make contact with the hospital in the usual manner?

This process of articulating the issue, interpreting it and reflecting back what has been said can be a useful learning method and is also part of the critical dialogue strategy of critical companionship. For example, in her seventh session, I reflected back to Andy 'being in company?' and later 'her behaviour was a problem for the night staff?'. Here, I was asking Andy to think more deeply about what a patient's need for being in company might mean. I was also asking Andy to question the idea that a patient's behaviour can be seen as being a problem, because of the labelling implied and the negative connotations underpinning the statement.

Perhaps many dilemmas are rooted in misunderstandings of what the real issue is, rather than in an actual conflict between core principles. Sometimes, when supervisee practitioners have heard the supervisor repeat back (as part of reflecting the issue to the supervisee), they hear what they have said in a different perspective. Sometimes they then recognize the limitation of their understanding, or that what they have said, or what they believe, does not make sense or fit comfortably with their philosophy for practice.

Learning to think for oneself, whilst keeping the phenomenological experience of the patient central, takes time and effort. Good decisions are not natural. Much of the effort is unseen, as it takes place inside the heads and hearts of clinical nurses and they do not usually talk their way through these processes as a matter of course. Colleagues do not always have the opportunity to see or hear about the ways in which an expert colleague weighs up options and consequences, or how or why values and beliefs may be influencing what is happening. Therefore, less experienced nurses find it difficult to learn ways of developing their decision-making skills. Supervision, or structured guided reflection, appears in some cases to have parallels with the framework of critical companionship. Titchen (1998, 2000) sees critical companionship as a methodology for clinical supervision. She found that if the experienced supervisor articulates her reflections to the supervisee, as part of the 'articulating craft knowledge' strategy within a critical dialogue, then the less experienced practitioner is exposed to this usually hidden knowledge and becomes able to critique it.

## Andy's evaluation of supervision

The reader may find it helpful to find out what Andy thought of supervision. At the time this chapter was written, she had moved into supervision with another experienced member of the team, someone who was more of a peer than a manager or clinical leader. Thus, she now has the experience of supervisors with different styles of supervision and in different roles. Andy says about her supervision or structured guided reflection:

Initially I found supervision nerve wracking, partly due to the underlying feeling that the result of these sessions would be to reinforce my view that I had not dealt with practice situations correctly . . . and partly due to the nature of the sessions, whereby my personal feelings were revealed to my manager, leaving me feeling vulnerable. I would work through Johns' model of reflection, but still feel negative about my ability to work therapeutically with patients and their families. Jan worked hard with me to help me to recognise for myself that I did something positive in each situation. Through these sessions I became more confident in my ability to explore my practice in a more realistic way – to view situations in a more balanced way and not to start from the basis that what I did would be wrong.

At first, the sessions seemed very separate to my practice, but after a few months I realised that this was not how it was supposed to be. The aim of the sessions was to apply what was learnt in the sessions into my practice and also to develop my skills in reflection, so that I could begin to reflect in action and not just in retrospect. I feel reflection has linked theory and evidence to enhance my practice development. Recognition of my own development was very positive and supervision with Jan mobilised my ability to assess my development and my natural tendency to be overly self-critical. Thus increased self-awareness is another benefit of clinical supervision. One of the greatest benefits gained from supervision is that it encouraged me to challenge practice without feeling negative or disloyal about doing it. It has helped me to realise that although I may lack years of professional experience in practice, in comparison to some of my colleagues, I have acquired skills necessary to develop my own learning. I now also recognise that my own life experiences and the values and beliefs I have acquired are, in themselves, important in the development of humanistic nursing. In recognising this, I can now challenge others and myself about practice in a productive and developmental way.

Changing supervisors resurfaced some of the anxieties I had when I first started supervision. The need to get to know the supervisor before revealing inner feelings seems to me to be extremely important and highlights the fundamental issue of the relationship between the supervisee and supervisor. The relationship has to be therapeutic for supervision to be of benefit in exploring the nature of the nurse patient relationship. I now feel ready for the challenges of group supervision.

## Summary

This chapter has provided an insight, through the experiences of one nurse, into the way in which clinical supervision or structured guided reflection can support the development of practitioners. The philosophical and theoretical approach underpinning clinical supervision may lead practitioners on a variety of journeys. For example, the values and beliefs at Burford and of the clinical supervisor who, in many ways, modelled critical companionship, supported Andy in developing her professional craft knowledge and skilled companionship skills. The kind of learning that Andy describes and the integration of this learning into her being and practice is something that few formal education courses in the classroom could offer.

## Notes

1 See Titchen's Chapter 10 in this book, which offers a conceptual framework for an expert in humanistic (patient-centred) nursing to help a less experienced practitioner develop these skills.

2 See the Royal College of Nursing's (1999) Open Learning Pack for practical assistance on how to introduce clinical supervision in this way.

## References

Benner, P. and Wrubel, J. (1989) *The Primacy of Caring: Stress and Coping in Health and Illness*. London: Addison-Wesley.

Bennis, W. and Nanus, B. (1985) *Leaders: Strategies for Making Change*. New York: Harper & Row.

Binnie, A. and Titchen, A. (1999) *Freedom to Practise: The Development of Patient-Centred Nursing*. Oxford: Butterworth-Heinemann.

Bond, M. and Holland, S. (1998) *Skills of Clinical Supervision for Nurses*. Buckingham: Open University Press.

Burns, S. (1994) Assessing reflective learning. In *Reflective Practice in Nursing* (A. Palmer, S. Burns and C. Bulman, eds), pp. 20–34. Oxford: Blackwell Scientific Publications.

Butterworth, T. and Faugier, J. (1992) *Clinical Supervision and Mentorship in Nursing*. London: Chapman & Hall.

Carper, B. A. (1978) Fundamental ways of knowing in nursing. *Advances in Nursing Science, 1*(1), 13–23.

Carr, W. (1989) Introduction: Understanding quality in teaching. In *Quality in Teaching* (W. Carr, ed.), pp. 1–20. Lewes, Sussex: The Falmer Press.

Hawkins, B. and Shohet, R. (1989) *Supervision in the Helping Professions*. Buckingham: Open University Press.

Heron, J. (1975) *Six Category Intervention Analysis*. Guildford: Human Potential Resource Group, University of Surrey.

Johns, C. (1993) Professional supervision. *Journal of Nursing Management*, **1**, 9–18.

Johns, C. (ed.) (1994) *The Burford Nursing Development Unit Model: Caring in Practice*. Oxford: Blackwell Scientific Publications.

Johns, C. (1995) The value of reflective practice for nursing. *Journal of Clinical Nursing*, **4**, 23–30.

Kikuchi, J. F. (1992) Nursing questions that science cannot answer. In *Philosophic Inquiry in Nursing* (J. F. Kikuchi and H. Simmons, eds). London: Sage.

Kohner, N. (1994) *Guidelines for Developing Clinical Supervision*. London: Kings Fund Centre.

Kouzes, J. M. and Posner, B. Z. (1988) *The Leadership Challenge*. San Francisco: Jossey-Bass.

Lauder, W. (1994) Beyond reflection: Practical wisdom and the practical syllogism. *Nurse Education Today*, **14**, 91–98.

Montgomery, C. L. (1993) *Healing Through Communication: The Practice of Caring*. London: Sage.

Pearson, A. (ed.) (1988) *Primary Nursing: Nursing in the Burford and Oxford Nursing Development Units*. London: Croom Helm.

Platt-Koch, L. M. (1986) Clinical supervision for psychiatric nurses. *Journal of Psychosocial Nursing and Mental Health Services*, **24**(1), 6–15.

Royal College of Nursing (1999) *Realising Clinical Effectiveness and Clinical Governance through Clinical Supervision: An Open Learning Pack*. Abingdon: Radcliffe Medical Press.

Schön, D. (1983) *The Reflective Practitioner*. London: Basic Books.

Titchen, A. (1998) *A Conceptual Framework For Facilitating Learning in Clinical Practice*. Occasional Paper No. 2. Sydney: Centre For Professional Education Advancement.

Titchen A. (2000) *Professional Craft Knowledge in Patient-Centred Nursing and the Facilitation of its Development*. DPhil thesis, University of Oxford; Oxford: Ashdale Press.

# 17

# Using reflective group supervision to enhance practice knowledge

**Clare Amies and Shane Weir**

This chapter outlines an approach to group supervision utilizing a reflective approach, and explores ways in which this approach is used to enhance practice knowledge. We have developed this approach to supervision based on a peer support approach to learning from experience and generating practice knowledge. It has arisen from our individual and collective experiences in this field, including: Clare's studies with Jan Fook and exploration of Jan's reflective approach to practice; Shane's interest in Michael White's work in narrative therapy; and our experiences in management within human service organizations.

Over the years of working in the field of social work we have often had discussions with people about their work and found that we had some shared experiences in our assumptions and values. The approach to **reflective group supervision** began as an attempt to get in touch with our assumptions about the service system and how these assumptions impact on the way we work. Reflective group supervision has been used in our practice for the last five years and has developed and grown with the collaboration and experiences of many of our colleagues. We have found this approach to have a profound impact on how we get in touch with our work, and how people can be helped to pursue this goal in a supportive, non-judgmental manner. Reflective group supervision recognizes and accepts that people have different approaches to their work.

## The context of the current work environment

Because of demands on time and resources and the need to fulfil funding-body requirements, attention is often paid to service targets, throughputs, outputs, goals, objectives, and various forms of data collection to justify what workers are doing. Organizations often use supervision as a procedure to hold workers accountable to the duties required in performing their jobs. A major dilemma currently facing many human service organizations is the profound impact the lack of worker support and accountability can have on the provision of services to the people who require these services.

The emphasis for supervision in this case is on outcomes and not on the process of doing the work. In this environment supervision often becomes a top-down exchange, emphasizing the organization's expectations rather than exploring what workers are actually doing, how they do what they do, and what informs the way they do it. In such a context people may be the passive recipients of (limiting) supervision rather than active participants in organizational activities. In the former case, valued knowledge can be transferred only one way and the practice wisdom of supervisees is not effectively utilized in the broader context of organizational life. Accountability becomes extrinsically based and advice can quickly become direction. Although advice or direction may at times be required, advice can be easily ignored and the philosophy and intention behind the direction discarded.

Effective supervision is achieved by combining support and accountability. The word **support** is used here to describe a way that assists workers to be accountable. By accountable, we mean the ability to develop one's practice standards. Inherent to practices of accountability is workers' exploration of their value systems and workplace ethics. The process of group supervision presented in this chapter enables workers to think past the limitations of their individual world view. It is a process of inquiry that provides an opportunity for people to extend themselves in relation to their work, and to think outside the parameters they would usually consider.

## The five-stage process

The five stages of reflective group supervision include: the presentation, reflective questioning, group discussion, presenter's feedback, and summing up. These are described in detail below.

### The presentation

The presenter chooses a practice example to present to the group. The example is not a case presentation. It is a focus on the practice of the presenter and does not include detailed information about the service user. The worker undertakes to describe an example of his/her practice.

The presentation may be:

- an intervention that really made a difference;
- an interaction that went particularly well;
- an incident where things did not go as planned;
- an example which captures the intent of the work generally;
- an example which is typical or demanding about the job;
- a situation where the person feels stuck in his or her work.

The practice the person chooses to describe might include any activity the person performs or experiences as a worker, for example how they responded to a particular interaction, the implementation of a programme, or a particular incident that occurred or was observed. The person's choice about what to present may be directed by what they wish to learn, change, evaluate or explore from a situation as it relates to their practice. Members of the group find it useful for the presenter to provide a brief written summary of the example, including what she or he wants to focus on or hopes to gain from the session. The following example demonstrates this phase in action.

**'Rita's' presentation: Rita works in a psychiatric disability support service**

**Background:**

I have been working with Gary *[name changed]* for about a year. He has been very reluctant to stipulate much in the way of clear goals and has been reluctant to make any commitments. We have made a number of medical and dental appointments together, but when due, Gary has not followed through. Gary seemed unable and unwilling to look at the underlying reasons for this. He went two or three times to a recreation group and appeared to enjoy some aspects of this, but did not want to continue. After some discussion over a lengthy period of time, Gary went twice to a podiatrist. An appointment was also made for follow-up with a physiotherapist.

**Incident:**

Gary did not keep the appointment with the physiotherapist. I felt very let down, as I had begun to feel that we were starting to make some progress. I also felt resentful. Then I started to think about whose goals I was following and why? What role should I be taking? I seemed to be pushing my own agenda.

**What I hope to gain from this session:**

To be clearer about how I can offer options and help increase a client's motivation, whilst ensuring we are working towards the client's goals and not mine.

### Reflective questioning

In this stage group members ask a series of reflective questions that are designed to assist the presenter to reflect on the account. It is not a forum for advice-giving or directions on how the person could have approached the situation. The reality of what works for one person does not always work for another. Telling people what they could or should have done quite often does not acknowledge what they did or are actually doing. Through this activity, presenters have the opportunity to explore their practice fully in a way that acknowledges the strengths of their current work and also provides an opportunity to explore further possibilities with their work. These reflective questions go beyond 'what else might you have done in this situation?' Reflective questions are questions that elicit and focus on the presenter's thoughts, feelings, assumptions, language used, and contradictions between espoused theories and theories in use. Karl Tomm (1988) suggests that reflective questions facilitate intent; they generate reflection and choice that invariably lead to action.

The group seeks to gain a thorough understanding of the experience of why the person acted in a certain way and what contributed to that action. We have discovered that questions that are laden with the interpretations and hypotheses of individual group members are often not useful. Each group member may have a particular theory about the presenter's example that will more than likely have a disparate influence over conversations with the presenter. An air of curiosity often assists group members to stay in touch with what is important for the presenter. The conclusions that the presenter forms are the ideas that must be given prominence. Reflective questions may seem unusual at first, but when people become familiar with a reflective approach their questioning is limited only by their imagination. A variety of questions are asked during this stage of the process, all of which elicit different sorts of information. We have found it useful to identify certain types of question and to formulate working lists of questions to assist people in this endeavour. The examples below are not exhaustive and represent a small sample of what is possible. It is important to remember that questions must be relevant to the aims stated by the presenter and should not be asked in an interrogatory manner.

Types of question include:

- *Clarifying questions that establish the context for the presenter's example*: Was this your first interaction for the day? What had been put in place before this occurred? What were the events preceding the interaction you have just described? How long had you known this person?
- *Inquiring into the actions of the presenter*: What was your intention in saying what you said? What do you think the impact of that conversation was? Were you tempted to do or say something and then decided not to? What knowledge or experience informed your decision to follow that direction with the person? What was your main purpose throughout the interaction?
- *Questions that inquire into the effects of the situation on the presenter*: Were you satisfied with how you responded during this situation? What outcome did you hope for? What impressions did you think the person had of you? Do you recall how you were feeling at the time? How will this contribute to how you will work with people in the future? Are you aware of anything now that you weren't at the time?
- *Getting in touch with assumptions and values*: What motivated you to use that intervention? How did you decide? What were you taking into account? What influences informed your assessment of the situation? How did this situation reinforce or challenge your existing ideas about the work? Do you have any notion of how the person using your service may have viewed it?
- *Questions that locate practice in relation to workplace culture*: Is that a standard procedure within your team? What effect does that procedure have on the way people use or view the service? Is there orthodoxy about the way things are done here? How does this affect your practice?
- *Questions that locate the issues discussed in a broader theoretical or sociopolitical context:* How does talking about boundaries in your work shut out possibilities for other descriptions of what you did in your work? Does the process of engagement that you have been taught help or hinder your practice in this example? Are there ways that you have been able to stay true to your philosophy about the work while having to work within the constraints you have just described?

## Group discussion

Michael White has provided the inspiration for a structure where colleagues can bear witness to the presenter's explanation of events. It is White's (1995, 1997) concept of the 'reflecting team' that we have used here as the structure for the group discussion. Rather than the group offering advice or problem-solving, they can share in ways the issue presented might affect them in the performance of their own duties. This is done in a way that honours the presenter's journey to find ways to make sense of his or her work and the problems associated with it, in a way that has meaning for him or her.

In the discussion section, the presenter observes a conversation between the other team members about their impressions of the previous discussions. Some presenters have found it useful to move physically outside the group's seating arrangements, so that they are external to the group discussion and are in a position to observe the group discussion from a discreet perspective. Conversations among group members are encouraged to contemplate how the presentation has affected their ideas about their own practice. It is important to concentrate on how the presenter's example has contributed to some new thinking or reinforced similar ideas. This provides an excellent opportunity for participants to create practice knowledge from their experiences and understandings and from the experiences of others (e.g. the presenter). Inevitably, as group members ask questions of the presenter they start privately reflecting on what the conversation means in relation to their own work experiences. In this stage of the process group members have the chance to speak publicly about aspects of the presentation that held particular significance for them. It is the responsibility of group members to conduct conversations that link what is being discussed to the presentation. Since the aim is to enrich the presenter's practice experience and application, the focus should remain on the presenter's example.

Often a group member may wish to speak of potent feelings or thoughts the presentation has aroused. When this occurs, group members have the responsibility to ask questions of their colleague that link the memories, feelings or thoughts back to the presentation that helped elicit them. In this way it is unlikely for group members' conversations to represent homilies.

We have found some of the following questions useful to consider during group conversations:

- What is being evoked for me after listening to the presentation?
- What has the presenter contributed to the memories and thoughts I am currently reflecting on?
- What will I take away from the presentation today?
- How will this conversation contribute to my work in the future?
- What do you think the people mentioned in the presentation might think if they witnessed the presenter reflecting on her work in this way?

Conversations that highlight themes, values or broader sociopolitical ideas about the work may also be possible in this stage.

### Presenter's feedback

In this section the presenter gives feedback to the group about their questions and discussions from the previous two sections, i.e. the reflective questions and the group discussion which they have just observed. The presenter may include what was useful and not useful about the process, or may clarify a particular point with group members. The presenter may wish briefly to question a group member about a particular response.

### Summing up

This is a time for all team members to draw out any patterns or themes that have future practice implications for their service or programme. The focus is on emerging patterns, practice knowledge generated or at times rejected/discarded, workers' interpretations, and the underlying assumptions that may be present about the work. Finally, some attempt may be made to link practice to relevant theory. This stage becomes the vehicle to commit to further action or take some of the ideas that have emerged to other group forums.

## Reflective group supervision in practice

Reflective group supervision is a peer approach to fostering support, professional development and accountability. The reflective approach allows workers:

- the possibility of documenting or describing practice in a way that keeps alive what workers actually do;
- to develop and improve practice that can have a developmental and educative component;
- to be accountable for their practice in an intrinsic rather than extrinsic manner, which highlights responsibility in a way that is not just ceded to a manager;
- to examine the theoretical assumptions implicit in their practice;
- to establish the possibility of a co-construction of meaning between colleagues; i.e. to provide an opportunity for workers to join together in

recognizing that we often encounter similar problems in our work even though we may make sense of and deal with them in different ways.

Reflective group supervision has certain guidelines which we have found useful in the delivery and the subsequent questions relating to the presentation. Stages assist in giving workers direction rather than allowing the process to meander aimlessly.

### Creating an atmosphere

It is a challenge for many organizations to set up an environment in the workplace where workers are encouraged to explore their practice in a way that bolsters confidence and enhances quality service provision. Reflective group supervision requires workers to talk about their practice in a group environment. The atmosphere for this approach must be supportive, trusting, non-judgmental, honest and considered.

When people agree to answer questions about the way they work, they open their practice to scrutiny and potential criticism from their colleagues. It must be acknowledged that there is a certain vulnerability that comes with this process. To this end, practices must be employed within the group to monitor the effects of the power relations associated with people opening their practice to be scrutinized. The responsibility for ensuring the environment is supportive and constructive, not criticizing or destructive, is a dual one shared by the presenter and his or her colleagues. We have found that a supportive atmosphere is attainable where workers volunteer rather than are directed to participate, are familiar with each other, and where it is clear that there is no redress from management. Where there are serious ethical concerns, they should be addressed through a separate forum or process.

For reflective group supervision to work within the spirit of a supportive atmosphere we have found that certain practices can be useful in encouraging the care of our colleagues. Some of these practices are:

- allocating sufficient and regular time to the process;
- seeing reflective group supervision as an important, integral and valuable part of organizational culture, not as an isolated activity;
- combining other rituals in the process, e.g. a shared meal (breakfast, lunch, morning or afternoon tea) before or after the group meeting;
- attending to the agenda of the presenter rather than to the agendas or interests of others in the group (who will be the focus of the agenda on other occasions).

We have found the following strategies or questions assist in the maintenance of a supportive atmosphere:

- Asking the presenter permission to ask certain questions.
- Accepting that someone does not wish to follow a particular line of questioning.
- Asking the presenter:
  - are the questions we are asking helping your aim for the session?
  - are there other questions or conversations that we could be having that would be of assistance?
  - how is it going for you?

## Worker knowledge and experience

Reflective group supervision is an approach that can be used in a variety of human service organizations that recognize the value of a worker's subjective experience and practice wisdom. Whether it be a clinical procedure performed by a podiatrist (chiropodist) or counselling by a therapist, there is usually more than one way to produce the desired outcome for all involved. The process that facilitates reflection is different from statements that instruct people about what to do. Reflection is facilitated by questioning workers to gain an understanding of how and why the work is done in a particular way. Paulo Freire (1973) asserts that action without reflection and reflection without action are unjustifiable.

A complaint that seems to resonate loudly through the halls of many universities concerns the lack of apparent answers to the question 'How does the theory relate to what I'm about to be doing?'. In the corridors of many workplaces, the talk is often about discarding or reorienting one's thoughts from the impracticalities of the theories that are taught. Reflective group supervision provides an avenue to link theory and practice together and to share practice wisdom. It assumes that what informs a person's practice may have a lot more to do with a theoretical stance than is acknowledged. The other side of this coin is that this process can uncover interesting and unusual marriages and contradictions between a worker's espoused theory and the theory in use. Reflective group supervision is an attempt to start from the ground up by uncovering workers' direct practice knowledge.

The reflective approach acknowledges the following three points:

1 People bring particular knowledge to their work which may have certain theoretical assumptions or may be based on intuition (Fook, 1996). By investigating what informs our work and what influences us in the course of performing certain duties, and by understanding why we choose certain procedures or make particular decisions over others, we can take responsibility for locating our decisions within a value system, a frame of reference and a particular cultural influence. When people begin to understand what influences their work some startling things begin to happen. People find clarity around why they do what they do. They begin to define or identify the impact of their value system on others, leading to a greater understanding of power relations between client or patient and worker. To respect the rich diversity of people who require services from us we must also learn to acknowledge our cultural influences in terms of the way these factors affect our work; similarly we must learn to respect the influence of culture in others, particularly our colleagues.
2 Personal and professional experience or knowledge affect the ways in which people create the meaning that guides their practice. This is not only something to be recognized in our work, but also is something to be celebrated. It is important to notice how our work and thought are influenced within the realms of the taken-for-granted notions of particular professional discourses. We use 'discourses' to mean language and ideas that describe people in certain ways, ways that often become truisms. We can then start to question the idea of what information we choose to share with clients; we can investigate how we describe the people who want our assistance.
3 Examining practice issues in a group enriches the experience of the participants by expanding their understanding of the practice experience of colleagues. Sharing with one's colleagues can provide powerful consciousness-raising possibilities. The shared awareness of peer learning provides satisfaction in creating new ways of relating to one's experience via the realization that we are not alone in grappling with workplace or work-practice dilemmas.

Workers, and how they do what they do, in part determine the culture of an organization. This seems obvious, yet the fact is often hidden behind official ways of describing programme or clinic service delivery. Our approaches to the work are never cast in stone. The scrutiny afforded to our work, as it is influenced by funding and organizational requirements, theoretical perspectives and political agendas, takes on a different position when it is the responsibility of all of us to dissect what it is we do. This practice can be liberating and can create openings for us to collaborate with our colleagues and think about our work in new ways.

## Conclusions

Working with people who are customers of human service organizations is often a complex and challenging task that requires ongoing critical reflection. Supervision provides a vehicle for that reflection. The immediate and most obvious benefits for developing and embracing this approach include:

- workers joining together around common workplace dilemmas;
- an understanding that there is no single way of responding or intervening in dilemma situations;
- providing an opportunity for workers to formally discuss and deal with practice issues as a team;
- developing shared understandings, expectations and philosophy about work.

Reflective group supervision enables workers to become familiar with their reasons for doing things in a certain way and with the ways they make decisions about their work. It also provides an avenue to celebrate the diversity of approaches and experiences various people bring to their work. There are a number of useful side benefits to using reflective group supervision. It provides a means for articulating practice within the workplace. Providing the opportunity and time to reveal and examine practice and practice knowledge through reflection allows workers to deliberate, change and analyse taken-for-granted actions and ideas. This approach can enhance quality assurance in organizations by enabling workers to expand on their understanding of the tasks they perform, revise their knowledge base and gain greater insight into why they do what they do.

## References

Fook, J. (1996) Developing a reflective approach to practice. In *The Reflective Researcher* (J. Fook, ed.), pp. 1–8. St Leonards, NSW: Allen & Unwin.

Freire, P. (1973) *Pedagogy of the Oppressed.* New York: Seabury Press.

Tomm, K. (1988) Inventive interviewing: Part III. Intending to ask lineal, circular, strategic, or reflexive questions? *Family Process*, **27**, 1–15.

White, M. (1995) *Re-Authoring Lives: Interviews and Essays.* Adelaide: Dulwich Centre Publications.

White, M. (1997) *Narratives of Therapists' Lives.* Adelaide: Dulwich Centre Publications.

# 18

# Professional craft knowledge and ethical decision-making

**Karolyn White**

This chapter focuses primarily on the significance of professional craft knowledge to ethical decision-making and the ethical importance of professional craft knowledge to quality professional practice. I argue that professional craft knowledge, which includes an appreciation of the context in which clinicians make ethical decisions and their understanding of particular patients,[1] is ethically significant and must be taken into consideration when making good ethical decisions. The key arguments in this chapter are also applicable to other professional areas, particularly where the well-being of clients is an immediate concern.

## Professional knowledge

To recognize the importance of professional craft knowledge in the process of making good ethical and clinical decisions we first need to recognize the importance of knowledge to the professions. Firstly, as discussed in Chapter 2, professional knowledge comprises propositional (research and theoretical) knowledge and professional craft (experiential) knowledge. Both these forms of knowledge are informed by the professional's personal knowledge. Higgs and Titchen (1995) suggest *inter alia* that effective professional practice relies on all these ways of knowing.

Secondly, knowledge is centrally important to the concept and status of professions. This is because professionals and professional organizations obtain much, though not all, of their expertise, authority and autonomy from the possession of knowledge, which is inculcated via a lengthy tertiary education. Since knowledge confers legitimacy on professions, professional knowledge must be qualitatively different from other types of knowledge.

Knowledge which is accessible to, and assessable by, ordinary persons will not count as professional knowledge. Professional knowledge is exclusive knowledge which involves the use of professional judgment. Judgment is required, not only for the effective and appropriate use of knowledge, but also in the construction, testing and development of a profession's and a professional's knowledge base.

Members of professions draw upon discipline-specific and generic professional knowledge, and exercise their judgment in the effective use of this knowledge. Moreover, this knowledge must be used in ethically sensitive and appropriate ways, for example for the good of society and individual patients. Professionals are also obligated to act professionally, i.e. to act and behave ethically.

## Professional craft knowledge

Professional craft knowledge refers to non-propositional, often tacit knowledge (Higgs and Titchen, 1995). This type of knowledge is often unarticulated because it involves knowledge and judgment which are intuitive and which, further, are gained through experience rather than being taught. Importantly, this knowledge is not reducible to formal scientific knowledge. Liaschenko (1998), in a paper discussing nursing epistemology in the context of testimony, provides some useful illustrations of what we, in this book, would class as professional craft knowledge. She has identified four types of knowledge used by nurses. The first type is the knowledge of therapeutic effectiveness, which is essentially scientific. The other types of knowledge are 'knowledge of how to get things done, knowledge of patient experience, and knowledge of the limits of medicine' (Liaschenko, 1998, p. 11). It is the last three types of knowledge that can be classified, for our purposes, as examples of professional craft knowledge.

### Experiential know-how

The first type of practical knowledge described by Liaschenko, experiential know-how, includes connecting patients to resources and services in the context of complicated and fractured health care systems. Liaschenko argues, and I would agree, that it requires skill and knowledge of the available resources, negotiation and communication expertise and competence and, importantly for our purposes, an understanding of 'the significance [of this know-how] to the well-being of patients' (Liaschenko, 1998, p. 15). We could also include in this category knowledge of what to do, and how to improvise, in an emergency. These skills and 'know-how-to' knowledge are also deployed by nurses in other ways. Liaschenko cites a case study reported by R. Jacques (see Liaschenko, 1998) in which a nurse:

> spent approximately 2 hours trying to get a pain medication increased for a post-surgical patient. She finally reached the physician and got the order increased. However, what is publicly represented to the world is that the physician ordered an increase in medication and the nurse followed the order.

(Liaschenko, 1998, p. 16)

Liaschenko points out that what is missing from the above description is 'the knowledge involved in locating the physician and presenting the case, the time involved and the skill of attending to this while doing multiple things simultaneously. These things have no status as work, they are not recognised as knowledge' (Liaschenko, 1998, p. 16).

This form of 'knowing-how' described by Liaschenko is distinct from simply knowing the local routines and practices. Knowing-how, in our and Liaschenko's sense, is gained by understanding how the system works, knowing which people to contact, knowledge of alternative resources, the ability to set priorities, and knowing the needs of particular patients: whether they require home help, whether their case is urgent, and so on. It also involves improvisation, and it is knowledge gained and used **for the good of and in the best interests of the patient**. For this reason, ethics plays an important part in this type of decision-making. Ethical principles as well as practical or therapeutic considerations should drive action.

### Knowledge of patient experience

Knowledge of patient experience is the second type of practical knowledge described by Liaschenko. This knowledge involves understanding the meaning of illness in the lives of specific patients.

> People generally do not live their lives in the discourse of medicine. Rather, they live in the language of everyday life, in the places and temporal rhythms that make up that everyday life, connecting them to others and generating a history. Knowledge of patient experience requires a reportioning of the nurse so that her or his gaze moves from the body as an object of medical intervention to the body of someone living a life

(Liaschenko, 1998, p. 16)

It is critical to note that knowledge about our patients' experience – understanding what it must be like for a particular patient in a particular situation and even being open to the idea that people are more than the sum of their medical conditions – requires that practitioners be receptive to such knowledge in the first instance, and secondly that they have well-developed sensibilities in order to understand the implications of this knowledge **for the patient**.

Lawler (1991) also stresses the importance of nurses' knowledge of patient experience. Lawler found that nurses not only know **that** and **how to**, they also know and understand people. This knowledge is not irrelevant or inconsequential; nurses must know and understand people in order to perform the technical/scientific side of nursing work or, in Liaschenko's terminology, they must have the knowledge of therapeutic effectiveness. This 'knowing and understanding people' knowledge includes recognition of feelings like vulnerability, dependency, embarrassment, horror and fear, and recognition of how these feelings influence each and every patient. Nurses must then judge how their patients can be helped to accommodate and/or integrate these experiences. The individual patient's feelings about the situation (and its physical, emotional and environmental elements) are then accommodated and integrated into nursing practice. Lawler (1991) demonstrates the complexity of nursing knowledge and ways of understanding, and, further, how this must be learnt by practical experience.

The work of Brody (1987, 1997) can be used to illustrate the importance of knowing the patient experience. Brody argues that 'suffering is produced, and alleviated, primarily by the meaning that one attaches to one's experience' (Brody, 1987, p. 5). It follows that in order to relieve suffering, practitioners need to understand the meaning particular patients attach to their experience of illness or disability. A patient's experience and the meaning affixed to it cannot be known scientifically; it can be known only by constructing a narrative. 'The primary human mechanism for attaching meaning to particular experiences is to tell stories about them. Stories serve to relate individual experiences to the explanatory constructs of the society and culture and also to place the experiences within the context of a particular individual's life history' (Brody, 1987, p. 5). Knowing how to construct a narrative with and for a patient, and knowing how to use this story for a patient's benefit, are epistemic skills partly constitutive of professional craft knowledge and are therefore ethically significant.

### *Knowledge of how patients manifest illness*

Professional craft knowledge also includes knowledge embedded in experience of how particular patients manifest illness and, in addition, how subtle changes to their medical condition are exhibited. Expert practitioners are able to learn from their experience because they are able to relate to other people's experiences. Because of this ability, experts can often notice subtle alterations to a patient's condition before less experienced practitioners are able to do so and often before there is any obvious sign of a patient's deteriorating condition (see also Benner, 1984).

Let me illustrate this point with a personal experience. Many years ago I was working as a nurse in a neurosurgical intensive care unit. It was my first placement as a registered nurse and I was working under the supervision of a very experienced neurosurgical nurse. We were caring for an unconscious patient, admitted with head injuries. My colleague noticed something was wrong with our patient and began to assess him. 'He will need a tracheostomy very soon, he is deteriorating,' she claimed, 'I'll call theatres and the resident.' The resident doctor came quickly and also examined the patient. 'There is nothing wrong with this man, nurse,' he rather contemptuously stated. 'Haven't you ever heard a man snore before?' At this stage I was confused and embarrassed. I trusted my nursing colleague, but I could not detect anything wrong with our patient. Yet within the hour the patient was transferred to theatre for an emergency tracheostomy. My nursing colleague was right, and although she could not explain why she knew the patient's condition had deteriorated, she knew, on the basis of experience and a deep understanding of this particular patient, that it had.

This example illustrates two major challenges facing professionals when using professional craft knowledge as part of professional decision-making and action, particularly when these processes are driven by important ethical considerations such as patient well-being. Firstly, the professional craft knowledge of health professionals needs to be respected as a legitimate form of knowledge. This requires that the clinician is able to articulate and credibly defend the position adopted and knowledge espoused. Secondly, health professionals need to explore the knowledge underpinning and supporting experiential knowledge as part of the transformation of professional experience into knowledge and the articulation of tacit professional craft knowledge.

### *Knowing and empathy*

Knowing the patient experience requires knowing how to empathize with patients by seeing things from their perspective. Code (1994, p. 81) argues that some degree of 'feeling with' others is necessary for appropriate care. Empathy:

> at its best resists closure, invites conversation, fosters and requires 'second person' relations. And empathy, moreover, is a self-reflexive skill. When it is well developed, well practiced, it incorporates a capacity to assess its own aptness: a capacity that enables its practitioners to judge the kind and degree of empathy a situation, a person, or a group requires; and to hold back at places where their habitual empathetic practices may be inappropriate, excessive, or inadequate. Empathy at its best calls for a finely tuned sensitivity both in its cognitive moments (working out how much one can/should know) and in its active ones. And neither 'moment' is self-contained: they are mutually constructive and inhibiting.

(Code, 1994, p. 81)

Code (1994) convincingly argues that the skills of empathy and empathetic knowing are marginalized in scientific epistemology. 'Scientific – and, derivatively, social scientific – knowledge is better, so the prevailing wisdom goes, to the extent that it eschews empathy, with its affective (hence not objective) tone, and its concern with the irrelevancies of human particularity' (Code, 1994, p. 77).

### Knowledge of medicine's limits

Liaschenko's third category of non-propositional knowledge is knowledge of the limits of medicine. Nurses, Liaschenko argues, 'by witnessing the experience of patients . . . recognize that medicine is not omnipotent' (Liaschenko, 1998, p. 17). Nursing's understanding is, however, silenced because such knowledge cannot be accommodated. Nurses are not 'heard, understood, (or) taken seriously' (Liaschenko, 1998, p. 18).

Arguably, such knowledge is implicit in other ways of knowing as described above. In my experience both as a teacher of ethics to health care practitioners and as a registered nurse, I would agree that nurses' knowledge and ways of knowing are either marginalized or not counted as knowledge. Lawler (1991), again, provides examples of this point. Terminally ill patients, for whom there is no hope of cure and no medical reason to try to prolong their lives, are deemed 'not for resuscitation' (NFR). This means no active medical treatment will be instigated in the event of a cardiac arrest and possibly that all burdensome treatment will be ceased. This is sometimes described as 'doing nothing' for the patient (Lawler, 1991). One of the nurses Lawler interviewed stated:

> I personally hate it, because I think there's still stuff we *[nurses]* can do for them, but it is a term that's frequently used when no more curative work can be done, like whatever you give them isn't going to cure the disease, but I think it's very erroneous and very bad to say we can do nothing for them because there is a whole heap you can do and should be doing for them.
>
> I perceive it purely as a medical thing . . . Some days they [patients] would ask you questions, they would want to talk to you. You could sit down for 2 or 3 or even 4 hours with somebody. That's not doing nothing. Even though their treatment might have been ceased, you're still doing something.

(Lawler, 1991, p. 187)

I have argued that what we are calling professional craft knowledge includes: know-how; understanding the importance and meaning of illness in the lives of particular patients; knowing how particular patients manifest illness; the significance of knowing how to construct a narrative about a patient's life; knowing the importance of empathy; and knowing the limits of medicine. Clearly not all these skills will necessarily be involved in every clinical situation. Universally, however, the use of professional craft knowledge will involve professional judgment. By 'judgment' I do not mean a mechanical means–end rationality; rather I mean a coming to a decision or a resolve, which is dependent on professional craft knowledge and the constitutive skills concerning ways of perceiving, feeling and learning in situ.

## Professional craft knowledge and ethical decision-making

The primary role and commitment of health care practitioners is to help maintain and improve the health of patients, as far as is legitimately possible. To achieve this end practitioners need to have not only theoretical/scientific knowledge but also knowledge of patients as people who are at times dependent and vulnerable. Moreover, practitioners must have knowledge of patients as individuals. Knowledge of patients as being dependent enhances the prospect of meeting the basic ethical commitments to them; indeed, I would argue that it is a prerequisite for making good ethical decisions.

From the previous section it will be evident that professional craft knowledge is situationally dependent. You cannot develop the know-how described by Liaschenko unless you have worked in the health care system. You cannot know the meaning of illness or disability in the lives of certain patients unless you meet with them, talk to them, and are open to their experience. Thus professional craft knowledge is not an abstract body of knowledge, but knowledge relating to ill, dependent persons in clinical circumstances. Moreover, professional craft knowledge, embodied in knowing how to get things done, how to construct an appropriate narrative with and for the patient, how to empathize, etc., will generally lead to better ethical decision-making. Because without professional craft knowledge ethically important things about particular patients will be overlooked.

Johnstone (1994, pp. 398–401) cites a case which can be used to illustrate the above point. It is the case of Mr H, a 60-year-old man admitted to intensive care with septicaemia. His past history included 'severe coronary artery disease and a malignant condition' which was in remission. Given the patient's past history and current condition he was ordered to be listed as NFR by his doctors. The patient was not consulted about the NFR order.

Ordering NFR for a patient has obvious ethical implications. We are not only saying that no further medical treatment will be efficacious, we are also saying that the patient would be better off dead, or, at least, that it would be all right if the patient were to die. The first obvious ethical point to make is that medical officers make this ethical decision based on their notion of the 'good' or the best interests of the patient. Secondly, in not discussing the order with Mr H his doctors were clearly not respecting his autonomy.

A further ethical point can be made here. By not discussing the NFR order with Mr H, the doctors had no idea what such an order would mean to and for Mr H. They had no knowledge, no deep understanding, about the context within which they had made the decision, nor the ethical implications of enforcing their notion of what was good for Mr H without either consulting him or even knowing what his notion was; for example, what this medical decision would mean for Mr H as a husband. Nor did they appear to understand why involving him in this decision might be important.

The nurse caring for Mr H spoke with him and discovered his viewpoint:

> 'I'd do anything to buy some time. You see, my wife's very ill at home. She has cancer which can't be operated on. She's always been totally dependent on me – even more since she's been sick. She doesn't have very long to live, and all I want is to live long enough for her, because she's so afraid of being left alone. We can't do much, and we stay in separate rooms at home. But at least we're reasonably independent and together. I can bring her a cup of tea when she wants it and things like that. I don't care about me, but I want to live long enough for her . . . she's so afraid of being alone . . .' Smiling, Mr H. concluded: 'It's such a comfort knowing that you and the doctors are doing all that you can for me here . . .' (Johnstone, 1994, p. 399)

The nurse attempted to get the NFR order changed, but it still stood when Mr H was discharged home six days later. The doctors could defend their decision medically and possibly ethically by appealing to abstract principles, particularly beneficence or doing good. Such explanation, however, only shows the importance of professional craft knowledge to making good ethical decisions and the inadequacy of overly general and abstracted approaches to ethics.

## Care, ethics and professional craft knowledge

The Gilligan–Kohlberg debate is germane here. Kohlberg (1981) found that moral maturity develops hierarchically and becomes more abstract. Kohlberg maintained that progression to moral maturity occurs through a culturally universal, invariant sequence of three levels, each with two stages. Progression is from the cognitively lower, less moral level to a higher stage, without regression. Pre-conventional morality is heteronomous and egocentric, conventional morality involves heteronomous adherence to rules and laws. Post-conventional morality, the highest stage of moral maturity, is the application of **abstract and generalizable principles**. What is important to note, for our purposes, is that Kohlberg's theory of moral development is the application of formal theory and is consistent with a scientific approach to clinical practice.

Carol Gilligan (1982), whilst collaborating with Lawrence Kohlberg in developing a theory of moral development, noticed that Kohlberg's theory was *inter alia* inadequate as a theory of moral development for girls. Her own research indicated that Kohlberg's model either excluded the different moral responses of women or devalued their voice. Gilligan then advanced the idea that women have a different moral voice, as opposed to an inferior moral voice. This different voice, or ethic of care, reflects women's concerns about maintaining relationships, care, affection, connection and love. Women, she argues, attempt to avoid hurting others, and try to resolve conflict by compromise and accommodation. Women's morality contrasts with 'masculine' morality (the justice perspective) as defined and described by Kohlberg.

The moral voice Gilligan has identified is compatible with professional craft knowledge. Care, for Gilligan (1982, 1987), is situational and local. Relationships, especially the identities of people involved (parent, wife/husband, friend) are of central importance in the care framework, as is the context in which these relationships occur. The care orientation, with its emphasis on relationships, particularity and detail, requires a range of skills and ways of attending to people, including sensitivity, receptivity and empathy, in order to secure morally appropriate understanding of the particular persons, problems, relationships and so on. These skills concerning knowing, perceiving and feeling are precisely those exemplified as professional craft knowledge in the professional health care setting.

Gilligan's (1982) work is particularly relevant to the practice of health care. Lawler's (1991) study identified that nursing is contextual, particular and practical. Nurses respond to, and are involved with, particular people in the context of their experience of illness, loss or disability. Exemplary nursing occurs within a relationship and requires that the nurse be sensitive, attentive and responsive, not only to the articulated needs of patients, but also to the covert signs of their discomfort and vulnerability. This requires certain skills, knowledge and expertise, a moral attentiveness, and way of being. Harbison (1992, p. 203) also argues that 'Gilligan's emphasis on caring and relationships accords with nurses' common experience'. She uses the work of Benner and Wrubel (1989) and Gilligan (1982) to show that caring is a moral experience and that care has value.

> The basic activities of caring are being there, listening, being willing to help and able to understand. These take on a moral dimension, reflecting the imperatives to pay attention, and not turn away from need. For example, one nurse might discern, in casual conversation with a patient, a disguised plea for help, where another nurse might not. From Gilligan's perspective, the sensitivity and attentiveness to another's need demonstrated by the first nurse are moral qualities.
>
> (Harbison, 1992, pp. 203–204)

These points show that the interaction of caring and professional craft knowledge in the nurse or health care worker establishes a fundamentally sound basis for appropriate ethical understanding and decision-making.

### An instructive story

The attentive relationship with patients often defines the moral boundaries for nurses. Recently a story was related to me. An experienced neonatal intensive care nurse encountered a situation which was a moral dilemma for her. She had been caring for a very sick premature neonate for several months. The situation from the outset was dire, but all hoped for the best. During the months she became close to the baby and his parents. Eventually it became obvious that medical treatment was not working, and the baby would certainly die. It was also obvious by this time that the baby was in great pain, and any nursing care or medical treatment, including changing the nappy, was unbearable for the baby. The parents had trouble accepting the situation. They insisted that all treatment should be done. They were older parents and the baby was conceived through in vitro fertilization. Caring for this sick neonate was difficult for the nursing staff, including my student. Treatment, the nurses argued, was a form of child abuse. At the same time my student recognized why the parents so desperately wanted this baby to live, even to the point of denying the pain their baby was experiencing and the futility of further treatment.

The doctors (and some of the less experienced nurses), possibly because they spent less time with the baby and the parents and therefore did not see how the parents loved the baby, were more likely to condemn the parents. They construed the problem both in terms of competing and contradictory rights (baby's right to die with dignity vs. parental autonomy and right to decide for their baby) and in terms of competing and contradictory interests (best interests of the baby vs. best interests of the parents). The moral bind, as the experienced nurse saw it, was how best to accommodate all involved. The experienced nurse could see and wanted to accommodate the parents' perspective. At the same time, since she had cared most for the baby and spent most time with him, she was alive to the pain and distress suffered by the baby, and wanted all medical treatment (but not nursing care) to cease. The parents finally agreed to cease mechanical ventilation which, as the baby was ventilator dependent, would ensure death. My student disconnected the ventilator and held the baby in her arms until he died. Ideally the parents should be the ones to do this, but in this case they were too distressed. While it was a difficult decision for the experienced nurse, she argued that she was the next best choice. In her experience doctors commonly would have turned the ventilator off and left the baby in his cot to die. And, in this case the other nurses did not have the same relationship with the baby and his parents. She felt that since she had cared for the baby while he was alive, she would continue to care for him while he died. It was the last caring thing she could do for him.

The caring relationship this nurse developed with the baby and his parents set the moral boundaries. This case, for her, was not defined in terms of rights or who was in the right; the moral problem was embedded in and defined by relationships. Her connection to the parents and their baby, her sensitivity to their situation, enabled her to see the moral problem in a different and more complex way. Being a 'non-Cartesian' knower[2] enabled this nurse to come to know the relevant things about the parents, the baby and the other carers involved in the case.

While these skills and ways of knowing and feeling would be realized and expressed differently in a non-professional, non-technical, non-clinical setting, they would broadly be the same range of skills and dispositions. Therefore, professional craft knowledge, while it is one specific realization of a range of skills and capacities for morally important knowing, feeling and so on, is nonetheless not knowledge which can be acquired independently of clinical professional experience.

## Implications

Thus far I have discussed the local implications of professional craft knowledge on ethical decision-making: how this knowledge is an ethically important consideration for practitioners and how professional craft knowledge can be usefully invoked by practitioners to make ethical decisions. There are also broader implications. Professional craft knowledge underpinning ethical decision-making can be applied to our law, local policy, policy reform and improvement of health care practices.

There are also educational implications. We need to incorporate into professional education a recognition of the reality and the value of professional craft knowledge in order to enable managers and practitioners to see that it is artificial and inappropriate to divorce ends (goals) from means in health care. The practice of leaving **ends** decisions to the managers and **means** decisions to the practitioners is ethically inappropriate. Professional craft knowledge cannot be properly understood except as implicitly embodying, firstly, knowledge of appropriate ends of health care practice and, secondly, knowledge of how such goals can be realized in the case of the particular patient. Therefore, professional craft knowledge is essential to ethical decision-making and to resolving and maintaining the integrity of the health care practitioner.

## Acknowledgement

I want to thank Dr Michael Carey for his help in the preparation and writing of this chapter.

## Notes

1 I use the term 'patient' to include 'client'. I know the term 'patient' is out of favour with some health care professional groups; however, in the interests of clarity as much as for philosophical reasons, I will continue with 'patient'.

2 By comparison, for a Cartesian knower, knowledge is attained by individuals, exercising reason, isolated from others and their own feelings and senses. The knower is autonomous, in the sense of being self-sufficient, detached from feelings and sensibilities (with respect to the quest of knowledge), alone, yet connected to others by the common ability to reason.

## References

Benner, P. (1984) *From Novice to Expert: Excellence and Power in Clinical Nursing Practice*. Menlo Park, CA: Addison-Wesley.

Benner, P. and Wrubel, J. (1989) *The Primacy of Caring*. Menlo Park, CA: Addison-Wesley.

Brody, H. (1987) *Stories of Sickness*. New Haven, CT: Yale University Press.

Brody, H. (1997) Who gets to tell the story? Narrative in postmodern bioethics. In *Stories and Their Limits: Narrative Approaches to Bioethics* (H. L. Nelson, ed.), pp. 18–30. New York: Routledge.

Code, L. (1994) 'I know just how you feel': Empathy and the problem of epistemic authority. In *The Empathic Practitioner: Empathy, Gender, and Medicine* (E. S. More and M. A. Milligan, eds), pp. 77–97. New Brunswick: Rutgers University Press.

Gilligan, C. (1982) *In a Different Voice: Psychological Theory and Women's Development*. Cambridge, MA: Harvard University Press.

Gilligan, C. (1987) Moral orientation and moral development. In *Women and Moral Theory* (E. Kittay and D. Meyers, eds), pp. 19–23. New Jersey: Rowman & Littlefield.

Harbison, J. (1992) Gilligan: A voice for nursing? *Journal of Medical Ethics*, **18**(4), 202–205.

Higgs, J. and Titchen, A. (1995) Propositional, professional and personal knowledge in clinical reasoning. In *Clinical Reasoning in the Health Professions* (J. Higgs and M. Jones, eds), pp. 129–146. Oxford: Butterworth-Heinemann.

Johnstone, M. (1994) *Bioethics: A Nursing Perspective*. Sydney: W. B. Saunders.

Kohlberg, L. (1981) *Essays on Moral Development Vol. 1: The Philosophy of Moral Development*. San Francisco: Harper & Row.

Lawler, J. (1991) *Behind the Screens*. Melbourne: Churchill Livingstone.

Liaschenko, J. (1998) The shift from the closed to the open body – ramifications for nursing testimony. In *Philosophical Issues in Nursing* (S. Edwards, ed.), pp. 11–30. Basingstoke, Hants: Macmillan.

# 19

# Gaining knowledge of culture during professional education

**Maureen H. Fitzgerald**

## Let's talk story

I have a diploma in nursing. After 14 years of nursing I decided to return to university to complete an undergraduate degree. I supported myself by working as a 'rent-a-nurse', a 'temp'. I did staff relief for agencies that supplied nurses to cover staff shortages in local hospitals.

One evening I was assigned to a medical-surgical unit in a large teaching hospital. I had never worked there before so everything took twice as long as it should have. I did not know the local customs or where the unit stored standard supplies, although based on previous experience in other hospitals I could figure a lot of things out for myself and did not have to constantly ask questions. Each unit might be laid out a little differently and there might be differences in how the staff organize themselves, but there are also a lot of commonalities across hospitals in different parts of a city, or even a country.

In this unit nurses were assigned a set of rooms. You took care of all the patients in those rooms. One of my rooms, a private room, was empty. Several hours later I was told 'we' were getting a transfer from the Intensive Care Unit (ICU) and the patient would be admitted into 'my' empty room.

I waited and waited for the patient. I regularly checked the room in case I had been in with another patient when the patient arrived and everyone 'forgot' to tell me she had arrived. These things do happen, especially when you are the 'temp'. Some places put temps through a period of testing to see how they respond. If you handle things 'well' then they will ask to have you back the next time they need an extra nurse.

Finally, about two hours before the end of the shift the patient arrived. I helped transfer her from the ICU bed. The ICU nurse who had accompanied her rattled off some information about the patient and, as she turned to leave, asked, 'Any questions?'

'Yeah. Are you sure she should have been transferred? Are you sure she is stable enough?'

'We wouldn't have transferred her if she wasn't! I forgot her chart. I'll bring it down in a couple of minutes.'

I introduced myself to the woman, took her vital signs, and tried to make her comfortable. But I wasn't comfortable. Something was wrong here, but I did not know what it was.

For the next hour I went back to check on the woman about every 15 minutes. Something was wrong but I could not figure out what it was. My sense of discomfort was so strong that I told the resident that I had an uneasy feeling about this woman. I asked him if he would mind taking a look at her. But I could not tell him what was wrong. He told me he was busy and if I could not give him something specific what did I want him to do. He told me he had seen her when she came from the ICU. He had helped transfer her into bed. She was fine.

I kept going back into her room. I checked her vital signs. They remained stable. I looked her all over. Nothing seemed to have changed but suddenly I knew what was wrong. I did not know how I knew what was wrong but I would have staked my life on it. This woman was having a gastrointestinal (GI) bleed and if we did not do something soon she would have a massive and life-threatening bleed.

I went and told the resident. His response was: 'How do you know?' I could not tell him how I knew. All I could say was that I knew because I had taken care of many people with GI bleeds. When I worked in the emergency room and the ICU I was the one that always took care of these people and I could 'tell a GI bleed from a mile away'. He did not think that was a good enough explanation. He was busy, her vital signs were stable, and I could give him no 'objective evidence' to support my claim so he refused to check her for me.

It was almost time for my shift to end. I signed off all my charts and gave my report to the charge nurse. But I just knew I could not leave until I checked this lady one more time. This time I was sure. I could smell the bleed. When someone is having a GI bleed there is a very distinctive smell. Her abdomen was distended, she was restless, and she desperately wanted a bedpan. I wished I had measured her abdomen earlier so I would have some 'evidence' to give the resident. I put her on the bedpan and went to get the resident.

This time I told him he better 'get in there and check her now! She is about to blow!' With extreme reluctance, complaining all the while, he got up and started towards her room. I ran back.

Just as the resident walked into the room the woman vomited a huge amount of blood. It covered the bed and hit the wall. From the smell I could tell she had probably passed nearly the same amount from her rectum. Within seconds she went into shock and cardiac arrest.

The resident just stared at me. 'How did you know? How did you know?'

As I went into action I told him: 'I just did! Maybe next time you will believe a nurse when she tells you a patient is in trouble, even if she can't tell you why. Now don't just stand there, call a code!'

I have begun this chapter with a story or narrative. In some cultures it would be considered quite rude to go straight to the point. To use a phrase from Hawaii, you 'talk story' first to establish relationships with others. You use talking story, the exchange of stories, to work towards the real point of the conversation. Talk story is also used to talk about things, especially important things, without appearing to talk about them. Talking story or talking through stories is a way to come at things in a more indirect, often less confronting, way.

Western health professionals and educators also talk story. In fact, like people in most societies, they commonly use story-telling as a means to communicate. As Brody (1987), Mattingly (1998) and others note, people communicate, try to understand, problem-solve, and often teach using stories or narratives. They use stories to explain things that are difficult to explain, often because they do not have the necessary vocabulary. They also use stories, in particular dramatic stories, as a way to illustrate a point or add emphasis. Stories or narratives give coherence and meaning to events in people's lives. People may even use them to construct and reconstruct, 'shape and even create' (Kleinman, 1988, p. 49) experiences and events to make them more meaningful, or in some cases more satisfying. This is consistent with what Clark (1993) and others call 'story making', a process which can also be used as a form of therapy or a research method.

There is a large and ever growing body of literature on the use of narratives in therapy and research. In this chapter I focus on the use of narrative as a means for acquiring knowledge and making sense of experiences. I suggest that much of the knowledge people gain about culture during their professional education comes about through the formal and informal use of narratives and story-telling, that story-telling is a way to share professional craft knowledge and a means for acquiring it. I draw attention to the way in which a particular kind of narrative, critical incidents, can be consciously used to help develop professional cultural craft knowledge. In doing so I suggest that not only the process of story-telling and story-making but also the content of stories, all stories, are cultural. I suggest that by understanding ourselves as cultural beings who work within a cultural system, and using stories and the analysis of stories to do so, we can develop a better understanding of how culture affects health, illness, healing, and the behaviours and interactions associated with them.

## Narratives and story-telling as cultural process

Narratives and story-telling are used to relate 'social dramas' (Turner, 1974) using plot lines, metaphors and rhetorical devices that are culturally, personally and symbolically meaningful and effective for communicating that meaning (see also Kleinman, 1988). Generally narratives, as renditions of social dramas, follow a standard course. They begin with an introduction that sets the scene, establishes the plot, and provides essential information. The story then develops following a culturally logical sequence that builds to a climax, which is then resolved (Turner, 1974).

Stories, especially those with a moral message, are used to socialize others, to teach them cultural (and professional) norms and expectations. They are used as a way to ground knowledge and experience in their context, highlight the potential consequences of particular behaviours, and help people remember. Contextualized information is easier for many to remember than decontextualized information. This is why lecturers tell stories in their teaching and why learners like to hear them. Story-telling is a culturally familiar and cognitively effective teaching strategy.

People learn not only from listening to stories, but also through story-making and story-telling. This is especially true when the story involves a situation to which the learner needs to attach meaning. The learning occurs during both the process of constructing and relating the story and the process of interpreting or making sense of that story, a process which often involves others – peers, teachers, supervisors. This form of narrative can be called a 'critical incident'.

## Critical incidents

A critical incident is a story with a climax, dilemma or issue to be addressed, but no clear resolution. When it ends there is still a need to attach meaning before the story can be resolved. As a result, the story is open to alternative interpretations. This makes it particularly useful for encouraging the development of reflective thinking and problem-solving skills. (For more detail on critical incidents see, e.g., Brislin et al., 1986; Brookfield, 1990; Sue and Sue, 1990; Brislin and Yoshida, 1994; Fitzgerald et al., 1995, 1997a, 1997b; Mullavey-O'Byrne and Fitzgerald, 1995; Edwards, 1999; Fitzgerald, 2000.)

The opening story is then actually a critical incident. You still do not know how I knew that this woman was going to have a crisis. Why did the doctor behave the way he did? Why was he so surprised that I had successfully predicted the crisis? Why did I feel so frustrated? You have some hints about why the event transpired the way it did, but nothing to confirm your interpretation. However, to answer these and other questions you need to engage in reflective analysis using the information in the story and your existing knowledge. In the process, you identify what additional information you need to interpret the story, how you can acquire that information, and then you critically analyse the quality of that information and apply it to the next stage of analysis. At each stage you should move closer and closer to what Geertz calls 'thick description' (Geertz, 1973).

## Is this a culturally based critical incident?

As explicated in the work of people like Benner and Tanner (1987) and Agan (1987), there should be little difficulty in identifying the introductory story as an example of craft or intuitive knowledge. I 'intuitively' knew that there was something seriously wrong with this woman based on many years of experience. At that point I had more than 14 years of expert experience, much of it in the area of critical care, to draw upon. But despite my expertise I did not always know why I knew what I knew. In the past, especially when I was Head Nurse of an ICU, I had not often needed to justify my 'gut' feelings. I had a reputation for the kind of 'sixth sense' that Benner and Tanner (1987) talk about. The staff, including the doctors, knew me and trusted my 'instincts' because they had enough evidence to believe me if I said something did not 'feel' right. We communicated on a different level than I did with the doctor in the opening story because we had some shared knowledge. When pressed for an explanation of why I knew what I knew or why I did something the way I did, I could usually come up with a reasonable explanation, but that ability failed me on this occasion.

It took several hours to get the woman stabilized so she could be transferred back to ICU. I left the hospital at about two in the morning and spent much of the rest of the night trying to figure out 'How did I know?' If I could figure out how I knew then maybe next time I could come up with an explanation that would meet the kinds of evidence the doctor sought in order to act.

Although it actually took me a couple of years of this reflective analysis before I decided I had fully identified all the factors that made me 'know', that night I was able, in hindsight, to identify the key factors. For example, without being consciously aware of it, I was responding to things like smell, which initially were quite subtle.

OK, so this is an example of craft knowledge, but this chapter is supposed to be about culture and gaining cultural knowledge. Is this a story about culture? Is it a culturally based critical incident? Is it about gaining cultural knowledge? How can we use it to help people gain cultural knowledge and identify and address cultural issues in professional practice? How do we learn to identify cultural issues? And how do we help others to do so? The rest of this chapter addresses these questions. I will argue that the same processes that I used to understand this situation from a medical perspective can be, and later were, used to understand it from a cultural perspective, that they can be used with both inter- and intra-cultural situations. In fact, the very processes I used were themselves cultural; I used analytical processes that I learned from others, processes typical of people from a particular cultural background. I would also suggest that if I had possessed a better understanding of the concept of culture at the time, I might have been able to develop a more effective strategy to get the doctor to act, a strategy that would not have required knowing how I knew from a medical perspective. At the very least, I might have better understood why past strategies were not effective on this occasion.

## Culture

Before we can decide if this is a culturally based critical incident we must ask, 'What do we mean by the term culture?' There is no single definition of the term culture. In the 1960s two famous anthropologists, Alfred Kroeber and Clyde Kluckhohn, showed this when they identified and critically analysed more than 160 anthropological definitions of culture (Kroeber and Kluckhohn, 1963). However, although there is no single agreed definition, as the Kroeber and Kluckhohn work and the selection of definitions offered in Table 19.1 show, there are some factors that are inherent in most definitions.

| **Table 19.1 Some anthropological definitions of culture** |
|---|
| Standards for perceiving, believing, evaluating and acting.<br>(Goodenough, 1981) |
| Culture is a set of guidelines (both explicit and implicit) which individuals inherit as members of a particular society, and which tells them how to *view* the world, how to experience it *emotionally*, and how to *behave* in it in relation to other people, to supernatural forces or gods, and to the natural environment. It also provides them with a way of transmitting these guidelines to the next generation by the use of symbols, language, art and ritual.<br>(Helman, 1990) |
| The totality of man's learned, accumulated experience. 'A culture', say 'Japanese culture', refers to those socially transmitted patterns for behaviour characteristic of a particular social group.<br>(Keesing and Keesing, 1971) |
| Patterns, explicit and implicit, of and for behaviour acquired and transmitted by symbols constituting the distinctive achievement of human groups, including their embodiments of artefacts; the essential core of culture consists of traditional (i.e., historically derived and selected) ideas and especially their attached values; culture systems may, on the one hand, be considered as products of actions, on the other, as conditioning elements of further action.<br>(Kroeber and Kluckholn, 1963) |
| An organized body of rules concerning the ways in which individuals in a population should communicate with one another, think about themselves and their environments, and behave towards objects in their environments.<br>(LeVine, 1982) |
| The acquired knowledge that people use to interpret experience and to generate social behaviour.<br>(Spradley and McCurdy, 1975) |

Culture is the learned and shared patterns of perceiving and adapting or responding to the world characteristic of a society or population. Culture is reflected in such things as a society's learned, shared beliefs, values, attitudes and behaviours. Although culture is dynamic and ever changing, it maintains a sense of coherence. (For more detailed discussions of the concept see, e.g., Ember and Ember, 1988; Krefting and Krefting, 1990; Fitzgerald and Mullavey-O'Byrne, 1996; Fitzgerald et al., 1996, 1997a; Haviland, 1997; Keesing and Strathern, 1998.)

Culture is rather insidious. Much like professional craft knowledge, we know it without necessarily knowing we know it. We learn it without necessarily realizing we are learning it. We use it without necessarily recognizing that we are using it. This is because it is something we acquire as part of a lifelong learning process. Health professionals do not enter into their professional education as culturally blank slates. They bring with them cultural knowledge, values, beliefs, ways of doing things, and a particular world view or way of conceptualizing and adapting to the world around them. They bring knowledge of their own culture, and often some knowledge of other cultures. And they go on learning and acquiring cultural knowledge.

What many health professionals do not bring to their professional education is an awareness that everyone, including all health professionals and all clients, is a cultural being. They may recognize that other people, especially those who are distinctively different in some way (e.g. language, dress), are cultural beings, but often they do not see themselves as cultural beings, particularly when they are in their professional role (Fitzgerald, 1992). They often do not recognize that medical systems are a product of the cultures in which they occur. Frequently they fail to appreciate that medical knowledge, even what constitutes medical 'fact' or evidence, is a cultural construction that makes sense to people within the system because they share a particular way of thinking about, communicating about, and conceptualizing the world around them and the events that happen within that world.

## Culturally based critical incidents

So is the opening story a culturally based critical incident? It is, but not because the woman was Black. Her ethnicity and cultural background are not of central importance in this particular version of the story. They may help explain why she had diabetes and why it was so out of control that she ended up in the ICU. They may or may not help explain why she had this GI bleed or why the staff chose her to be transferred out of the unit when they needed a bed for another patient. At this point we should note that people often confound the terms ethnicity and culture. (See, for example, Fitzgerald, 1992; Fitzgerald and Mullavey-O'Byrne, 1996; Fitzgerald et al., 1996, 1997a, 1998.) Ethnicity, like culture, is a culturally constructed concept. Ethnicity may be based on shared culture, but ethnicity and culture are two distinctively different concepts. Ethnicity is a sense of shared 'peoplehood' which can be based on many factors other than shared culture (language, country of origin, physical features, etc.).

However, this is not a story about ethnicity or racism; it is not even about this patient. It is about the experience of a nurse within a particular cultural context and her interactions with a doctor. It is a culturally based critical incident for many reasons, including the following. It is about cultural ideas of what constitutes knowledge and evidence. It is about cultural conceptions of what constitutes and who holds expert knowledge. It is about status, role, power, and the organization of social systems and social institutions like a society's medical system and the health care agencies that might be found within it. It is about the way in which culture influences the structure and content of the events and interactions that occur within these systems and institutions. This is a story about how health professionals communicate with one another and the rules for inter-professional communication. It is about the socialization of health professionals and the kinds of rites of passage that occur within social institutions. This is a story about a particular view of the world and how that view of the world influenced the way people behaved and interacted with one another. It is cultural because it is culturally based and it reflects the culture in which it occurred. Had this incident happened in another cultural context it might have transpired in a very different way.

The opening incident is, in fact, culturally dense. It could be analysed in many ways and such analyses could focus on different aspects. The cultural analysis of the incident is not the purpose of this chapter. **Rather, in this chapter, I suggest that deep, reflective interpretive analysis of incidents and experiences like this one can be used as a strategy for helping health professionals gain cultural knowledge and knowledge about culture.** In fact, situations involving people from similar cultural backgrounds can be equally or more useful for this purpose than a concentration on situations in which the key protagonists are from different cultures. Such analyses can help people take off their cultural blinkers so they can identify their cultural biases and assumptions before they look at intercultural situations. Cultural analyses can be integrated into all aspects of a professional education programme and applied in any subject.

## Using critical incidents to develop professional cultural craft knowledge

Critical incidents can be used in several ways to enhance critical reflection and cultural competency or cultural knowledge and expertise – professional craft knowledge in the area of culture. (See, for example, Brislin et al., 1986; Brookfield, 1990; Fitzgerald, 2000; Fitzgerald et al., 1995, 1996, 1997a, 1997b.) They can be used as models or examples or they can be used as the foundation for exercises that encourage the acquisition of critical reflective and interpretive thinking skills. We use all these approaches with the Intercultural Interaction Project in the School of Occupation and Leisure Sciences at the University of Sydney. (For detailed descriptions of this project see Fitzgerald et al., 1997a, 1997b; Fitzgerald, 2000.)

As a model or example, a critical incident can be presented followed by a previously developed detailed analytical discussion of the incident based on the published theoretical literature, one that might also draw on the presenter's professional craft and personal experience knowledge, to identify the cultural issues. In other words, the presenter would present his or her critical analysis of the incident highlighting issues the presenter believes are important in that context. This is the approach commonly used in textbooks, research reports and classroom lectures. This would tell others what some of the issues are, and perhaps they could transfer this knowledge to another situation and use it to help identify cultural issues in other situations. But there are other ways in which this and other stories can be used that increase the likelihood that people will be able to transfer knowledge and skills to new situations, a hallmark of professional craft knowledge.

Critical incidents can be used as the stimulus for focused discussion, data collection and critical reflection exercises. (See, for example, Brislin et al., 1986; Brookfield, 1990; Fitzgerald et al., 1995, 1996, 1997a, 1997b; Edwards, 1999; Fitzgerald, 2000.) In other words, critical incidents can be used as experiential learning exercises in a 'learn by doing' approach. Initially, especially with people with minimal clinical experience, it is useful to use critical incidents drawn from the professional practice of others, like the one offered above. At the next level, people can draw on and develop critical incidents from their own practice. However, this should be done with some caution and only with a skilled facilitator, one who is culturally competent and has the skills to address the emotional issues that can arise with analysis of personally experienced incidents. There is a risk of reinforcing cultural stereotypes. More importantly, all critical incident-based educational programmes need to be conducted in culturally and psychologically 'safe' contexts, as this approach involves confronting one's cultural and personal beliefs, values and assumptions, and in many cases one's past behaviours in similar situations.

A third approach is to use critical incidents as the focus for a research project directed at illuminating cultural issues in professional practice. This experiential learning approach can be used with individual learners, but is especially useful with groups where discussions of the project process and outcomes are part of the learning experience. This approach involves assisting groups of learners to develop a culture-related research question based on their own experiences, that can be addressed using critical incidents as a stimulus and/or a response. In other words, learners select a topic they want to explore in more depth. As a stimulus, respondents are asked to respond to a video or printed version of a critical incident. As a response, respondents are asked to tell a story, a critical incident, in which the respondent thought culture was an issue. Learners are generally encouraged to use ethnographic interviewing (Spradley, 1979) and to tape record the interview. We also ask them to keep fieldnotes and/or a research journal. Projects can also involve or focus exclusively on the re-analysis of a dataset of existing transcripts or critical incidents, although most learners do not find this to be as rich a learning experience.

Learners then transcribe their interview tapes and analyse the interviews in terms of process and content. The transcription process helps to focus on details of the interview and encourages reflective analysis. The analyses are then shared with the other group members through short verbal presentations. Thus, although each individual may conduct only one or two interviews, indirectly they participate in more. Finally, the interview data, data from the presentations, and the literature are used to prepare an analytical (a critical, reflective and interpretive – thick descriptive) essay related to the research topic.

In all approaches, the critical incident approach assumes some cultural and professional knowledge among learners. The critical use of this knowledge can help them analyse the situations depicted in the critical incidents. Interviewing 'cultural experts', expert clinicians and other experts, like members of various cultural groups, also provides the opportunity to draw on the professional craft knowledge and personal experience of others. The story-telling and the dialogue surrounding the telling and reporting of the story allow the sharing of cultural and professional knowledge and critical reflective analysis on the part of both respondent and listener.

The approach provides a model for interacting with clients/families and expert clinicians, and legitimizes story-telling as a valid way to collect and share information. It encourages learners to look for the cultural meanings in people's stories, especially the stories people tell in everyday interactions, like clinical interactions. This perspective helps learners begin to recognize that the stories their clients tell them are not digressions or ways to avoid answering the professional's questions, but are in fact a way of answering such questions. Such stories are culturally and personally meaningful and in telling such stories the clients are communicating with health professionals – if only they would listen. This approach helps people to learn how to listen to and interpret such stories in a way that can also be meaningful for the professional.

## Conclusions

One of the responsibilities of health professional educators is to help their students recognize themselves as cultural beings, recognize others as cultural beings, and recognize that culture influences all aspects of health and illness, including interactions between health professionals and health professionals and their clients. But how can this be done? How can this kind of cultural knowledge be incorporated into the craft knowledge of health professionals as part of an ongoing process? How can professionals be moved from a reliance on 'cookbook' approaches for addressing cultural issues in professional practice to developing the skills to deal with common and uncommon cultural events?

Early work in the area of cultural awareness and sensitivity was often based on propositional knowledge. It was based on a behaviourist cognitive framework that focused on rote learning of cultural facts about people from 'other' cultures. More recently, there has been a transition towards a more integrative and assimilationist approach to learning about and incorporating cultural knowledge. Early in this phase, 'cultural training' focused on developing a particular kind of experiential knowledge through activities like cultural simulation exercises, where people engage in classroom exercises in which they experience a simulation of what it is like to be the cultural 'other'. This stage was followed by a move towards the use of strategies like the critical incident approach, which initially focused on intercultural interactions and incidents.

Each of these approaches addresses a different aspect of cultural knowledge: one is cognitive and the other affective. Both have a tendency to encourage an 'us and them' mentality, where only the 'other' is viewed as a cultural being. Both assume that people can learn about culture in context, with all its complexity, by taking it out of context. Neither addresses the question of how health professionals acquire cultural knowledge and use it in practice.

In the newest phase, or perhaps what I hope will be the newest phase, the focus includes a significant emphasis on the self, and not just the other, as a cultural being. It places learning about culture into a cultural context by making it experiential and by drawing on the experiences of health professionals. In this approach the health care system is recognized as a cultural context in which cultural dramas get played out, reported and analysed, and much of it is done through story-telling. It recognizes that health professionals learn from listening to and analysing these everyday stories, and therefore they need the appropriate skills to do so. In this phase there is a greater recognition that we constantly communicate with one another and constantly teach one another about culture and other professional issues through the cultural processes of story-telling, story-making, interpretive reflection and the search for meaning. Professional craft knowledge comes not just from experience, it comes from the ability to analyse critically that experience in culturally meaningful ways. It is not the search for facts or propositional knowledge that is important in professional craft knowledge; it is the search for meaning.

So what is your cultural analysis of the opening critical incident? How would you make it culturally meaningful for you?

## References


Agan, R. D. (1987) Intuitive knowing as a dimension of nursing. *Advances in Nursing Science*, **10**, 63–70.

Benner, P. and Tanner, C. (1987) Clinical judgement: How nurses use intuition. *American Journal of Nursing*, January, pp. 23–31.

Brislin, R. W. and Yoshida, T. (1994) *Improving Intercultural Interactions: Modules for Cross-Cultural Training Programs*. Thousand Oaks, CA: Sage.

Brislin, R. W., Cushner, K., Cherrie, C. and Yong, M. (1986) *Intercultural Interactions: A Practical Guide*. Newbury Park, CA: Sage.

Brody, H. (1987) *Stories of Sickness*. New Haven, CT: Yale University Press.

Brookfield, S. (1990) Using critical incidents to explore learners' assumptions. In *Fostering Critical Reflection in Adulthood: A Guide to Transformative and Emancipatory Learning* (J. Mezirow, ed.), pp. 177–193. San Francisco: Jossey-Bass.

Clark, F. (1993) Occupation embedded in a real life: Interweaving occupational science and occupation therapy. *American Journal of Occupational Therapy*, **47**, 1067–1078.

Edwards, M. (1999) Critical incidents and perspective transformation: A comparative media study. Honours thesis, University of Sydney.

Ember, C. R. and Ember, M. (1988) *Anthropology*. Englewood Cliffs, NJ: Prentice Hall.

Fitzgerald, M. H. (1992) Multicultural clinical interactions. *Journal of Rehabilitation*, April/May/June, pp. 1–5.

Fitzgerald, M. H. (2000) Establishing cultural competency for health professionals. In *Anthropological Approaches to Psychological Medicine* (V. Skultans and J. Cox, eds), pp. 184–200. London: Jessica Kingsley.

Fitzgerald, M. H. and Mullavey-O'Byrne, C. (1996) Analysis of student definitions of culture. *Physical and Occupational Therapy in Geriatrics*, **14**, 67–89.

Fitzgerald, M. H., Mullavey-O'Byrne, C., Twible, R. and Kinebanian, A. (1995) *Exploring Cultural Diversity: A Workshop Manual for Occupational Therapists*. Sydney: School of Occupational Therapy, The University of Sydney.

Fitzgerald, M. H., Mullavey-O'Byrne, C., Clemson, L. and Williamson, P. (1996) *Enhancing Cultural Competency*. Sydney: Transcultural Mental Health Centre.

Fitzgerald, M. H., Beltran, R., Pennock, J., Williamson, P. and Mullavey-O'Byrne, C. (1997a) *Occupational Therapy, Culture and Mental Health*. Sydney: Transcultural Mental Health Centre.

Fitzgerald, M. H., Mullavey-O'Byrne, C. and Clemson, L. (1997b) Cultural issues from practice. *Australian Occupational Therapy Journal*, **44**, 1–21.

Fitzgerald, M .H., Williamson, P. and Mullavey-O'Byrne, C. (1998) Analysis of therapist definitions of culture. *Physical and Occupational Therapy in Geriatrics*, **15**(4), 41.

Geertz, C. (1973) *The Interpretation of Cultures*. New York: Basic Books.

Goodenough, W. (1981) *Culture, Language, and Society*. Menlo Park, CA: Benjamin/Cummings.

Haviland, W. A. (1997) *Anthropology*. Fort Worth: Harcourt Brace.

Helman, C. G. (1990) *Culture, Health and Illness*. Oxford: Butterworth-Heinemann.

Keesing, R. M. and Keesing, F. M. (1971) *New Perspectives in Cultural Anthropology*. New York: Holt, Rinehart & Winston.

Keesing, R. M. and Strathern, A. J. (1998) *Cultural Anthropology: A Contemporary Perspective*. Fort Worth: Harcourt Brace College Publishers.

Kleinman, A. (1988) *The Illness Narratives: Suffering, Healing, and the Human Condition*. New York: Basic Books.

Krefting, L. H. and Krefting, D. V. (1990) Cultural influences on performance. In *Occupational Therapy: Overcoming Human Performance Deficits* (C. Christiansen and C. Baum, eds), pp. 101–122. Thorofare, NJ: Slack.

Kroeber, A. L. and Kluckhohn, C. (1963) *Culture: A Critical Review of Concepts and Definitions*. Cambridge, MA: Harvard University Press.

LeVine, R. A. (1982) *Culture, Behavior and Personality: An Introduction to the Comparative Study of Psychological Adaptation*. New York: Aldine Publishing.

Mattingly, C. (1998) In search of the good: Narrative reasoning in clinical practice. *Medical Anthropology Quarterly*, **12**, 273–297.

Mullavey-O'Byrne, C. and Fitzgerald, M. (1995) Disconfirmed expectancies in intercultural interactions. In *Abstracts of the 18th Federal and Inaugural Pacific Rim Conference: Australian Association of Occupational Therapists, Hobart, Tasmania*, p. 159. Melbourne: Australian Association of Occupational Therapists.

Spradley, J. P. (1979) *The Ethnographic Interview*. New York: Holt, Rinehart, Winston.

Spradley, J. P. and McCurdy, D.W. (1975) *Anthropology: The Cultural Perspective*. New York: John Wiley & Sons.

Sue, D. W. and Sue, D. (1990) *Counselling the Culturally Different: Theory and Practice*. New York: John Wiley & Sons.

Turner, V. (1974) *Dramas, Fields, and Metaphors: Symbolic Action in Human Society*. Ithaca, NY: Cornell University Press.

# 20

# Transferring professional craft knowledge across cultural contexts

**Robyn L. Twible and Elizabeth C. Henley**

## Background

The nature of practice at the dawn of the twenty-first century dictates that health professionals have markedly greater contact with people from other nations and various cultural groups from all around the world. Many countries are characterized by cultural, ethnic and linguistic diversity, especially the developed countries such as Australia, the UK and the USA, in which a substantial proportion of the population are migrants or children of migrants. Other countries, such as India, have historically been composed of diverse cultures (Henley and Twible, 2000).

As the world becomes a global village, driven by developments in information technology, ease of travel and the internationalization of business, we recognize the attributes and strengths that different cultural groups bring into this arena, which generate a mutual respect for diversity and difference. Within any country, diverse ethnic groups want their cultural uniqueness to be recognized and resist being placed into a homogeneous 'melting pot'. There seems to be little doubt that an increase in intercultural interactions is becoming the rule rather than the exception for most aspects of daily life and professional life.

At the same time, health policy throughout the world has shifted emphasis from institutional to community care, with an emphasis on health and wellness and universal access. These major changes have necessitated a shift in emphasis from the institutional medical model to alternative models of health care delivery. The reality is that institutional care is now limited to the initial management of acute conditions. It is not an appropriate environment for the management of chronic problems, the rehabilitation of people with disabilities or the promotion of health and wellness. Nor is it the right environment to address the determinants of health. This move from institution to the community has generated a significant change in many of the features of health care delivery, mostly to the benefit of the consumer. The impetus for change, coupled with the increasing economic constraints worldwide, has provided an urgent need to develop innovative ways of utilizing available health personnel.

Preparing health professionals to change practice from traditional institutional services to community services is a professional imperative, as is the need to ensure that professionals adopt strategies to maximize their skills and abilities to interact with clients from a variety of cultural backgrounds that are different from their own. Such preparation requires special consideration of complex contextual issues, as well as reorganization and reconceptualization of the philosophies underpinning the education of health professionals and the structural ways in which educationalists teach health professionals to provide care (culture, politics, environment, social structure, service delivery models, etc.). The most important factor to consider is that health professionals must undergo a major change in attitude both to service delivery modes and to their roles under these different models. If the concept of seamless health care is to succeed, encompassing a smooth transition of the client from the institution to the home environment, the complex nature of the interrelationship between the client's culture and the community will need to be successfully considered, negotiated and executed by all health professionals with whom the client interacts.

## Educational considerations

From an educational perspective there is a consistent rise in the number of students from other countries enrolling as part of exchange programmes in university campuses around the world. It is likely that academics will find that their students are from increasingly varied ethnic groups and diverse cultural backgrounds (Varney and Brislin, 1990).

Today, education programmes throughout the world should prepare health professionals to work in multiple environments, and a primary objective of educators should be to develop the required competencies in graduates. The interactions between the students and their learning environment as well as between the students' own culture and the cultures in which they develop their clinical skills are complex. Factors to consider include the country of origin and cultural background of the student, which may be the same as or different from the teacher's, and the learning environment, which could be on- or off-campus, learning or practice in focus, single or multicultural. In addition, the student may be being educated to return to another country and/or culture, or may be intending to live in the country of education, which may be native or foreign. It is in undergraduate education that attitudes are established and can be most readily influenced, so that graduate health professionals acquire the requisite knowledge, attitudes and skills to work in both institutional and community settings in a range of countries and cultures.

Consideration also must be given to the competencies of the education providers, for they are the ones who will undoubtedly exert influence over the learning of their students and graduates (Henley and Twible, 2000). Faculty members who are aware of the importance of intercultural interactions and different service delivery models are most likely to incorporate these approaches into their teaching activities; however, it is important for all educators to incorporate such information into their teaching, not just those who specialize in cultural and community issues. Education about culture and community needs to be embedded across the curricula and permeate all aspects of the educational process.

## Cultural considerations

In most societies the provision of health care involves many different interactions among people whose needs and views on what constitutes health care may be vastly different from each other and from the service provider. This difference can pose problems for both the provider and the recipient unless care is taken to facilitate the concurrent and interactive processes of health care and cross-cultural communication. When people from different backgrounds come together in a therapy interaction, that interaction is influenced by many factors, and the overlap of knowledge and influence between the participants will vary from one situation to another. In some cases, the amount of overlap or sharing will be great; in others, especially if one or more of the participants comes from a culture with a very different medical system, the overlap will be much less. The example in Fig. 20.1 demonstrates a situation where there is a significant amount of cultural overlap (Fitzgerald et al., 1995).

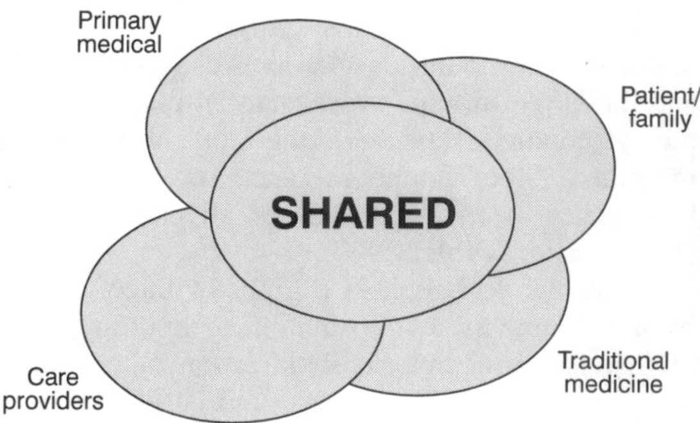


**Figure 20.1** Circle diagram of shared knowledge or influence (adapted from Fitzgerald et al., 1995)

Obviously, the greater the overlap, the easier the interaction; the less the overlap among participants, the more challenging will be the interaction for the health professional to effect a successful outcome. As in all situations, it is critical to put culture and models of practice into context. It is important, therefore, to determine a working definition of **culture** and its constituents.

Culture is a complex concept; it is not the 'kind of superficial, cookbook, rule ordered system of etiquette that some . . . seem to think it is' (Avruch and Black, 1991, p. 28). Everyone has a culture, which influences all aspects of daily life. It should not be seen as something 'other', as external to a person. Rather, culture is an integral part of each person; it is more than tradition and is not static but dynamic, evolving continuously. Another important factor to recognize is that the diversity **within** cultures is often as great as the diversity **across** cultures. Therefore, health professionals must be careful to avoid the trap of cultural stereotyping when dealing with clients from cultures other than their own. Each person must be viewed from an individual perspective; an open, sensitive reasoning process can be used to facilitate the client–therapist interaction. As Fitzgerald et al. (1995) point out, the influences of culture on each individual will vary from one situation to the next; 'everyone does not know everything, nor do they necessarily understand all aspects of their culture in the same way' (p. 6).

In developing the concept of culture, it is essential that health professionals understand the distinction between culture and concepts of ethnicity and race. **Race** refers to the biological characteristics of people, involving genetic, anatomical and structural differences (Riggar et al., 1993; Fitzgerald et al., 1995). **Ethnicity** is distinct from race in that ethnicity describes those characteristics of a group of people that provide the group with common markers or a sense of belonging. These markers may include linguistic, behavioural or environmental factors (Fitzgerald, 1991). **Culture**, on the other hand, is:

> an abstract concept that refers to learned, shared patterns of perceiving and adapting to the world which is reflected in the learned, shared beliefs, values, attitudes and behaviours characteristic of a society or population.

(Fitzgerald et al., 1995, p. 6)

The term 'cultural competency' has become more commonly used to describe the knowledge, skills and attitudes that health professionals develop in order to successfully interact with clients from cultures other than their own. Walker (1991, p. 6) defines cultural competency as:

> the ability of individuals to see beyond the boundaries of their own cultural interpretations, to be able to maintain objectivity when faced with individuals from cultures different from their own and be able to interpret and understand behaviours and intentions of people from other cultures non-judgementally and without bias.

The culturally competent person is one who is willing to explore personal values, beliefs, attitudes and emotions, and understands how these affect interactions with other people. Cultural competency develops and evolves with continued exposure to information on culture, communication and involvement in intercultural interactions. Most importantly, it involves critical reflection (Fitzgerald et al., 1997).

## Developing professional craft knowledge across cultural contexts

### Issues related to culture and practice

Although the need for health professionals to address issues of culture is addressed in the literature from a theoretical perspective (Dyck, 1989; Krefting, 1991; French, 1992), there is limited information relating to strategies to be employed for successful integration of cultural awareness in practice or how it should be taught in an educational setting. The amount of attention paid to cultural considerations in health service delivery and education varies across health professions. For example, there is a paucity of literature dealing specifically with physiotherapy and issues of culture, whereas much information on culture comes from the fields of occupational therapy, rehabilitation counselling and medical anthropology (Lightfoot, 1985; Dyck, 1989; Meadows, 1991; Kinebanian and Stomph, 1992). A workshop manual for occupational therapists exploring cultural diversity (Fitzgerald et al., 1995) contains an extensive bibliography of over 150 articles dealing with issues of culture in rehabilitation.

An important and insightful study undertaken by Robison (1996) highlights some of the deficits demonstrated by physiotherapists in their management of clients from another culture. His findings may also be of value to other health professionals. Robison (1996) perceived that problems in intercultural interactions were related to differences between the values of the health professionals and the clients – a fact that many of the therapists did not recognize. The therapists who recognized these differences were able to modify interactions appropriately. Interestingly, therapists from migrant backgrounds did not necessarily score higher on Robison's cultural competency index than those from non-migrant backgrounds. Generally, therapists with a poor understanding of their own value system created problems from both the client's and the therapist's perspective. Negative experiences produced negative stereotyping and bias towards people from different cultural backgrounds. In addition, therapists who expressed assimilationist or ethnocentric attitudes often lacked an understanding of the components of the human condition; and therapists who displayed dispassionate attitudes tended to display a fear or hesitancy towards treating people from different cultural backgrounds.

Fitzgerald (1992) concurs with Robison and suggests that the problem lies in a lack of health professionals' acknowledgement of alternative beliefs and awareness of cultural differences. The author points out that 'in every clinical interaction there are at least three cultures and medical systems involved: a) the personal or familiar culture to the provider; b) the culture of the client or patient, and c) the culture of the primary medical system' (Fitzgerald, 1992, p. 38).

In summary, cultural differences in intercultural interactions have the potential to create confusion and even conflict. Unsuccessful interactions may be characterized by a lack of satisfaction with the interaction in both the health professional and the client. Cultural values play an important role in influencing the reactions, beliefs and even outcomes of therapy (Robison, 1996). Successful intercultural interactions in health care are characterized by mutual satisfaction, effective communication and positive outcomes (Meadows, 1991).

## Client–culture–community interaction

There are several factors to be considered in the process of developing professional craft knowledge across cultural contexts. The first step is recognizing and understanding the basic human condition. From this starting point, health professionals must develop a compassion for their fellow human beings and a cultural sensitivity; their approach to practice should be client/family-centred (Robison, 1996).

Health professionals should have an understanding of disability and its effect on families. It is important that they understand the impact of disability in the context of the different environments in which they may be working, with the constraints that will be imposed on the clients, their families and their communities.

Further, it is important to recognize that the client comes from a community; whether health professionals are working in an institution or within the community they must consider the client as a cultural being (with all that it implies) and also consider the resources and limitations that exist within the client's community. Clients, their culture, their community and the therapy all interact with each other and will influence all aspects of health care delivery. Health professionals must be well aware of different models of service delivery and their relative strengths and weaknesses. This awareness entails a thorough understanding of and an affinity for community development philosophies and strategies, where the focus of attention lies in the community as well as in the individual client. In all health care services, it is crucial that all aspects of management, from problem identification to intervention, are directed by meeting the needs of the client and family carers (Clemson et al., 1999).

## Professional approaches to reasoning

Health professionals tend to have a profession-specific approach to their reasoning in service delivery. Since reasoning occurs in a cultural and a community context, it requires consideration of these contextual variables which are vital dimensions in effecting a positive outcome. Cultural awareness, acquisition of professional craft knowledge relating to culture, and use of knowledge about culture are critical elements of sound professional practice. Creating opportunities for learning related to these elements should permeate the education and practice of the health professional. Therefore, learning experiences must be provided which establish knowledge-seeking behaviours in health professionals who routinely explore clients' stories in order to understand the client's and family's problems (Clemson et al., 1999). Culture needs to be considered routinely in every aspect of provision of health services to clients. In addition, culture and the context in which services are delivered are intimately related. Health professionals must be sensitive to these interdependent factors when providing service, whether in an institution, an outpatient centre or in the community.

It is important to consider people's beliefs about health and illness, including beliefs about the cause of any illness they experience, what kind of illness it is, the natural course the illness will take and how it should be treated. Some explanations are common to groups of people and may be seen as having a cultural basis. The sources we draw upon to inform us about our state of health and to explain it to others are popular, professional and traditional. Authors use the term 'explanatory models' to describe the explanations for illness and disability given by health practitioners and their clients and to distinguish between lay explanatory models and the clinical models used by health practitioners.

It is often difficult to match the health professional's perception of a particular illness or disability with the client's understanding and experience of it. The disparity is likely to be even greater when the client and the health professional come from different cultural backgrounds. It is evident any therapy interaction can involve perspectives from multiple cultures and from several explanatory models within each culture. Narrative reasoning ('the client's story') and history-taking exercises are an integral part of the therapist–client interaction, and consideration of cultural and other influences should be routinely considered as part of this process.

Enhancing self-monitoring skills is a way of improving reasoning in any situation (Boud and Walker, 1991; Carnevali, 1995; Refshauge and Higgs, 1995). One way to facilitate self-monitoring is to systematically apply a series of questions or a reflective framework (i.e. a series of concepts followed by a systematic set of questions) which encourages this conscious reflection and metacognition (Bridge and Twible, 1997). For example, a framework that may be used to facilitate problem-sensing may include the concepts of identifying key words, knowledge of the key word, functional implications and therapy hypothesis. Because reasoning occurs in a given community and cultural context, health professionals must be 'prompted' to consider culture and other contextual factors routinely throughout their interactions with clients (i.e. through the assessment, intervention and evaluation phases of service provision).

Novice therapists often make reasoning errors because cues are missed or underpinning knowledge is absent. Having some means of checking current knowledge and understanding is essential; in practice it is not acceptable to interact with a client without any idea of what the client's potential dysfunction might be (Bridge and Twible, 1997). Awareness of the local context is crucial to the health professional's ability to function in a particular environment. For example, a health professional who lacks knowledge of the importance of specific role tasks of a female carer within a particular family group may make incorrect assumptions; these assumptions may lead to inappropriate therapy strategies for the carer (such as requiring practice three times daily of a functional task like feeding a disabled child, when the mother works full time). In some client interactions, such lack of awareness may result in the health professional omitting a component of the rehabilitation programme that is important to the client's everyday life. For this reason, therapists need to become sensitized through repeated exposure to real-life case studies for critical analysis and proposed solutions.

Once awareness has been established, the health professional can identify the knowledge that needs to be acquired. For relevant cultural information there are important sources, such as peers, cultural informants or brokers, as well as clients, family members and other community members; these sources are often more valuable than the professional literature (see Fig. 20.2) (Henley and Twible, 2000).

Having accessed available sources of knowledge, the health professional further needs to validate the information for the current clinical situation.

This knowledge can then be used to decide the form of client assessment, through observation of

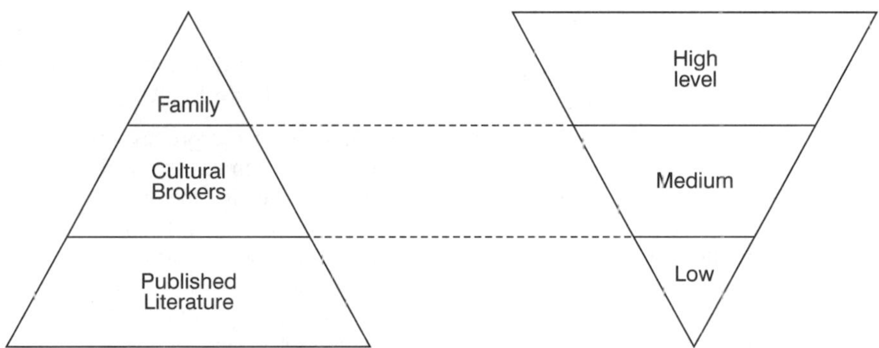


**Figure 20.2** Hierarchy of knowledge sources for cultural decision-making

performance of the physical examination and functional activities. One of the most useful tools for a therapist in a community setting is a model of functional assessment. This model, adapted from an occupational therapy model (Reed and Sanderson, 1980), has been used successfully for the past five years by students and therapists in rural community-based rehabilitation projects in southern India (Twible and Henley, 2000). The model sets the client at the centre of the assessment process, so that all decisions about management are made from the client's perspective. Using local knowledge, the therapist begins to develop working hypotheses, validates assessment findings, and selects and implements a management programme, having considered the implications, assessed the risks and determined the expected outcomes. The focus in problem validation is on examination of discrepancies between the original clinical image and the real and gradually unfolding scenario (Bridge and Twible, 1997), including the application of local knowledge.

No single experience will be adequate to ensure that learners acquire the requisite skills to influence their practice comprehensively. It is the type and method of education that is the crucial factor in improving competence (Carpio and Majumdar, 1992; Robison, 1996). Workshops and other small group activities have been a useful means of facilitating cultural competency and reasoning skills, as they challenge the values, preconceptions and biases of health professionals as well as providing opportunities for application of knowledge and skills to expanded case studies derived from real encounters; these case studies are designed to provide detailed cultural, social, geographical, and physical information about clients and the environments in which they live (Henley and Twible, 2000).

## Strategies for action

Many health professionals regularly face dilemmas when dealing with clients from cultures other than their own. As previously mentioned, the issues relating to these dilemmas are complex and can arise from many sources. There is no simple way to overcome such problems. Instead, a series of different approaches should be used to try to identify the critical incident(s) which triggered the dilemma.

The 'critical incident' theory of Brislin et al. (1986) and the methodology based upon it have been valuable tools in workshops to develop cultural competencies in health professionals (Fitzgerald et al., 1995). Critical incidents are situations for which there is a need to attach meaning. In that sense, critical incidents are closely related to client stories or narratives. For example, in a workshop environment, clients and health professionals are asked to tell a story about a situation in health care in which they believe culture was an issue. These stories provide the basic material for developing critical incident scenarios, which are analysed to develop potential explanations. Reasonable explanations then provide the foundation for developing strategies for action. Fitzgerald et al. (1995), in their intercultural interaction project, list a number of key questions to assist in the analysis of critical incident scenarios. They include:

- Is culture the key issue in the incident?
- If not, what was the key issue?
- Is culture a secondary issue?
- If culture was an issue, what was the cultural issue or issues involved?
- Were the assessments offered reasonable? Was the solution reasonable?
- What could have been done to address the needs of the client, family and the others in the story in an appropriate and sensitive manner?
- What other issues or ideas come to mind as you read the story?

In addition, Fitzgerald et al. have identified key principles to consider in acquiring local knowledge and provide frameworks for exploring local issues relevant to individual practitioners and the client population, as well as suggested guidelines for developing policy for the management of clients from diverse backgrounds (Fitzgerald et al., 1995, pp. 20–27). Readers are recommended to read the reference in full for more specific details.

### A case study to develop cultural competency in undergraduate health professionals

An example of the process of developing cultural competency comes from the project we have conducted during the past five years through interdisciplinary student fieldwork placements in community-based rehabilitation projects in rural and remote villages in southern India. In the preparatory phase, students participated in a series of workshops and other activities designed to further develop their professional reasoning and cultural competency so that their fieldwork experience in India would be enriched and their learning enhanced.

When students were interviewed after their placement, it was apparent that the Indian fieldwork experience highlighted for them the impact that their interaction with the Indian culture had on their cultural competencies. Although Lightfoot (1985) suggests that experience with diverse cultures is important, findings from India suggest that it may be the type of experience that results in an enhancement in aspects of cultural competency. Students reflected that in order to provide effective therapy, they had to seek knowledge specific to Indian culture and to consider which cultural factors would have an impact on therapy. Examples included: feeding activities occur with the use of the right hand only; the procedure for toileting involves squatting; the clothing which students wore had an impact on the level of respect gained from the staff and villagers. Students reported that personal values and assumptions were often in conflict with Indian values concerning health care. For example, Australian students and Indian people had different expectations of independence in activities of daily living for children. This disparity led to a critical incident, in that the students were initially unaware of the cultural norms and identified a 'deficit' which they felt was detrimental to the development of the child. They initially urged the Indian therapists and parents actively to encourage children to do as much as possible for themselves. However, they noticed that this suggestion was not perceived as a reasonable therapeutic intervention. Upon questioning the Indian CBR workers (cultural brokers), the students were informed that a cultural norm of Indian parenting is fully to assist the child with many activities of daily living until about the age of five, at which time more independence is allowed. To mediate a successful therapy outcome, students had to accept that their attitudes towards independence were not culturally applicable.

## Conclusions

The varied situations in which health professionals work heighten the importance of understanding the unique nature of people from different environments, recognizing that each individual is different and that assumptions cannot be applied to all people associated with a particular group. Clinical competencies, communication skills, innovative strategies, a person-oriented attitude and compassion are significant factors in intercultural interactions whether at home or abroad. If health professionals develop good reasoning skills and cultural competence they can function well in any context by thinking through the issues related to the particular situation.

## References


Avruch, K. and Black, P. W. (1991) The culture question and conflict resolution. *Peace and Change*, **16**(1), 22–45.

Boud, D. and Walker, D. (1991) *Experience and Learning: Reflection at Work.* Geelong, Australia: Deakin University Press.

Bridge, C. and Twible, R. L. (1997) Clinical reasoning: Informed decision making in practice. In *Occupational Therapy: Enabling Function and Well-Being*, 2nd edn (C. Christiansen and C. Baum, eds), pp. 158–179. Thorofare, NJ: Slack.

Brislin, R. W., Cushner, K., Cherrie, C. and Yong, M. (1986) *Intercultural Interactions: A Practical Guide.* Newbury Park, CA: Sage.

Carnevali, D. L. (1995) Self-monitoring of clinical reasoning behaviours: Promoting professional growth. In *Clinical Reasoning in the Health Professions* (J. Higgs and M. Jones, eds), pp. 156–173. Oxford: Butterworth-Heinemann.

Carpio, B. A. and Majumdar, B. (1992) Experiential learning: An approach to transcultural education for nursing. *Journal of Transcultural Nursing*, **4**(1), 4–11.

Clemson, L., Fitzgerald, M. and Mullavey-O'Byrne, C. (1999) Families' perspectives following strokes: Unheard stories. *Topics in Stroke Rehabilitation*, **6**(1), 60–77.

Dyck, I. (1989) The immigrant client: Issues in developing culturally sensitive practice. *Canadian Journal of Occupational Therapy*, December, pp. 248–255.

Fitzgerald, M. H. (1991) The dilemma – race? Ethnicity? Culture? *The Rehab Journal* (Pacific Basin Rehabilitation Research and Training Centre and the Rehabilitation Hospital of the Pacific), **7**(2), 5–6.

Fitzgerald, M. H. (1992) Multicultural clinical interactions, *Journal of Rehabilitation*, April/May/June, pp. 1–5.

Fitzgerald, M. H., Mullavey-O'Byrne, C., Twible, R. L. and Kinebanian, A. (1995) *Exploring Cultural Diversity: A Workshop Manual for Occupational Therapists.* Sydney: School of Occupational Therapy, Faculty of Health Sciences, University of Sydney.

Fitzgerald, M. H., Mullavey-O'Byrne, C., Clemson, L. and Williamson, P. (1997) *Enhancing Cultural Competency/ Training Manual.* North Parramatta, NSW: Transcultural Mental Health Centre NSW.

French, S. (1992) Health care in a multi-ethnic society. *Physiotherapy*, **78**(3), 174–179.

Henley, E. C. and Twible, R. L. (2000) Teaching clinical reasoning across cultures. In *Clinical Reasoning in the Health Professions*, 2nd edn (J. Higgs and M. Jones, eds), pp. 255–261. Oxford: Butterworth-Heinemann.

Kinebanian, A. and Stomph, M. (1992) Cross cultural occupational therapy: A critical reflection. *American Journal of Occupational Therapy*, **46**(8), 751–757.

Krefting, L. (1991) The culture concept in the everyday practice of occupational and physical therapy. *Physical and Occupational Therapy in Pediatrics*, **11**(4), 1–16.

Lightfoot, S. C. (1985) The undergraduate: Culture shock in the health context. *Australian Occupational Therapy Journal*, **32**, 118–121.

Meadows, J. L. (1991) Multicultural communication. *Physical and Occupational Therapy in Pediatrics: The Quarterly Journal of Developmental Therapy*, **11**(4), 31–42.

Reed, K. and Sanderson, S. (1980) *Concepts Of Occupational Therapy*. Baltimore: Williams & Wilkins.

Refshauge, K. and Higgs, J. (1995) Teaching clinical reasoning in health science curricula. In *Clinical Reasoning in the Health Professions* (J. Higgs and M Jones, eds), pp. 105–116. Oxford: Butterworth-Heinemann.

Riggar, T. F., Eckert, J. M. and Crimando, W. (1993) Cultural diversity in rehabilitation: Management strategies for implementing organizational pluralism. *Journal of Rehabilitation Administration*, **17**(2), 53–61.

Robison, S. (1996) Exposure and education: The impact on the cultural competency of physiotherapists. Honours thesis, School of Physiotherapy, Faculty of Health Sciences, University of Sydney.

Twible, R. L. and Henley, E. C. (2000) Preparing occupational therapists and physiotherapists for community based rehabilitation. In *Selected Readings in Community Based Rehabilitation* (M. Thomas and M. J. Thomas, eds), pp. 109–126. Series 1, CBR in Transition. Bangalore, India: Asia Pacific Disability Rehabilitation Journal.

Varney, S. and Brislin, R. (1990) Using the culture general assimilator to prepare for multicultural exchanges. *HERDSA News*, **12**(1), 9–13.

Walker, M. L. (1991) Rehabilitation service delivery to individuals with disabilities: A question of cultural competence. *OSERS News in Print*, pp. 6–11.

# 21

# Learning together: fostering professional craft knowledge development in clinical placements

**Dawn Best and Helen Edwards**

> Long after physical therapists forget what was taught in which course during academic preparation, they remember their clinical education experiences.

(Paschal, 1997, p. 169)

How can we foster the development of professional craft knowledge in clinical placements? Given that a large proportion of professional craft knowledge has traditionally not been articulated, documented or valued, there is little clarity about how best to conceptualize and implement the process of acquiring such knowledge. In this chapter, we advocate adopting two strategies within clinical placements. First we suggest using the social learning or apprenticeship model to understand better how learning occurs in clinical settings. Second, we recommend adapting the critical companionship model to enhance the learning of both teacher and student. The clinical placement is an ideal setting in which to adopt these approaches, because it provides a rich and varied environment where professional craft knowledge is a key aspect of clinical activity and of the lived experiences of participants.

Taken together, these two strategies will add value as well as depth and understanding to learning professional craft knowledge in clinical settings. The social learning or apprenticeship model highlights the social act of becoming a professional and belonging to a health profession. During the clinical placement, the value of informal social learning processes can be acknowledged and the importance of role modelling emphasized. Further, we advocate that clinicians should 'learn together' with students during clinical placement, to enhance the value of the teaching/learning experience. This can be achieved through adapting the critical companionship model to clinical education. By learning together in this social way, both students and clinicians will develop their professional craft knowledge.

## Understanding learning in the clinical placement: a powerful experience

Learning in clinical settings is a complex, multifaceted process. To understand and explain such learning requires a model which will take account of the nature of professional learning and the complexity of the situation in which that learning occurs. The model also needs to incorporate some individual characteristics of teachers and learners because clinical practice, the vehicle for clinical learning, is a process heavily dependent on interpersonal interactions.

Clinical learning is far more than application of theoretical knowledge in clinical settings. Best et al. (1999) highlight the effect that the professional socialization process in clinical settings has on student perceptions of learning. As students begin to understand the essence of their profession they become aware of what they need to experience and learn in order to attain that essence. Their learning becomes focused and powerful. As they shift identity from student to therapist (or therapist-in-training), they assume markedly greater responsibility for their learning.

The clinical environment has a strong influence on students' learning. In the authors' experience, the role models which clinicians as teachers provide have a powerful effect on how and what students choose to learn in clinical settings. The influence of clinicians far outweighs that of academic staff from the university, even though both may be members of the profession. What is it about the clinical environment that accounts for this power?

Motivation is important in student learning. A major advantage of learning in clinical settings is that students are motivated by the nature and location of this setting. The clinic is the real world; the clinic is where students 'give their best'. An educationally created clinical learning situation, such as an in-house clinic in a university, does not have the edge of real **practice** (e.g. consequences, temporality, busy-ness, confusion, complexity). From research on clinical education in different settings, Edwards (1997, p. 150) made the following comments about in-house university clinics:

> The emphasis on the educational aspects of the clinical encounter is clear to teacher, students and patients. Service to the patient is considered a by-product of the clinical teaching process, and not a necessary objective. This creates a somewhat artificial contrived environment. While it is seen by the students as a useful learning process it is not seen as 'the real thing'.

Learning in and through practice in a clinical setting can be construed as a type of apprenticeship. Rogoff (1990) described apprenticeship as a guided participation in social and cultural activity with companions who support and stretch understanding. Although health science educators may be uncomfortable with the term 'apprenticeship', this definition is one that fits well with a number of aspects of current educational philosophy. Lave (1996) uses the concept of socially situated practice theory to describe the nature of learning in and through practice. Her theory highlights the relationship between person and environment. In these aspects Lave's theory has particular relevance to students in health-related areas, since she acknowledges that it is impossible to separate the person acting from the social world in which the activity takes place. Her theory also highlights the notion that environments are constantly changing. The idea of changing participation in changing communities of practice (Lave, 1993, 1996) provides the key to a new understanding of learning in the clinical environment by helping us to make sense of our experience and our observations. It is always difficult to predict how students with different backgrounds, personalities and life experiences will make the transition from the academic environment to the clinical environment. What is a rewarding, challenging learning experience for one may not have the same outcomes for another. The examples (e.g. apprenticeship of tailors in Liberia) used by Lave to illustrate her theory are very different from clinical placements in the health professions. Yet her insights into apprenticeship, focusing as they do on community and the real 'lived in' world, force us to review our conception of apprenticeship.

It is commonly accepted that health science education has progressed beyond the apprenticeship model. However, denigration of the **traditional** apprenticeship model assumes that apprenticeship consists of training for repetitive tasks and rule-bound behaviours and that, as such, it is inadequate for accommodating the advances in scientific knowledge and the complex requirements of professional practice in today's health care settings, including the employment of professional judgment and demonstration of accountability arising from professional autonomy. Another concern with apprenticeship learning in the traditional model involved its dependence for success on how expert the 'master' was and how committed the master was to provide quality learning, assessment and feedback to the 'apprentice'. Rejection of the apprenticeship model certainly coincided with the move to university-based education and the consequent valuing of the abstractions and generalizations of propositional knowledge above more personal and informal learning.

Lave (1996), on the other hand, portrayed apprenticeship rather differently. Her observational study of 250 master tailors and their apprentices in the poor and marginal districts around the central business district of Monrovia in Liberia provides a new perspective on learning. These tailors made a few pairs of trousers a day and used the day's profits to buy more material for the next day. Contrary to the assumption that the apprenticeship model merely encourages reproduction of a specific set of skills, Lave's research demonstrated that the apprentices learnt far more. They certainly learned how to make clothes. However, it was a powerful learning environment which enabled apprentices to learn many complex lessons concurrently.

> They were learning relations among the major social identities and divisions in Liberian society which they were in the

business of dressing. They were learning to make a life, to make clothes, to grow old enough, and mature enough to become master tailors, and to see the truth of the respect due to the master of their trade. It seems trivially true that they were never doing only one of these things at a time.

(Lave, 1996, p. 151)

This concept of apprenticeship ascribes value to the social act of becoming and belonging; to the construction of identities in practice. It highlights the importance of guides and role models as exemplars of practice and presents a wider view of learning goals which encompass development of professional identity and self-evaluation skills as well as the mastery of technical competence. This optimal apprenticeship model presents a useful framework through which we can develop strategies for fostering professional craft knowledge. In the apprenticeship model:

a novice gets to be an expert through the mechanism of *acculturation* into the world of the expert. Actual participation in this world is critical for two reasons: a) much of the knowledge that the expert transmits to the novice is tacit and b) the knowledge often varies with context.

(Farnham-Diggory, 1994, p. 466, author's italics)

Fostering professional craft knowledge development requires teachers to acknowledge and value the informal social learning processes which impact on students as they develop professional identities in practice environments. It is during the clinical placement that health science students learn 'the stuff of the profession'. They learn what the profession is, how to act as a practitioner, what the attitudes and beliefs of the profession are, and how to modify practice to meet the needs of the specific situation. They refine skills to become more efficient, more proficient, more flexible and more professional.

Using the social learning approach encourages us to focus on the essence of professional craft knowledge and to think of clinicians as embodied exemplars of what students are striving to become. This approach assumes that the learning process is a reciprocal one and that what is learned continues to be modified by the learning process and the context. It can explain some of the power of learning in clinical settings.

Although there were differences between the individual tailors and their apprentices, there were similarities in the learning outcomes for the apprentices. They learned how to be tailors and all that entailed. Lave (1996, p. 153) asserts that 'there are common parts in all effective learning practices, breaking down distinctions between learning and doing, between social identity and knowledge, between education and occupation, between form and content'.

The social learning approach is compatible with the development of expert practice as described by Benner (1984) and with education of the reflective practitioner (Schön, 1987). Both these writers acknowledge the profound effect which ongoing experience in a practical environment, coupled with modification of actions, has on the practitioner's developing understanding of practice. This approach also fits the hermeneutic understanding of staff and education development as advocated by Webb (1996). We cannot understand a situation unless we become a part of it. By becoming a part of it, we change the situation. All these writers suggest that practitioners develop understanding through ongoing experience and a continual search for meaning. 'Situated learning always involves changes in knowledge and action and changes in knowledge and action are central to what we mean by learning' (Lave, 1993, p. 5).

## The importance of personal knowledge in the placement

Professional knowledge encompasses propositional knowledge, professional craft knowledge and personal knowledge (Higgs and Titchen, 1995). In clinical practice the distinction between professional craft knowledge and personal knowledge is blurred (Higgs and Titchen, 1995). For example, personal moral stance and professional ethics are closely related. The clinician's personal knowledge and personal frame of reference are important in framing and determining the clinician's approach to practice, which in turn impacts on his/her generation and use of professional craft knowledge. Personal knowledge and professional craft knowledge are closely connected in the novice, and personal knowledge is critical for effective functioning in any clinical environment. Students need to know themselves, to have an understanding of their attitudes, beliefs and responses, before they can achieve competence in clinical practice. The following reflective comments from physiotherapy students (from Best, 1993) after their first significant clinical placements indicate that the experience of being in clinics for eight weeks had fundamentally changed them.

> My placements have been a valuable learning experience and have taught me a lot not only about the physiotherapy profession but also about myself.
>
> I feel that I am growing emotionally as a result of my clinical experiences which will be invaluable to my future growth as a physiotherapist.
>
> I am often reminded about how well one must know oneself to be a physiotherapist. Knowing one's self means knowing one's body as well as one's mind. We all react differently to pain and illness. This can affect interactions with patients.

Such understanding of self helps students become empathic to their patients and adopt a holistic approach to practice.

As they develop professional craft knowledge, students become able to relate to people as individuals in their specific situations.

> During the course everyone who passes must develop skills and textbook type knowledge . . . However there are more subtle skills which I feel that I am presently gaining which are probably equally important in becoming a physiotherapist. One of the most important is treating patients as whole individuals with expectations and fears and being able to communicate effectively with them.
>
> The most important aspect of the clinics for me was the growing appreciation for the patient's individual needs and the need to look at each patient as an individual with a unique condition. They require treatment at this level with an understanding of their body, mind and soul.

Personal knowledge and the understanding of self heighten students' ability to self-evaluate, to engage in critical appraisal of their practice and to acknowledge their strengths and weaknesses.

> After these 8 weeks I have become more aware of my weaknesses and can concentrate on improving these areas. I also have come to realise my strong points and can use these to my advantage.

Clinical placements encourage students to assume responsibility for their learning and to become that most desired of professionals, one who engages in lifelong learning.

> Perhaps the largest realisation that I came to was the necessity of continuing my own education over and beyond that which I will learn in this undergraduate course. In the first and second year it was easy to assume that by the time I had finished the course I would be excellent at absolutely everything. Now I am satisfied with being competent at everything with a commitment to improve my knowledge and skills as long as I am a physiotherapist.

## Using the clinical placement to foster professional craft knowledge: some pointers

### Use existing resources

There is considerable literature directed towards promoting student learning in the clinical environment which provides more than adequate starting points. It includes Stengelhofen's (1993) *Teaching Students in Clinical Settings*, which applies the deep and surface learning paradigm to clinical contexts. In *Facilitating Learning in Clinical Settings*, McAllister et al. (1997) provide both an adult learning perspective and an experiential learning framework in which to ground clinical education. Higgs and Edwards (1999), in *Educating Beginning Practitioners*, cover a wide range of educational trends, from individual strategies to society-wide changes. Best and Rose (1996), in *Quality Supervision*, skilfully integrate theory with practice to provide a user-friendly guide to supervision. Titchen and Higgs (1995) explicate educational strategies for facilitating the use and generation of knowledge in clinical reasoning. These strategies include observing, listening, questioning, story-telling, keeping reflective diaries, and developing concept maps.

### Plan and prepare

Fostering student learning in clinical settings requires teachers to plan and prepare thoroughly. First it is necessary to have clinical placements available where students can learn to become beginning practitioners. To achieve this requires an enhanced and cooperative arrangement between universities, health authorities and the professions (Ferguson and Edwards, 1999).

Considerable thought, planning and organization is required to foster learning for both students and their teachers. Fostering professional craft knowledge through the clinical placement requires attention to be paid to the relationship between clinician and learner as well as to maximizing experiential learning opportunities. Strategies include:

- planning the student learning experience;
- briefing and preparing the student to optimize learning from the experience;
- allowing the experience, the student–patient encounter, to occur;
- revisiting the experience afterwards for reflection and debriefing;
- supporting all participants.

Through these strategies, teachers can encourage students to become aware of and develop their emerging professional craft knowledge. It is vital to optimize student learning during the placement. Paschal provides the following excellent summary for clinical teachers:

> Good clinical teachers enable student learning. They begin by inviting students to participate in the community of . . . practice, then they plan, model, coach, question, encourage, instruct, supervise and evaluate to optimize the learning experience.

(Paschal, 1997, p. 182)

Preparing and supporting both students and their supervising practitioners will enhance the outcomes from the clinical placement. Both are engaged in a change process which can be stressful. A supportive, relatively stress-free environment is required where the focus is on changing identity and on the personal and social aspects of learning. Students need to be 'primed' for placements. Supervising clinicians need an understanding of how students learn in clinical settings, of the expectations placed on students and of the standards expected from students (Baird and Edwards, 1999).

## Be flexible

Fostering learning in a clinical setting must remain an essentially flexible process. Flexibility is necessitated by the variety of students and placements, and by the complexity that is professional craft knowledge. The real clinic does not replicate textbook or classic cases; there are no average or ideal students. Good clinical practice entails dealing smoothly and efficiently with the unpredicted and unpredictable. Fostering learning in clinical settings requires the capacity to extract educational value from any situation, however unexpected, and from any patient episode, however difficult or atypical.

Fostering student learning in clinical settings requires both clinicians and students to have the capacity to react flexibly to unexpected and serendipitous situations as they arrive; to seize the moment. Different clinical settings and different supervising clinicians have unpredictable effects on individual students. Similarly, the journey which individual students make in the affective domain of learning is unpredictable. For instance, some students are challenged, excited and motivated by the opportunity to take responsibility for the assessment and management of a client with little supervision. Other students may be so paralysed by the responsibility or fear of failure that they are unable to perform simple activities which are normally well within their capabilities. Students' expectations of the task and their subsequent performance are influenced by their prior knowledge and experience. Since learning is so individualistic, it is essential that clinicians find out about their students and get to know them as people. This requires both the development of a trusting relationship and an investment of time.

## Learn together

The placement is vital for fostering the development of professional craft knowledge. Seeing real examples of practice helps students make sense of the abstractions of theory and propositional knowledge taught in universities. Watching clinicians actually practise helps students create meaning and become aware of professional craft knowledge in use. However, to achieve understanding and meaning, students need more than just observation of practice. To the observer, skilful practice appears smooth, simple and coordinated. But beneath that smoothness there are hidden depths and complexities. Students need to be made aware of these hidden aspects of practice. Clinicians need to articulate their understanding of all that is happening as they practise, to foster optimally the development of students' professional craft knowledge. They need to highlight the 'knowing how' of their own professional practice. When clinicians model this process, students come to be aware of and understand the complexity of professional craft knowledge (its situation-specificity, nuances and contextual subtleties). Such understanding emphasizes for students the depth and importance of the learning which occurs during clinical placement.

Typically, students in clinics are so preoccupied with performing the technical skills associated with practice that they fail to appreciate other aspects of professional craft knowledge. Explicating practice and cueing students to its subtlety and complexity helps them become aware of practice requirements. It assists students through the stage of becoming aware of the task required, and the difficult stage of learning to coordinate all elements of the tasks. Even when students understand what is required in clinical practice, the actual coordination of simultaneous tasks may be problematic:

I am so busy thinking up my next question that I rarely hear the patient's answers

(Best, 1993)

Clinicians can work together with students to develop their awareness of relevant clinical signs. Students need to recognize, make sense of and ascribe meaning to data obtained through all their senses. Initially students need guidance in linking this incoming data to the concepts of clinical practice in their profession (e.g. recognizing the feel of increased or decreased muscle tone).

Reflection and feedback are necessary to encourage students to improve clinical practice during their experience in the clinical placement. The professional craft knowledge which students are acquiring in clinical settings is mainly regarded as tacit knowledge. It accrues over time, primarily through practice. Typically there is no attempt to generalize beyond the practitioner's own experience (Titchen, 1998). Thus, one of the difficulties which arises with helping students acquire professional craft knowledge is that, traditionally, 'professionals cannot say what is the basis of their professionalism. They do not have the wherewithal to understand their practice. They never have had' (Fish and Coles, 1998, p. 9). One of the goals of education today is to help clinicians and students move beyond these limitations, to learn to articulately and credibly explicate the rationales and bases for their interventions.

The largely tacit nature of much of professional craft knowledge used in clinical practice today is graphically illustrated by Fish and Coles (1998) with the metaphor of an iceberg to describe professional practice. The behaviour which can be observed in the clinic is the visible tip of the iceberg. Below, hidden from observers of the practice and often from the practitioners themselves, are knowledge, feelings, expectations, assumptions, attitudes, beliefs and values. In developing professional craft knowledge, students need to become aware of this 'hidden 90 per cent' of practice.

Titchen (1998) advocates using a collaborative relationship to develop professional craft knowledge through a process she calls **critical companionship**. (See Chapter 10.) Critical companionship is 'a metaphor for a helping relationship, in which the critical companion accompanies less experienced practitioners on their own very personal experiential learning journeys' (Titchen, 1998, p. 1). Within this supportive and trusting relationship the more experienced practitioner, the critical companion, facilitates awareness of practice and personal issues by observing, questioning, clarifying and providing feedback on performance. Through such dialogue and support, practitioners are enabled to explicate their practice.

The critical companionship model could usefully be adapted to foster students' professional craft knowledge in the clinical placement. The model provides the opportunity for clinicians and students to support each other, in spite of their different levels of expertise. With goodwill and effort, clinicians and students can honestly question and clarify practice while respecting personal and practice differences. Through the process of critically reflecting on their actions as part of teaching, clinicians can better understand their craft knowledge. They can discover words and language with which to explain their practice. Students are provided with authentic examples of the 'what' and 'how' of professional craft knowledge, through their mentors' explanations of practice. Clinicians model a description and analysis of practice which extends below the tip of the iceberg. In adapting the critical companionship model to work with students, clinicians can provide a living demonstration of how one comes to know practice, of how one develops professional craft knowledge. Through that very process of working with students, clinicians will gain a deeper understanding of their own practice. Over time, they will begin to construct a much needed research base of professional craft knowledge.

## Conclusions

Learning in clinical settings is a complex, multi-faceted process. This chapter provides a number of insights which will help clinicians foster the development of professional craft knowledge in the clinical placement. The clinical placement is a type of social and professional apprenticeship. It is an opportunity for both clinicians and students to learn in and through practice. Clinicians can construe their task as enabling students to be ready for changing participation in changing communities of practice. Clinicians must plan and prepare carefully, yet be flexible, in order to foster the development of professional craft knowledge through the placement. The placement is an opportunity for clinicians to learn together with their students. Adapting the model of critical companionship has benefits for both the experienced clinician and the novice student. The process of modelling practice and explaining its rationale reveals professional craft knowledge to students and deepens clinicians' understanding of practice. Using the apprenticeship model and the critical companionship approach to foster professional craft knowledge in the clinical placement can thus become a personal research process which will in time form the basis for a new understanding of the very essence of professional practice.

## References


Baird, M. and Edwards, H. (1999) Supporting clinical supervisors: How smart are we really? *Proceedings of the 3rd Biennial Conference of the Foundation for Quality Supervision*, pp. 36–52. Melbourne: La Trobe University.

Benner, P. (1984) *From Novice to Expert: Excellence and Power in Clinical Nursing Practice.* Menlo Park, CA: Addison Wesley.

Best, D. (1993) Perceptions of learning in clinical placements: A study of third year physiotherapy students. MEd thesis, La Trobe University.

Best, D. and Rose, M. (1996) *Quality Supervision: Theory and Practice for Clinical Supervisors.* London: W.B. Saunders.

Best, D., Cust, J. and Prosser, M. (1999) The implications of student learning research for health science education. In *Educating Beginning Practitioners* (J. Higgs and H. Edwards, eds), pp. 136–142. Oxford: Butterworth-Heinemann.

Edwards, H. (1997) Clinical teaching: An exploration in three health professions. PhD thesis, University of Melbourne.

Farnham-Diggory, S. (1994) Paradigms of knowledge and instruction. *Review of Education Research*, **64**, 463–477.

Ferguson, K. and Edwards, H. (1999) Providing clinical education: The relationship between health and education. In *Educating Beginning Practitioners* (J. Higgs and H. Edwards, eds), pp. 52–58. Oxford: Butterworth-Heinemann.

Fish, D. and Coles, C. (1998) *Developing Professional Judgement in Health Care.* Oxford: Butterworth-Heinemann.

Higgs, J. and Edwards, H. (1999) *Educating Beginning Practitioners: Challenges for Health Professional Education.* Oxford: Butterworth-Heinemann.

Higgs, J. and Titchen, A. (1995) Propositional, professional and personal knowledge in clinical reasoning. In *Clinical Reasoning in the Health Professions* (J. Higgs and M. Jones, eds), pp. 129–146. Oxford: Butterworth-Heinemann.

Lave, J. (1993) The practice of learning. In *Understanding Practice Perspectives on Activity and Context* (S. Chaiklin and J. Lave, eds), pp. 3–32. Cambridge: Cambridge University Press.

Lave, J. (1996) Teaching and learning in practice. *Mind, Culture and Activity*, **3**, 149–164.

McAllister, L., Lincoln, M., McLeod, S. and Maloney, D. (1997) *Facilitating Learning in Clinical Settings.* Cheltenham: Stanley Thornes.

Paschal, K. (1997) Techniques for teaching in clinical settings. In *Handbook of Teaching for Physical Therapists* (K. Shepherd and G. Jensen, eds), pp. 169–197. Boston: Butterworth-Heinemann.

Rogoff, B. (1990) *Apprenticeship in Thinking: Cognitive Development in Social Context.* New York: Oxford University Press.

Schön, D. (1987) *Educating the Reflective Practitioner: Towards a New Design for Teaching and Learning in the Professions.* San Francisco: Jossey-Bass.

Stengelhofen, J. (1993) *Teaching Students in Clinical Settings.* London: Chapman & Hall.

Titchen, A. (1998) *A Conceptual Framework for Facilitating Learning in Clinical Practice.* Occasional Paper No. 2. Sydney: Centre for Professional Education Advancement, University of Sydney.

Titchen, A. and Higgs, J. (1995) Facilitating the use and generation of knowledge in clinical reasoning. In *Clinical Reasoning in the Health Professions* (J. Higgs and M. Jones, eds), pp. 314–325. Oxford: Butterworth-Heinemann.

Webb, G. (1996) *Understanding Staff Development.* Buckingham: Open University Press.

# 22

# Facilitating the development of professional craft knowledge

**David L. Smith**

As indicated in previous chapters, professional craft knowledge is the basis of all professional practice. Thus, it is the structured development of such craft knowledge that should be the basis of any preservice professional education curriculum. In Chapters 21 and 24, examples in physiotherapy education and teacher education, respectively, are discussed.

Being a professional, however, means much more than having an effective preservice education. The basis of continuing professional work is the commitment, skills and understandings to continue to learn from every experience of professional practice. Such lifelong learning is even more important in times of rapid social change. When change is slow, knowledge and solutions remain viable and can be taught through institutionalized teaching. When change is rapid and there are continually new problems emerging for which solutions do not exist, learning, not teaching, is the answer (Lovat and Smith, 1995). Thus it is imperative that, increasingly, professionals find ways to ensure that they are continually using the experience of their practice as a basis for the development of their professional craft knowledge.

Such learning may take place within a professional development programme offered by an employer or higher education institution. However, resources for such activities continue to decline, and ongoing professional learning is the responsibility of professionals themselves, either individually or as part of a learning organization (Senge, 1990; Leithwood and Seashore Louis, 1998). Thus, being an effective professional means continually examining your own practice.

A central feature of professional life is its dynamic intensity and interaction (Ewing and Smith, in press). While this provides much potential for learning, often such 'hot' action acts more as a barrier to learning than a facilitator. Rather, it is in times of quiet reflection on the action, in the recalling and reframing of events, interactions and circumstances, that the most powerful learning occurs. This chapter, then, examines different forms of engaging in professional learning, including action research, the use of critical friends and a number of strategies for reflection. Because of the limitations of chapter length, the review and discussion of each form is brief; however, references for those wanting further information are provided.

## Action research: investigating our own practice

Action research, developed by Kurt Lewin and others during the 1940s, is a strategy for increasing knowledge and bringing about social change through the systematic investigation of practice. It has a long history of use in areas of social practice including the professions, particularly in education (Kemmis and McTaggart, 1990; Elliott, 1991, 1993; Grundy, 1995).

Although action research may be undertaken successfully by an individual (e.g. Hussin, 1999), probably its strongest form is 'participative inquiry' (Reason, 1998). While there may be different modes of action research (Grundy, 1995), its major focus and purpose is for practitioners to change their practice through their own investigation, research and learning. Others may be involved as advisers, but one of the key features of action research is its emphasis on the responsibility of the practitioner for decisions relating to establishing the focus and parameters of the research, gathering data and deciding on the next steps in the process. This commitment is rooted in the well-evidenced principle that it is the practitioners who have to manage any change in their practice and change will only occur effectively if they are committed to making it happen, and if their beliefs and understandings are in concurrence with the change (Fullan, 1993; Lovat and Smith, 1995).

Thus, action research may be viewed as changing practice by 'pulling yourself up by your own bootstraps'. While there are those who argue that action research is not real research because it does not generate propositional knowledge, or comply with the canons of a narrowly defined view of scientific research, and its results are contaminated by the close involvement of the researchers, there is no doubt that it is, demonstrably, a powerful form for changing practice and for personal and professional learning (Kemmis and McTaggart, 1990; Zuber-Skerritt, 1996; Reason, 1998).

Action research may best be conceived as a continually expanding spiral (Kemmis and McTaggart, 1990). Thus, the action research process is dynamic and continuing: the result of investigating one problem or issue leads to further questions for investigation. In one sense, therefore, action research never stops. It can be seen as the very basis of professional practice and professional learning.

Each cycle of any action research programme begins by focusing on something that the practitioner would like to improve. All of us as practitioners have ideals about our practice that we have not yet been able to attain. It is these beliefs and the desire to achieve these ideals more closely that are often the beginning of a programme of action research.

The interrelated steps in each cycle of the action research spiral can be short or extended, and can be represented in different ways (Kemmis and McTaggart, 1990; Grundy, 1995). Simply, however, these steps may be described as planning, doing, reviewing and replanning.

## Planning

Planning usually involves several interrelated activities, as described below.

### *1. Reviewing what is happening now, or some form of situational analysis*

This may involve a group talking about their practice (Heron, 1992; Reason, 1994), possibly including gathering information and data. It may happen by having someone else observe what you are doing, by you reflecting on some part of your practice or on a student's comment/question, or through a patient's or client's reaction to some interaction or treatment. Alternatively, something that you read or that a colleague mentioned may trigger the investigation.

### *2. Deciding on the focus of what is to be improved*

This results from the step above. Whatever is identified should be quite specific and clear. If possible, you should specify what it is that you are trying to achieve in terms of concrete outcomes. Specifying the goal of your desired improvement in concrete ways that you or someone else can see, hear, smell or feel, should mean that it is much easier to examine data/evidence to see if you have achieved the desired result.

In deciding on a focus/question/issue it is better to choose something small which can be investigated within the parameters of a busy professional life. You need to think big, but start small. Try to break down the bigger picture of what you want to achieve into smaller incremental stages. With some aspects of professional practice it is easy to specify changes in concrete outcomes and in small stages. In others, it is more difficult. The principles outlined above, however, still apply.

### *3. Deciding what evidence/data will be collected, how and by whom*

One of the key elements of action research is the idea that the systematic gathering of information is central to providing a basis for decision-making. Memories of what you believe happened in a situation are often far from what actually occurred. While acknowledging the significant problems of observation, its subjectivity, and theorized basis (Denzin and Lincoln, 1998), it is argued that at least the systematic gathering of data, while the action is occurring, has the potential for greater accuracy than memory.

While different forms of action research adopt different positions in relation to who should be responsible for gathering evidence (Reason, 1998), often, for many different reasons, the practitioner may not be the best person to undertake the observations or collect the data. Sometimes this is because it is simply not practically possible. In addition, we are often simply too close to ourselves to be able to see ourselves and our practices in any detached manner. Thus, in making decisions about how the data/evidence will be gathered, it is often useful, if possible, to include others apart from those attempting to improve their practice. These could be colleagues or researchers assisting in the project. They could equally be clients, patients, family members or students, depending on the context of the practice.

In making decisions about what data will be collected and the means to do it, it is again best if these decisions can be made in concrete terms. The results of activity 2 above will give guidance to the results and will be interactive with the processes and decisions of activity 3. Generally, some form of recording of the data/evidence is advisable, for example pencil and paper, laptop computer or audio/videorecording or photographs (Grundy, 1995). Each of these has limitations and, if possible, multiple forms of records are usually desirable.

In some contexts, records of practice or of evidence gathering may take forms other than those mentioned above. For example, different forms of narrative have been used in investigating teaching (Connelly and Clandinin, 1990; Knowles et al., 1994). Installations, models, role plays, dramatic presentations and performances (Cole and Knowles, 1999) may all be appropriate methods of gathering and providing evidence.

These are the main activities in the planning stage of the action research.

## Doing

The next stage of the action research cycle is the doing, or the putting into operation the decisions that have been made in the planning stage. As indicated, this stage involves some form of observation of practice, including recording of the observations/experiences, using some of the methods discussed above, so that data/evidence are available for the subsequent stage. In one sense, it is this stage that is the most important of all: it is the attempt to deliberately gather information in an organized and systematic manner about one individual's or a collective's practice for the purposes of its improvement that clearly separates action research from the anecdotal and superficial evaluation of daily practice. It is the former rather than the latter that is the basis of powerful professional learning and development.

## Reviewing

In this stage all the evidence/data are brought together, along with the practitioner's and observer's experience of the practice, to examine the results of the action. The main task is to examine the data/evidence, reflect on it and determine the extent to which the pre-specified desired change or outcome was achieved. Generally, for reasons already outlined, the reviewing is more effective if it involves at least one person other than the practitioners. If possible, and if there are no problems of confidentiality or dealing with sensitive evidence, it is often useful to have someone in this stage who has not been part of the previous stages, an outsider who comes fresh to the data/evidence and the discussion of it. Again, different proponents of action research advocate differently in relation to this issue (Reason, 1998).

Usually the review stage results in one of two decisions. The first possibility is that, based on analysis and discussion of the data, it is accepted that the outcome was achieved and there are new foci and outcomes to set. Alternatively, it is decided that the outcomes specified in the cycle were not achieved, or were not achieved fully, and it is necessary to repeat the cycle, possibly with some adjustments to the previous outcomes and/or the data and means to collect it. In either case, the action research cycle moves to the final stage, that of replanning.

## Replanning

It is this stage that is the link from one cycle to the next in the action research spiral. Replanning derives from the previous cycle, its aspirations and results, and begins the next cycle of research activity. This stage employs the same activities as activity 1 above in gradually moving the actions of the practitioners towards the desired improvement.

An important aspect of well-organized and successful action research is that it is a continuous learning spiral. Within the dynamic and accreting activities of each cycle the experience of action-researched practice provides powerful potential for professional learning. This potential is even more significant given that it is the practitioners who are establishing the goals and the parameters of their learning. Further, it is they who decide which aspects of what they learn from their research will be integrated into their practice and how it will be done. As already indicated, if individuals involve and share with others in their action research activity then the potential for learning is further magnified. It is this cooperative inquiry and collective learning that is the basis of the learning organization (Leithwood and Seashore Louis, 1998). For examples of action research in health care, see Meyer (1993), Hart and Bond (1995) and Binnie and Titchen (1999).

The importance of working with others in learning about and improving professional practice has been emphasized in both this and other chapters. This is because, arguably, each of us requires a mirror to reflect ourselves and our actions so that they are available for scrutiny. It is this challenge of self-examination and learning, resulting in increased self-knowledge and self-awareness, that is essential for continual professional and personal growth and development.

## Critical friends

One successful strategy to increase the potential for personal awareness and knowledge is through the use of **critical friends**. A critical friend, as the name suggests, is someone who is both your friend and your critic. The person is a friend in that there exists a relationship between you that provides for a reasonably high level of risk and trust, and that allows you to feel comfortable in confiding and talking openly and honestly, not only about perceptions of events, but particularly about beliefs and feelings. Most important, however, is that your relationship is not so close nor so intimate that either party feels it must never be threatened. This is essential since the equally central role of the critical friend is to act as critic. This may be the more difficult of the two interrelated roles. It includes not only listening and clarifying understanding but also being prepared to identify inconsistencies and contradictions in beliefs, ideas and actions: to challenge and confront, if necessary. It is also concerned with active listening, listening not only to the words but to the feelings, and identifying them to the speaker. A trusted critical friend, one with whom a professional practitioner can authentically risk and share at the deepest confidential level, is perhaps the most powerful stimulus available for learning that not only is deep and lasting, but also is the basis for improved professional practice.

Critical friends come in many different shapes, sizes and configurations. They can be singular or they can function as interconnected dyads or networks. Some writers have argued that, at least in some contexts, critics should be connoisseurs (Eisner, 1979), i.e. they should be highly knowledgeable in the field in which they are a critic. Following this line, dentists would be critical friends for dentists, maths teachers would be critical friends for maths teachers, paediatricians would be critical friends for paediatricians, and so on. While there is some logic and advantage to this, it should also be recognized that in these cases, it is unlikely that either party would be forced to re-examine fundamental principles, beliefs, assumptions or practices, since both parties have most likely been educated, trained, indoctrinated even, in the same paradigms, the same ways of thinking. Thus it is my strong belief, based on research and experience (Smith, 1998) in attempting to implement a critical friend approach to working with final-year student teachers in a university setting over the last ten years, that some of the most powerful questions for learning and change are those that demand a re-examination of taken-for-granted beliefs, assumptions, principles and practices. These are what I call 'stupid questions', questions that an expert in the same field would not ask: they are the questions that challenge and break the *presumed consensus*, that disrupt the accepted and unquestioned reality. These questions are most likely to be asked by someone who is not expert in the same field. In my experience, matching a maths teacher with an English or social science teacher is likely to produce 'stupid' questions and thus holds the potential for powerful re-examination of professional knowledge and the opportunity for new learning and development.

One of the most important characteristics of the concept of critical friends is that it does not take a great deal of resources. There are many examples in education, in the health professions and in business, of programmes of mentoring, or 'shadowing'. Any school, hospital, agency, company or organization can implement an effective structure for professional learning using critical friends. Generally, within such contexts, there is sufficient flexibility to enable such a structure to operate effectively. As already indicated, if an organization is able to implement a collective structure of critical friends, then this can be the basis for the development of a learning organization, an organization in which all members are committed not only to their individual learning and professional growth but also to that of each other and of the entire organization. It is such an organization that will be successful in times of increasing change, ambiguity and uncertainty (Leithwood and Seashore Louis, 1998).

In arguing for the use of critical friends, however, it should be remembered that being an effective critical friend demands a high level of skill as a listener and in forming and sustaining the interpersonal relationship that is the basis for critical friendship. These skills also include the ability to confront in constructively supportive ways, and to resolve conflict. Such skills are not necessarily developed naturally. Any effective critical friends programme must be supported by professional development activities that facilitate the development and maintenance of these skills and understandings.

## Reflection: learning from experience

As already indicated, although each of us as a professional engages in a wide variety of intense experience daily, we do not necessarily learn as much as we can from the experience. It is only in the relative quietness of thinking back on, reflecting, recreating in our mind, reframing, and thinking of alternative actions and their possible consequences, that we are able to bring meaning and understanding to the experience. As also indicated above, such reflection is likely to be more powerful when undertaken with others. In this last section, then, some ideas related to reflection and its relationship to professional learning and the growth of professional knowledge are examined.

Reflection, as with action research, is not a new concept. It originates in practices of both ancient Eastern and Western civilizations (Sumsion, 1997) and continues with the ideas of Dewey and, more recently, Schön (1983, 1987). While there are many definitions of reflection and many arguments about these definitions (Hatton and Smith, 1995), put simply, reflection refers to an active and deliberate attempt to make sense and meaning of experience: to understand what we do and why we do it, and the beliefs, perceptions and assumptions upon which our actions depend (Smith, 1999). As such, it has a central place in professional learning and the development of craft knowledge.

There is no doubt that we can mount training programmes which result in practitioners providing evidence of being reflective (Hatton and Smith, 1995; Sumsion, 1997; Smith, 1998; Hussin, 1999). While there is as yet little, if any, empirical evidence to suggest that a reflective practitioner is more effective than one unreflective, the anecdotal and the passionate creed (Laboskey, 1994) is that being a reflective professional is important, if you are going to understand your practice and the reasons for it (Smith, 1999).

One of the key elements of reflection is the capacity to step back from the immediacy of the practice, reflecting either *in* or *on* action (Schön, 1983), providing the opportunity to make sense of the practice in a new or different manner. There are many strategies that can be employed to facilitate reflection and it is not possible to discuss these in depth here (for a more detailed discussion readers are referred to Hatton and Smith, 1995; Smith, 1999). The strategies include oral strategies, possibly prefaced by some re-creation through imagination or visualization. Such oral strategies include conversations with critical friends; various forms of structured discussion; story-telling and performances such as dramatic presentations and role plays (Cusworth and Simons, 1997), possibly recorded for later discussion, even supported by installations and artworks (Cole and Knowles, 1999). Written strategies, often based on oral work, include diary and journal writing (Sumsion, 1997; Hussin, 1999), and narratives (Connelly and Clandinin, 1990). Poetry, various art forms and more formal reports (Smith, 1991) can also be powerful stimuli for reflection and professional learning. While some form of reflection is essential in the reviewing and replanning stages of action research, it is necessary to consider carefully the particular strategy or strategies which are most appropriate to the purposes and context of the desired reflection. For examples of reflective practice in health care, see Mattingly (1991), Palmer et al. (1994) and Rolfe (1997).

## Conclusions

Continuing professional growth and the development of craft knowledge are central to being an effective practitioner. Such lifelong learning is even more imperative, given the increasingly rapid rate of change and the associated increasing uncertainty and ambiguity of much professional life and its demands. While limited opportunities still exist for professional development provided by higher education institutions and employing agencies, the most ubiquitous and powerful opportunities for learning lie in the ongoing systematic investigation of daily practice.

Action research is one of the oldest and most validated forms of systematic investigation of practice by practitioners themselves, with the goals of learning about and understanding better their own practice, and effecting its improvement. In this chapter I have outlined the nature and processes of action research as a basis for professional learning. It has been argued that engaging critical friends in these processes increases the potential for such learning. Finally, it is essential that, to optimize the learning from experience and action research, opportunities for reflection, for reframing and for considering alternatives for action must be provided. The chapter has suggested some possible strategies for such reflection and processing.

## References


Binnie, A. and Titchen, A. (1999) *Freedom to Practise: The Development of Patient-Centred Nursing*. Oxford: Butterworth-Heinemann.

Cole, A. and Knowles, G. (1999) Arts based inquiry. Installation presented at the American Education Research Association Meeting, Montreal, April.

Connelly, M. and Clandinin, J. (1990) Stories of experience and narrative inquiry. *Educational Researcher*, **19**(5), 2–14.

Cusworth, R. and Simons, J. (1997) *Beyond the Script: Drama in the Classroom*. Sydney: Primary English Teachers' Association.

Denzin, N. and Lincoln, Y. (eds) (1998) *Strategies of Qualitative Inquiry*. Thousand Oaks, CA: Sage Publications.

Eisner, E. (1979) *The Educational Imagination: On the Design and Evaluation of School Programs*. New York: Macmillan.

Elliott, J. (1991) *Action Research for Education Change*. Buckingham: Open University Press.

Elliott, J. (1993) *Reconstructing Teacher Education: Teacher Development*. London: Falmer Press.

Ewing, R. and Smith, D. (2001) Doing, being and becoming in professional practice. In *Professional Practice in Health, Education and the Creative Arts* (J. Higgs and A. Titchen, eds). Oxford: Blackwell Science.

Fullan, M. (1993) *Change Forces: Probing the Depths of Educational Reform*. London: Falmer Press.

Grundy, S. (1995) *Action Research as Professional Development*. Occasional Paper no. 1, Innovative Links between Universities and Schools for Teacher Professional Development. Western Australia: Murdoch University.

Hart, E. and Bond, M. (1995) *Action Research for Health and Social Care*. Buckingham: Open University Press.

Hatton, N. and Smith, D. (1995) Reflection in teacher education: Towards definition and implementation. *Teaching and Teacher Education*, **11**(1), 33–49.

Heron, J. (1992) *Feeling and Personhood: Psychology in Another Key*. London: Sage.

Hussin, H. (1999) Learning to be reflective. PhD thesis, University of Sydney.

Kemmis, S. and McTaggart, R. (1990) *The Action Research Reader*. Victoria: Deakin University Press.

Knowles, G., Cole, A. and Presswood, C. (1994) *Through Preservice Teachers' Eyes: Exploring Field Experiences Through Narrative and Inquiry*. New York: Macmillan.

Laboskey, V. L. (1994) *Development of Reflective Practice: A Study of Preservice Teachers*. New York: Teachers' College Press.

Leithwood, K. and Seashore Louis, K. (eds) (1998) *Organisational Learning in Schools. Contexts of Learning*. Netherlands: Lisse: Swets & Zeitlinger.

Lovat, T. and Smith, D. (1995) *Curriculum: Action on Reflection Revisited*, 3rd edn. Wentworth Falls, New South Wales: Social Science Press.

Mattingly, C. (1991) Narrative reflections on practical actions: Two learning experiments in reflective storytelling. In *The Reflective Turn* (D. Schön, ed.), pp. 235–257. London: Teachers' College Press.

Meyer, J. (1993) Lay participation in care: A challenge for multidisciplinary teamwork. *Journal of Interprofessional Care*, **7**, 57–66.

Palmer, A., Burns, S. and Bulman, C. (1994) *Reflective Practice in Nursing: The Growth of the Professional Practitioner*. Oxford: Blackwell Scientific Publications.

Reason, P. (ed.) (1994) *Participation in Human Inquiry*. London: Sage Publications.

Reason, P. (1998) Three approaches to participative inquiry. In *Strategies of Qualitative Inquiry* (N. Denzin and Y. Lincoln, eds), pp. 261–291. Thousand Oaks, CA: Sage Publications.

Rolfe, G. (1997) Beyond expertise: Theory, practice and the reflexive practitioner. *Journal of Clinical Nursing*, **6**, 93–97.

Schön, D. A. (1983) *The Reflective Practitioner: How Professionals Think in Action*. London: Temple Smith.

Schön, D. A. (1987) *Educating the Reflective Practitioner: Toward a New Design for Teaching and Learning in the Professions*. San Francisco: Jossey-Bass.

Senge, P. (1990) *The Fifth Discipline: The Art and Practice of the Learning Organization*. Sydney: Random House.

Smith, D. (1991) Educating reflective practitioners in curriculum. *Curriculum*, **12**, 115–124.

Smith, D. (1998) Facilitating reflective practice in professional preservice education: Challenging some sacred cows. In *PEPE: Practical Experiences in Professional Education*, Research Monograph No. 2 (A. Yarrow and J. Millwater, eds). Brisbane, Auckland: University of Technology.

Smith, D. (1999) *The what, why and how of reflective practice in teacher education. Invited keynote address presented to Faculty of Education staff, Auckland College of Education, February 2*. Auckland College of Education.

Sumsion, J. (1997) Early childhood students' reflection on their professional development and practice: A longitudinal study. PhD thesis, University of Sydney.

Zuber-Skerritt, O. (1996) *New Directions in Action Research*. London: The Falmer Press.

# 23

# Professional craft knowledge and curricula: what are we really teaching?

**Sherrill A. Conroy**

Professional craft knowledge (PCK) refers to the practical know-how needed to practise within a chosen profession. Educators develop curricula with a goal of sharing practical strategies for students to implement PCK. Explicit curricula are available to students in the form of course outlines, course notes, and lectures. However, perhaps even more powerful than explicit material in shaping future health professionals are values, assumptions and PCK taught through implicit means, such as role modelling, by educators in class and clinical practice. I explore some relationships between explicit, implicit and null curricula in this chapter. When two or more concepts are explicitly espoused, implicit curricula can act to promote the values of one concept to the detriment of the other(s). This chapter highlights the effects of competition rather than collaboration, between and across curricula.

Know-how for health care students resides in acquisition of several complementary domains of PCK, including competent, scientifically based health care delivery (scientific PCK, or attention to measurable, physical dimensions of people) and holistic practice (holistic PCK, or responsive attending to clients' physical, intellectual, social, spiritual and emotional needs). Explicit teaching in one domain should augment the other. However, problems occur if implicit teaching of reductionist values, such as those taught in basic sciences, is preferred by educators over the demonstration of holistic values in practice. The dominant valuing of reductionist approaches at a study university[1] may prevent students from acquiring and realizing practical strategies to implement holistic values. Two ways in which this dominant valuing is transmitted to students are:

1 educators implicitly demonstrating detached approaches to health care delivery when acting as role models in classroom and clinical areas;
2 distanced approaches resulting in an unacknowledged disregard for explicitly taught holistic health care concepts.

I describe three curricular influences and then look at how some of the underlying assumptions can affect teaching. Quotations from students' narratives illustrate the effects of the dominance of reductionist values on the acquisition of holistic PCK. Suggestions to develop synergy between and across curricular influences complete the chapter.

## Three curricular influences

Many influences shape what students learn. Three influences that stem from curricula (Eisner, 1985; Shepard and Jensen, 1990; Watson and Ashton, 1995) are:

- **Explicit curriculum** (includes formal instructional design). In health care programmes, it concentrates heavily on the acquisition of scientific PCK and skill, including discipline-specific knowledge such as anatomy and physiology, physical assessment skills (Wellard and Edwards, 1999) and procedures. People are viewed through a biological lens framed by specific diseased body parts. Explicit teaching in holistic PCK includes therapeutic communication skills and values, including the idea of the client being more than the sum of biological parts, and client self-responsibility for wellness.

- **Implicit curriculum** (sometimes called the **hidden curriculum**). Although not formally acknowledged, educators may, upon reflection, admit to it. Attitudes towards people, procedures, health care organizational proceedings, and authority, for example, are subtly passed on to students. Implicit teaching in clinical areas may negate principles taught in class (see Denscombe, 1982, 1985; Sinclair, 1997).
- **Null curriculum**. This refers to what is consciously or unconsciously excluded from students' education. It eliminates items not prioritized as having enough importance to teach in an overloaded programme. However, omission in teaching of certain concepts can mask deeply ingrained prejudices against particular ideas or groups of people.

As one student, Annie, perceptively noted:

> We're going to be learning by watching how they act to a certain extent and obviously some of it will be copying . . . what they do . . . We're not just going to be copying blindly but I think there is some transference that happens and we *will pick up* some of these behaviours. [her emphasis]

## Curricular influences and underlying assumptions in action

Explicit teaching in health care PCK includes: (i) scientifically based health care; (ii) 'principlism'-based ethical decision-making (see below); and (iii) holistic approaches to care. Two potential outcomes can occur in classroom/clinical practice if reductionist-based PCK jockeys for position with holistic PCK:

1. Values associated with reductionist scientific endeavours override those inherent in holistic health care. Scientific practitioners value technical competence, objective distancing from 'the problem', statistical proof for claims to 'best care'. Holistic practitioners value ethical principles such as compassion, caring, collaboration, particularity, reciprocity and practical connection to clients viewed as 'whole persons'(Berger and Williams, 1992; Rawlins et al., 1993).
2. 'Space' for holism is similarly overtaken by a more reductionist approach to ethics as expressed in Beauchamp and Childress's (1994) **principlism theory**. Principlism advocates the use of four particular principles as seemingly paramount over other ethical principles. Some values, such as truth-telling and autonomy, are common to the two ethical approaches of principlism and holism. However, when two reductionistic approaches to health care, as found in principlism and scientific investigation, are combined, holism runs the risk of being excluded or diminished.

I argue that reductionist approaches foster a lack of respect for and an objectification of persons. Distancing from people supports paternalistic modes of practice, wherein the attitude of the practitioner suggests that clinicians are the only authorities on health care. Such practice might be derived from at least three implicit assumptions, operationalized by educators, which mitigate against holistically therapeutic practice. These interrelated assumptions are:

- superiority of science;
- principlism will cover all aspects of everyday ethics;
- practitioners are arbiters of health knowledge.

Although these assumptions may be consciously rejected by educators, they sometimes imbue classroom/clinical practice. Whilst recognizing that many professionals deliver caring, compassionate, clinically competent, collaborative practice, I have selected the following excerpts from student narratives to illustrate counterproductive curricular influences on PCK acquisition. Thus, practitioners here do not appear in the best light.

### Assumption 1: superiority of science

This assumption advances the idea that modern science can understand and predict ways to cure disease. The comfortable feeling this 'certainty' engenders, accompanied by a drive for efficiency, helps to counter unease about the many 'unknowns' in the human side of health care. Modern biotechnological advances have helped to foster this assumption. Nevertheless, it is recognized in preliminary courses that the human element in health care must be addressed with students. One introductory course explicitly teaches ideals of holistic health care, such as:

- a person's value is greater than the sum of their bodily parts;
- practitioners facilitate the full expression of a person's physical, emotional, intellectual, social and spiritual potential;
- compassionate care for the person as a unified entity is a given;
- client-centred responsibility for health care is desirable.

The sheer volume of classroom hours devoted to subjects such as anatomy, pathophysiology and other scientifically related material, helps to push holistic concepts taught in the introductory course to the recesses of student attention. The human body is compartmentalized into organs and systems. Heavy reliance upon explicit and implicit teaching of scientific reductionism encourages a belief that application of research-based knowledge alone equals 'excellent' care. With an emphasis on what is statistically proven for the larger population, there is a risk of forgetting the art of responding with compassion and respect to the particular concerns and understandings of individual clients. In an environment where body parts are examined more intensely than the whole person, moral issues arise because people are categorized. Such objectification of people is incongruent with holistic ideals.

Animal experimentation is also used for explicit introductions to scientific health care. Repeated films showing the severing of cats' nerves unsettles Peter:

> Everything is based on animal research . . . pretty exclusively until it gets to clinical work where it's applied to . . . performed on human subjects in a different way and then you get human results and there is absolutely no acknowledgement whatsoever . . . from any of the profs, that there is even a moral issue in this fact . . . and even among the students who just accept . . . it seems normal to them that they don't even blink an eye.

Peter's last sentence suggests that despite the concomitant explicit valuing of holistic practice, educators implicitly transfer an atomistic model to first-year students. In addition, the professor may not consider the 'client as person', but only see the 'patient as a body part to be repaired'. Wider ethical implications of animal experimentation upon health care delivery are not addressed by the professor.

Students, expected explicitly to assimilate quickly huge amounts of scientific minutiae, do not have time to question the relevance of the information to a client's particular situation. Learning may become rote, a blur of pathophysiology and microbiology, rather than a critical, reflective experience. Fast-paced learning coupled with implicit emphasis on speed in client encounters encourages the objectification of clients and students alike. Peter recounts:

> Here I am, the first time in a hospital, the first time dealing with the patients, and *[the instructor]* is sitting over me going 'quicker, quicker, quicker' *[with my treatments]. [my parentheses]*

Brief, hurried encounters diminish chances of practising therapeutic communication and caring skills taught explicitly in introductory courses. Students are expected to be able to rationalize their time, their knowledge and their emotions. Absent is recognition of the moral dimension when treating people as objects on a statistical conveyor belt. Rowan tells a similar story to Peter's:

> You've never even seen the patient before. And they'd have like at least 1000 past medical problems, and I'm sorry. It's going to take me an, at least an hour to do this . . . He dumped, he dumped this . . . patient on me and said, 'I'll be back in seven minutes'. Like 'ask, find out what's wrong with her and I'll be back in seven minutes'. So I looked at her and I'm like, 'So tell me your entire life story in seven minutes'.

These accounts suggest that it is left to students to develop the artful know-how of interacting holistically in fast-paced practice settings. One can infer from this evidence, and from findings in other research studies of newly qualified practitioners (e.g. Lathlean, 1987; Dowling and Barrett, 1991; Sinclair, 1997; Binnie and Titchen, 1998; Titchen, 2000) that students need role models who articulate PCK in practice to help them, for example, to get to know the client as a person or to use the initial assessment as an opportunity to establish a therapeutic relationship.

Annie recounts a Dantesque scenario wherein all pretence of relating to the client as an autonomous, dignified participator in health care was dropped by physician and nurse. She outlines a situation where the client was seen as a 'diagnostic problem' and not as a person in pain. Client dignity was stripped by the situation and by practitioners' thoughtless exposure of her body to a roomful of students:

This person's screaming on the table . . . we felt powerless . . . watching what was happening . . . The doctor would just go on with this thing . . . 'We see this part of the colon and this and this and I don't see any problems' and describing how the endoscope works, as though everything was normal and fine . . . I think the major (problem) was that . . . he wasn't trained to show how this works . . . to students. He wasn't trained to . . . take care of his patient either. I think he was relying on the nurses to do that and they didn't . . . He was just trained to do an endoscopy and make sure that this person was fine or not fine or what the disease was.

This narrative suggests that educators explicitly teach the value of scientific knowledge. Implicitly, they can teach how to treat humans in an objectified, distanced way. Such objectification is reinforced when clients are referred to by their bed number or by a diseased body part. Strategies that respect the dignity and unity of persons are not taught by such practices.

### Assumption 2: principlism will cover all aspects of everyday ethics

Principlism, as espoused by Beauchamp and Childress (1994) and as taught in formal lectures, champions four ethical principles: autonomy, justice, beneficence and non-maleficence. Proponents of rule-bound, duty-based principlism reduce ethical debate to a balancing and prioritizing of these four principles when searching for universalizable solutions to ethical dilemmas. In emphasizing these particular principles or values, other values such as connection, caring, collaboration and community-oriented morality taught in holistic health care are excluded. Lecturers present case studies to students, framed within principlism's values, when considering what the practitioner should do in the client's best interest. In situations described to me, rarely was class time allotted for participatory discussion although that prospect was dangled tantalizingly in front of students. Such discussions might encourage exchanges between students and educators in consideration of practical strategies of how to use holistic principles in clinical settings. Interestingly, students did not report any instances of principlism being utilized explicitly in their clinical experience, in spite of the fact that up to three blocks of lecture time were allotted to teaching a principlism-based approach to ethical decision-making.

So what kind of ethical approach to clinical action was demonstrated if neither principlism nor holistic orientations were articulated explicitly in clinical practice? A reductionist, distanced approach, as encouraged in scientific work (see Sinclair, 1997), and as used when balancing principles in classroom lectures, shone through implicitly in many clinical encounters. Although principlism theory advocates client autonomy and dignity, the 'object of interest' for the scientifically oriented practitioner might comfortably 'default' to body parts or technical dimensions of care, rather than a therapeutic engagement with people's concerns. Thus, for the scientifically and principlism oriented practitioner, a quick acceptance of universal solutions to ethical decision-making can occur, resulting in practitioner-dominated decision-making and lost opportunities for connection with autonomous clients.

Holism favours personal, contextualized solutions to ethical dilemmas wherein the client is an active decision-maker. Collaboration between practitioner and client in health care is important. When role models implicitly pay close attention to technical/psychomotor skills, such as the respirologist in the following excerpt, opportunities are lost for holistic PCK building, such as practical strategies for connection to clients. The respirologist nullifies any particularized, holistic connection to the person to whose chest he is listening. Care-**to** overrides caring-**for**. Annie observes:

My doctor in particular doesn't seem to listen much to what the person says. I'm a little biased in the sense that I feel he's not a very good role model because he, he's not . . . doing the things *[implicit]* that we've been at least told so far *[explicit]* that seem to be good . . . but in any case, yes, he, he'll do the small things, like listen to the chest, check the oxygen pressure because he is a respirologist . . . and ask the person how they're doing a little bit. But . . . nothing . . . too important. Nothing too . . . caring *[null]*. *[my parentheses]*

### Assumption 3: practitioners are arbiters of health knowledge

An implicit assumption that practitioners are arbiters of knowledge in matters pertaining to health sits comfortably with reductionist scientific practice and decision models. The 'doctor knows best' belief promotes paternalistic practice vs. client self-responsibility for health care. Paternalistic practice may be an attempt by practitioners to avoid emotional over-engagement with clients and to ensure 'best care' for clients who have less medical knowledge than practitioners. However, the balance might swing easily towards under-engagement with and distancing from clients.

Evidence that students in the study acquired the PCK of power-differential-maintenance between professional and patient suggests that students are exposed to paternalistic communication in practice. Peter, in reflecting on his first year, notes that he prefers the use of the holistic term 'client' to the more patronizing 'patient'. He dislikes the common practice of referring to a person by their disease. However, by his third year, Peter also refers to someone as 'the Stroke'. As mentioned earlier, calling a person by their disease is a distancing technique frequently used in 'caring' professions. It reflects the importance placed on body parts and pathology over seeing persons holistically. How has Peter learned this practical strategy for maintaining the power differential and depersonalized care? It appears that subtle, disrespectful communication between clinicians and their students and their clients demonstrates a power imbalance that favours the clinician, in both relationships, and role-models the following strategies.

The power differential is maintained in various ways. For example, a typical instructional mode in medicine involves bedside rounds where up to eleven students encircle the bed, observing clinician and client. Annie notes:

> Often . . . consent from the patient for us to be there is asked once we're at the bedside . . . I don't think it's fair to assume that they know it's a teaching hospital so they should be all right with that and they know that you're a medical doctor, so it's 'okay'.

The power imbalance is exacerbated by implicit treatment of clients as objects of observation. Paying lip service to client autonomy can occur when educators fail to demonstrate strategies which uphold client dignity and partnership in their care. Annie is acquiring holistic PCK, demonstrated by her attention to the client's dignity, without the benefit of expert role-modelling:

> This person is very vulnerable and not necessarily happy or . . . not necessarily in a good state of mind or strong. I know every time I feel very uncomfortable and I have a tendency to . . . lag behind the group to thank the person personally before I leave.

Tutorial discussions, regarding accessibility of professionals to clients and knowledge sharing with them, are consistent with explicit holistic lecture content about client dignity and autonomy. However, that dignity is diminished in clinical areas if clients are perceived, implicitly, without evidence, as emotionally or intellectually incapable of digesting medical information. 'One doctor said, "Most patients you'll see are dumber than you are" . . . And that was just last week', reports first-year student Louis. There may be a failure to recognize that it is the use of medical language, and not the client's intellect, that might be building barriers to the client's understanding of health problems and solutions. Practical strategies to communicate scientific knowledge in everyday language at bedside teaching rounds were often absent. At the beginning of his programme, Rowan felt people should be more informed by staff about their diagnosis and prognosis. However, he agreed by the end of his third year that patients should not be 'confused' by telling them in the early days of investigation and treatment what their disease was or what the proposed course of medical action would be. He believed the average person could not contend with too many variables. Through adopting the implicit beliefs of his role models, he acquired the PCK used in paternalistic practice. He did not know how to put into action the principles taught in holistic class content, relating to client self-responsibility for health care and collaboration between practitioner and client.

Detached observation of clients, as if they were objects under a microscope, promotes emotional distancing from clients. 'I couldn't actually reach out to that person at that moment. Still feel like I was behind some glass wall observing', states Annie. She was semi-paralysed by hierarchical constraints and the implicit detachment personified in the 'clinician'. Sometimes practitioners capitalize on a client's inability to talk and therefore inability to convey consent to student presence and teaching. Rowan described the removal of a respirator so that the students could take turns listening to breath sounds in spite of obvious client discomfort. A strong implicit message is sent to students that the client is an object of learning, an abstract tool for instructive purposes. Similarly, when students are taken to see colonoscopies on a sedated person, consent may not be requested, leaving clients dimly aware of student presence. Informed consent, respect for the person, autonomy, compassion and caring appear disregarded.

The idea of the client as an active, willing, autonomous partner in a collaborative quest for health is not being transmitted in practice (null curriculum) to the student. Missing are practical strategies to realize collaborative ideals. In keeping both physical and emotional distance from people, an implicit message is sent to students and clients alike that detachment is acceptable practice in a hierarchical structure. In recognizing that implicit message, Shane and Annie hope they will experience positive, long-lasting learning to prevent them from objectifying clients through their own verbal and body language. They hope to remember not to maintain the physician–client power differential through being condescending and arrogant.

*Shane:* In my learning experience, I'm looking, watching and not doing all that much yet, mostly observing . . . When I see something that I like . . . whether it's the way a doctor talks to the patient or, which you see a lot of . . . I . . . put it away and when I see stuff I don't like, which I see a lot of – condescension, arrogance – and I'll file that away and also as a kind of caveat to myself that I didn't like it . . . so don't fall into that trap at age 35 when I'll probably be a doctor . . . I think . . . the doctor–patient relationship is . . . even more than the educator–student relationship, a one way street.

*Annie:* Having the whole group in there, makes the interaction seem . . . as though . . . there's this huge distance between us and them, as though we're observing this tiny little animal in a cage and I don't think that's fair. I think it's a great gift that they're giving to us . . . of sharing what they're living and their experiences . . . My first experience in the hospital was like that and it bothered me for the whole week after . . . I don't know if that'll change. I've been told that, that's the way it's going to be throughout my whole residency unfortunately.

In communication classes, students are taught to view the person in a holistic way. However, implicit curriculum presented in practice placements desensitizes students to patients' humanity, emotions and needs. Students' experiences of role models' behaviour, towards both themselves and clients, set the scene for disengagement from people who are suffering. They learn strategies to achieve disengagement, such as physical aversion to client contact. As suggested in the above excerpts, this desensitization occurs because students are exposed to repetitive 'stripping' of clients' dignity by practising professionals. Rowan had some troubles with emergency room doctors and nurses when trying to find out if a woman on a stretcher in the hallway could have some water:

So I go to the doctor. 'Is it OK if this woman has a glass of water?' 'Oh, why are you bothering us with this?' *[They reply]* . . . So then the next time I walk by the woman I avert my eyes . . . after 3 or 4 times this happens . . . that I get no help from the nurses or from the doctors, I don't want to help these patients any more that are lying in the hall.

Slowly Rowan is detaching himself from being connected to needy people and assuming the remote professional mode of the (implicit) role models around him. Louis comments: 'I think isolation in medical school helps exacerbate isolation in the hospital'. He observes that as a student 'you sit on your haunches and you analyse the world from a very distant point of view'. Practitioners may be fearful of becoming overly involved with clients. Nevertheless, they are not demonstrating practical strategies to achieve a balance between over- and under-engagement with others, as client-centred practitioners manage to do (see Binnie and Titchen, 1999; Titchen, 2000).

## Conclusions

To become rounded professionals, health care students need to acquire and integrate a number of PCK domains. In this chapter I have been concerned with the integration (and lack of it) of two of these domains, the practical strategies for delivering (i) scientifically based health care and (ii) holistic care. It has been shown that educators' implicitly held values and assumptions can shape students' ultimate learning through supplanting some explicitly taught concepts in favour of others. In this case, the concepts of holistic care (and its valuing of the client as a participant in care decisions) were overridden by those of scientifically based care (and its valuing of the superiority of science). This overriding was demonstrated by the kinds of practical strategy that students were exposed to and those to which they were not exposed. I conclude, therefore, that the values and assumptions explicated by practising professionals determine the substance of the PCK that students acquire in the clinical setting. The implicit teaching, offered through their role models' behaviour in the heat of clinical action, is likely to form the basis of students' most powerful and long-lasting learning.

The observations of this chapter suggest that students' clinical experiences often fail to furnish them with examples of practical strategies for bolstering client collaboration in health care. Instead, they are exposed to the strategies of paternalism, depersonalization, objectification and distancing. Distancing by professionals from their clientele is an implicit enactment of the scientific mode of disengagement with the 'object' of interest. The data suggest that, over time, it is these strategies that are acquired and practised by students.

The tensions and incongruities between explicit, implicit and null curricula need to be critically debated, if parallel curricular paths are to be articulated, integrated and implemented. Commitment to this debate presupposes a collaborative learning culture in the educational setting. In addition, it is likely that faculty and clinicians will need support in developing and implementing genuinely integrated curricula. The following suggestions, therefore, are offered for debate, critique of practice and development support:

- The philosophical and ethical bases of practice and of educational goals, as determined by faculty, should be examined.
- Kuhse's (1997) suggestion that ethics teaching should concern itself with the affective or dispositional aspect of ethical practice could be considered.
- Faculty and involved clinicians should be encouraged, individually and collectively, to critically reflect upon and articulate their fundamental values, assumptions and ideals.
- Faculty's commitment to the values and assumptions identified as desirable by the faculty in pursuit of excellent practice should be assessed.
- Faculty should be helped to identify differences between espoused values and values in action, perhaps by inviting students to share their experiences of clinical education and by really listening to what they have to say.
- Explicit curriculum should be re-examined in light of balance, approaches, emphasis and assumptions, such as those examined in this chapter, to consider what students are encouraged to value.
- Educators could engage in critical reflection upon their practice and upon alternative ways of teaching, involving clients and students in the process.
- Educators and practitioners could be helped to become aware of the nature of PCK and of how its acquisition can be facilitated. (See Chapter 5.)
- Critical companionship skills could be developed in good clinical role models. (See Chapter 10.)
- Opportunities should be provided for tutorial discussion about contradictory practices and about how students can (i) retain their beliefs and values about holistic, therapeutic health care and (ii) how they might change culture/world views in the future when they have the authority to change practice.

In all of the above, educators might find it helpful to work in partnership with their clinical colleagues by developing in-service education based on good practice and mutual learning. Titchen and Higgs (1999) suggest one such approach.

## Note

1 This chapter is based on selected findings from the author's work in progress. Sixteen medical, nursing and physiotherapy undergraduate students at a Canadian university gave multiple interviews, narrating reflections on their experiences and observations regarding their education to date. An interpretive phenomenological approach to the research offered an unprecedented glimpse into aspects of moral agency in these health science students. Pseudonyms mask their identities in this chapter.

## References

Beauchamp, T. L. and Childress, J. F. (1994) *Principles of Biomedical Ethics*, 4th edn. New York: Oxford University Press.

Berger, K. J. and Williams, M. B. (1992) *Fundamentals of Nursing: Collaborating for Optimal Health.* Norwalk, CT: Appleton & Lange.

Binnie, A. and Titchen, A. (1998) *Patient-Centred Nursing: An Action Research Study of Practice Development in an Acute Medical Unit.* Report No. 18. Oxford: Royal College of Nursing Institute.

Binnie, A. and Titchen, A. (1999) *Freedom to Practise: A Study of the Development of Patient-Centred Nursing in an Acute Medical Unit.* Oxford: Butterworth-Heinemann.

Denscombe, M. (1982) The hidden pedagogy and its implications for teacher training. *British Journal of Sociology of Education*, **3**, 249–265.

Denscombe, M. (1985) *Classroom Control: A Sociological Perspective*. London: Croom Helm.

Dowling, S. and Barrett, S. (1991) *Doctors in the Making: The Experience of the Pre-Registration Year*. Bristol: SAUS Publications.

Eisner, E. (1985) *The Educational Imagination: On Design and Implementation of School Programs*, 2nd edn. New York: Macmillan Publishing.

Kuhse, H. (1997) *Caring: Nurses, Women and Ethics*. Oxford: Blackwell Publishers.

Lathlean, J. (1997) Prepared transition. *Nursing Times*, **83**(37), 43–47.

Rawlins, R. P., Williams, S. R. and Beck, C. K. (1993) *Mental Health – Psychiatric Nursing: A Holistic Life-Cycle Approach*. St Louis, MO: Mosby Year Book.

Shepard, K. F. and Jensen, G. M. (1990) Physical therapist curricula for the 1990s: Educating the reflective practitioner. *Physical Therapy*, **70**(9), 566–575.

Sinclair, S. (1997) *Making Doctors: An Institutional Apprenticeship*. Oxford: Berg.

Titchen, A. (2000) *Professional Craft Knowledge in Patient-Centred Nursing and the Facilitation of its Development*. DPhil thesis, University of Oxford; Oxford: Ashdale Press.

Titchen, A. and Higgs, J. (1999) Facilitating the development of knowledge. In *Educating Beginning Practitioners: Challenges for Health Professional Education* (J. Higgs and H. Edwards, eds), pp. 180–188. Oxford: Butterworth-Heinemann.

Watson, B. and Ashton, E. (1995) *Education, Assumptions and Values*. London: David Fulton.

Wellard, R. and Edwards, H. (1999) Curriculum models for educating beginning practitioners. In *Educating Beginning Practitioners* (J. Higgs and H. Edwards, eds), pp. 61–69. Oxford: Butterworth-Heinemann.

## Additional reading

Gould, S. J. (1996) *The Mismeasure of Man*. London: Penguin Books.

Green, R. M., Gert, B. and Clouser, K. D. (1993) The method of public morality versus the method of principlism. *Journal of Medicine and Philosophy*, **18**, 477–489.

Veatch, R. (1973) The medical model: Its nature and problems. *Hastings Centre Studies*, **1**, 57–59.

# 24

# Using practical knowledge of the creative arts to foster learning

**Jennifer Simons and Robyn Ewing**

Professional practice today is quite different from the traditional model, where the client was knowledge-limited and therefore a passive recipient of knowledge transmitted by the in-command professional. Current practice involves knowledge-sharing between the professional and the client, with each developing metacognitive awareness of the learning process. This chapter takes a unique slant on the role of the professional in fostering learning. Learning in the arts prioritizes the practice knowledge of the professional and the life experience knowledge of the client. We recognize the often tacit, frequently non-communicated nature of this knowledge. This field is highly complex and incorporates both intuition and body language as part of the communicative process between professional and client.

In this chapter we place professional artistry under scrutiny. In our roles as educators, we use the creative arts to foster learning about learning, knowledge and professional practice. We explore two dimensions of knowing and the creative arts. One is knowing **in** the creative arts, the way practising artists come to know about their art. This form of embodied knowing is illustrated in three cameos in which the nature of knowing in the creative arts is portrayed through the eyes of artists. The second way of knowing explored here is knowing **through** the creative arts. We argue that the arts (e.g. drama, which is used as an exemplar) enable learners and teachers to engage with topics in a different way from other learning strategies, enabling a deeper form of embodied knowing to occur. Knowing **through** the arts can be used to learn the art itself (such as with music and drama students preparing for a career in these fields) or to learn about other topics (such as learning about complex issues related to living in society). In addition, the creative arts can be used to foster the development of generic skills such as interpersonal skills and creativity. Whether learners are coming to know **in** or **through** the creative arts, or whether they are learning about the arts, or about other knowledge or skill areas, what these activities have in common is embodied knowledge and embodied learning. This embodied knowledge, we argue, is the essence of knowing in drama particularly, and in the creative arts in general. Embodied knowledge is also a core dimension of the caring professions including teaching and health care. Titchen (2000), for instance, talks about graceful care, where grace, being a physical as well as an emotional, intentional attribute, is lived in professional practice.

The bulk of the chapter is presented through the eyes and minds of teachers (in this case primary school teachers) who are using the creative arts (particularly drama) to foster the development of embodied knowing and embodied knowledge. This strategy has provided a closer look at the essential connections between knowing and the creative arts. In preparing to help students learn about and through drama, the teacher has first to understand what it means to know in the creative arts. The teacher needs to learn from artists themselves what it is to know and practise in the creative arts. The following cameos bring this knowing to life.

## Valda Craig: knowing as a dancer

A great dance book has the title 'knowing in my bones'. Knowing occurs when you find the focus, the idea, the intention of the dance. You go into a studio and from an empty space play with music for images or an idea or even nothing and let the intention come. When it comes you just know – you feel it . . . I think the knowing is inside you – both head and heart; intellect and emotion have to come together. You know if it is 'there' or 'not quite there' . . . All the steps mean something to the dancer/choreographer; all belong to the focus or the theme or the feeling or the idea of the piece. Each movement belongs – it's not just a pretty step, not just a gap filler. (If it is a gap filler, there's a knowing that it is not quite right.) There is honesty and integrity. The colleagues, the dancers working with you, give material and ideas and the choreographer uses their material, adapts, adjusts, uses the techniques or the elements of composing, selects the spatial, temporal, dynamic according to the theme or intent – and refers back to them. Between them they *know* when it gels, when it belongs, satisfies, serves the intent. So I guess intuition is part of it as well . . . I guess feeling and knowing are as one. Playing with, taking risks, trusting self and the dancers, allowing changes, having guts to edit and to edit and edit, knowing that it has to be streamlined, not self-indulgent . . .

### Libby Gleeson: knowing as a writer

I think that I am somebody who is hooked on the notion of story – I think it's a fundamental thing that we do. I'm hooked on language. I actually believe that we can promote worthwhile reading and I want other people to share that so I write stories to make them read. If I have a mission at all it's to make readers think and to share the storymaking process with other people. Now I also happen to be a fairly moral person, I think, so a lot of my own personal ethics and so on are in the stories but I certainly don't set out to say: 'I want to write a book about "x" and that's my only purpose'. Issues and other ideas certainly are invested in all of those works but the most fundamental issue is about my need to explore my ideas through story and language. So much of my writing has come out of family life or a personal experience and at the same time I think none of it is autobiographical because it's all been fictionalised. So many ideas are generated by the writing process itself. To get these understandings you have to watch and watch. I think I agree with Kate Grenville that the difference between a novelist or a writer and those that don't write is that we all see the same things but the person who's writing sees the potential of a story in them. You see I think everyone's got stories to tell but it's a question of plucking it out and then fictionalising and constructing and putting a certain edge on them. I mean the birth of a baby in a family is both an ordinary, everyday event that happens to millions everyday as well as being the most significant thing that can happen in the life of that family. It just depends how you want to construct that story whether or not for a book or a poem or a play. There's a long phase where I edit. I rewrite as I go along the whole time and so much of this is intuitive, a type of knowing . . .

### Camilla Ah Kin: knowing as an actor

It (knowing) seemed to emerge slowly as I became conscious of the power and responsibility and ordinariness of this particular vocation. In terms of 'knowing' technically, perceptions of what is a good and edgy performance constantly develop and change; some of the acting produced from the Lee Strasberg school in the 60s would be considered old-fashioned now. What remains important is being conscious that one is in the middle of a process. When I first began my training and career as an actor I was able to saturate myself in the art form, its history and current content. Suddenly I became capable of assimilating much more, and at a faster rate than I ever had at school or in tertiary education. I found a 'language' that touched me profoundly, that took on a sacred quality. Instinctively I knew what to do with the language: I discovered a natural awareness of what various compositions of stage elements might give to an outcome, i.e. the story. Moreover this ability (though raw) was valued and nurtured in this environment. I finally unlocked my capacity to learn. A revelation of this type probably happens every couple of years; it may be a particular actor I work with, or a writer whose work I 'understand' or a political fury. I become aware that I am being bumped onto a new level of understanding humanity, a compassion, and for me that is the power of the storyteller, illuminator, actor, artist.

## Learning about knowing in the creative arts

There are different kinds of knowing just as there are different kinds of intelligence. Habermas (1972) has conceptualized three kinds of knowing; broadly, they are:

1 that which is scientifically provable and is technical and analytical;
2 that which is related to hermeneutics and negotiated through language;
3 that which is learned by experience and is self-reflective (Lovat and Smith, 1995).

Writing from a psychological perspective, Gardner (1993) has identified eight intelligences, several of which entail the concept of the body operating in space (e.g. kinaesthetic, intrapersonal and interpersonal intelligences). Each of the artists quoted above reflects primarily Habermas's second and third types of knowing, and all see intrapersonal reflection as crucial to their art.

Educational institutions, however, continue to overvalue scientific and technical ways of knowing and linguistic and mathematical/logical intelligences. Learning in the arts is often treated as a mere exercise of skills rather than developing a particular type of knowledge. Knowing in the creative arts encompasses the three kinds of knowing described by Habermas (1972), although it may not always be useful or even possible to compartmentalize knowledge in this way.

### Learning content through the creative arts

Knowing in the arts, and especially in drama, involves the whole person: body, mind, feelings and spirit (Morgan, 1998). As Peter Medway (1980) argued, all good teaching validates pre-disciplinary knowledge or 'knowledge we have acquired from the unsystematic processes of living' (p. 8). However, it is a feature of the arts that they take this knowledge, make it more conscious and help students reflect upon, understand and possibly change their relationship with the world.

Teaching and learning, particularly in drama, not only validate pre-disciplinary knowledge; they also validate the processes by which we accumulate this knowledge. This is especially true of primary age students, who learn so much through play. Their earliest knowledge is embodied knowledge. They use their story-telling or improvisations to make sense of an event or feeling from two to three years of age. They re-enact what they have observed and experienced in their past interactions with significant others, or project forwards with what they fear or hope **might** happen in the future.

Drama education often begins with dramatic play, where children simply act as themselves in an imaginary situation. For example, using Stanislavsky's 'magic if', they might visit in imagination an environment such as Antarctica to project how they might avoid environmental pollution. Older students might engage in different levels of role, enacting points of view not necessarily their own. This enactment may simply be sustaining the point of view of 'the other' in the face of challenge during improvisation, or it may entail presenting a different external appearance for some type of audience. The students may need to adopt costume, or accent, or different ways of moving in order to communicate this difference.

Trying out new possibilities in fictional contexts where nothing real is at stake is very important in learning to take risks and learning from mistakes. As Freire (1972) wrote:

> Learning begins with the learners in the here and now, the situation in which they are submerged, from which they emerge and in which they intervene ... They must perceive their state not as fated and unalterable but merely as limited and therefore challenging.

(p. 57)

With Freire, arts education rejects the 'banking' metaphor of knowledge, i.e. the concept of the expert knower, the teacher, transmitting his or her understandings and knowledge to the empty vessel learners. Rather, in arts education the teacher is more readily a facilitator of learning. How students learn is as important as what they learn. Typically, in drama, a problem is posed which teacher and students co-investigate, using content derived from the students' perceptions of the world. Often in drama the teacher adopts a low status role in an enactment where the students' status is elevated, helping them to consider the impact of power relationships in life.

Most forms of education seek to promote cognitive understanding, abstracting from examples of life frozen in textbooks, and reflection tends to be reflection after the event. However, in drama the classroom activity oscillates between enacting students' ideas and reflecting upon them, with knowledge being a pivot between action and reflection. Instead of freezing the processes of living, drama allows students to engage in reflection both in and upon action whilst they react spontaneously to other drama participants and to chosen stimulus material.

The creative arts encourage learners to deal with the ephemeral, entering into the feelings and experiences of others. In drama this may be done directly (adopting the role of 'the other') or indirectly (as an audience analysing as they watch others in role). Sometimes students do both, entering into the state that Bolton (1984, p. 162) describes as *metaxis*, where they are simultaneously **in** the action and **detached** from it. They experience feelings and reactions as a character, but also note and analyse what is happening in a distanced way. Drama thus develops metacognitive awareness while blending cognitive and affective learning. Knowledge is gained in all three of these areas.

Knowledge about metacognition is crucial. According to Bruner (1996, p. 161) 'going meta' includes students:

- becoming aware of intersubjectivity, i.e. knowing 'how people come to know what others have in mind and how they adjust accordingly' (p. 161);
- developing collaborative learning skills;
- being able to explain their beliefs and revise them in light of exchanges with others.

Another concept of Bruner's which is important for drama is 'distributed intelligence' (p. 154). The information explosion of recent times is so great that what any one person 'knows' is stored not only in his or her own head, but in books, computers, body habits, other people's minds and so on. We could say, for instance 'I'm content not to hold particular parts of family lore in my own head because Grandpa knows it and I can retrieve it from him when I need it'. Working as part of a social group is a way of developing this distributed intelligence.

## Learning in drama

In drama, as well as learning about content, students develop broader knowledge and ways of knowing, and also generic (e.g. interpersonal) skills. This section deals with the achievement of these outcomes by exploring learning to work collaboratively and creatively and by examining the notions of learning about self and aesthetic learning. Many of these skills and perspectives have wide application. Health professionals, especially, need to learn to work collaboratively, to use creative problem-solving, to address real world challenges and to understand self and others.

### *Learning to work collaboratively*

Almost all learning in drama involves a collaborative process. Students work as part of a group, and the material that is processed often involves ambiguity. The teacher may deliberately introduce material that is open-ended and unfinished in order to evoke from the group 'pre-disciplinary knowledge', which may be extremely diverse, depending upon the mix of people. The question for the teacher then becomes how to hold together this diversity. An important technique in the history of drama education has been the notion of 'universalizing'. Dorothy Heathcote (1988) pioneered this technique of looking below what seem to be dissimilar in situations and actions, to reveal common areas of meaning. The teacher structures activities, focusing firstly on a **general** idea of interest, narrowing to a **particular** and then **universalizing** to draw in the unique experience of the group at work on the idea.

So, for example, a group might appear to be investigating coach travel in the Australian colonial tradition (the general), focusing on a **particular** incident in the journey (e.g. an attack by bushrangers), but will really be testing the limits of a 'universal' trait, such as loyalty as it is understood by the drama group. Most often, the content of the drama work involves a concept that all group members hold in common. Sometimes, however, they may work with a point of view recognized as different, or arising from a perspective of one individual set against the usual view. Depending upon how the teacher structures the class, the knowledge developed may be a cultural value, may relate to minority views, or may be an evaluation of both dominant and minority perspectives.

### *Learning to use our creativity*

Young children begin life with vivid imaginations, which they learn to separate out from the 'real' world. As they are socialized into their own cultural traditions, many unfortunately also learn to bury their imaginative skills. The arts help students rediscover their imaginations and explore the many contradictions of the world in which they live. These abilities are vital for their successful negotiation of constant change in the world, enabling them to envision possibilities, ask new questions and solve difficult problems. In fact, Bruner (1996, p. 4) asserts that our ability to use our imaginations is pivotal to our capacity to create in both science and the humanities.

The drama class is very much about collaborative creativity, where it is the group rather than an individual who creates the art work. It involves risk-taking, because adding new ideas and directions in improvisation is a public act. As Boomer (1992, p. 35) writes, 'we will only take risks in a supportive and conducive environment – one in which we are challenged, but encouraged; we can feel the tension of the struggle, but not the fear; we can strive to get things right but not feel shame if we get it wrong'. An important decision for a drama teacher is balancing a level of ambiguity against the level of risk involved. Cutting back on ambiguity reduces risk, because students then become surer of 'the answer' or of what the teacher wants. A certain level of ambiguity is needed, however, to elicit unusual or creative responses. The more active students are in cognitive constructions, the higher the level of learning achieved, the more they come to know. Of course this involves a high level of risk for the teacher as well as for the students. Beginning teacher Jon Lane (1998) commented in his journal about his improvisation class:

> My directions were intuitions only, and at the time I couldn't have expressed them as I can now. It is an advantage of open ended improvisation that the teacher has to work out what the richest meanings are, along with the students. I wasn't consciously looking for anything in particular, so I was able to be surprised at what I found.

### *Learning about self and others*

At the core of the drama process is the concept of enactment or walking in someone else's shoes. When a particular point of view becomes embodied, not only do students dispassionately analyse, they experience in the body what it feels like to engage with others while holding that particular perspective. Entering imaginatively into someone else's life or experience in this way not only facilitates the development of empathy; relatively it helps us learn about ourselves and our lives with new eyes (Patterson, 1991).

At the same time, oral storying or narrative drama forms enable us to define who we are and celebrate our own lives. We tell stories to illustrate or understand or explain critical moments in our journey. Stories also help us understand the particular cultural group and family experiences in which our lives are embedded. Narrative is closely linked with our thinking, dreaming and being.

### *Learning about aesthetics*

Drama, dance, visual art, music and literature evolve differently in different cultures and social systems. The arts can reinforce the mores of those cultures and societies or can challenge their values. Often the artist sets out to question stereotypes or the way things seem to be. Knowing in and through the creative arts includes learning how to critique performances or works of art, and learning to become a connoisseur of different art forms, of how they heighten awareness or create a particular effect.

Gavin Bolton (Davis and Lawrence, 1986, p. 159) argues that raising a student's consciousness of form, of how a particular concept is expressed, begins a student's aesthetic education. When students structure their drama improvisations, the process of considering the form of expression moves the work into art. This awareness of form can be heightened with informal reflections upon their own work or that of their peers. They can also be taught to apply a more semiotic analysis, with an organized consideration of the signs employed by the artist to communicate with the audience.

Drama operates mostly through metaphor: the drama contexts are understood as representations of reality, not reality itself. Very young students engaged in role play will initially seek reassurance from the teacher: 'This isn't real, is it?' 'You're not really a witch, are you?' Ironically, the very question is evidence that the student holds the double world in mind (albeit shakily when beginning drama), the fictional context and the real world of the classroom.

## Teaching drama

The teaching of drama raises a number of pedagogical concerns for the teacher. Students are engaged in actively creating their own meanings (Wagner, 1995, p. 62) rather than guessing what the teacher has in his or her head, seeking a correct answer. Drama teaching is about letting go of the more traditional classroom interaction patterns in which the teacher controls the talk and activity. Effective management of learning in a drama class, where the talk and activity are less predictable, involves careful pre-planning but also rapid reflection-in-action, adapting to what the students actually do. Often a teacher abrogates the usual controls such as higher status, spatial organization and even a textbook. These controls need to be replaced by arrangements such as rules negotiated with the class, rituals (e.g. beginning with warm-ups or games), the formation of a focus circle, and strictly observed time constraints.

These teaching skills are best learned in practice; the teacher's knowledge needs to be embodied. Beginning teachers usually discover that even though they adopt a lower status role, their students (through metaxis) respect them as the teacher, and rarely need stronger management. When they do, the teacher can often do this in role, or can step out of role, and direct behaviour as the teacher. Usually, however, the freedom of their raised status role is sufficient recompense to keep students within their agreed classroom rules.

It is difficult to learn how to run a group enactment; it is best discovered by reflecting in and upon action. Beginning teacher Felicity Northcott (1998) commented in her journal on her growing confidence as a teacher:

> I was really starting to understand the distinction between direction and facilitation of students. It is a fine line . . . I was learning that the best, and really the only way, was to ask questions with embedded clues, to stimulate their thoughts and the development of their ideas.

She did this in role, and also through side-coaching from outside the improvisation. She also wrote responses in students' journals, warmly encouraging them to pursue ideas she saw as having creative potential.

## Conclusions

Knowing in the creative arts is a form of craft knowledge which is at once pragmatic, metaphoric and social through its use of semiotics and imagination (Morgan, 1998). It is embodied, holistic knowing. The notion of embodied knowing links knowing in the creative arts to other disciplines' professional craft knowledge, as examined in other chapters of this book. Through the eyes of learners and of the teachers helping them to know and to learn creative ways of knowing, we have sought in this chapter to make the embodied (craft) knowing of the creative arts come alive for readers. The creative arts can be used across a range of ages and learning situations to promote an understanding of many forms of practice knowledge including the nature of professional artistry, practice wisdom and embodied knowing.

## References


Bolton, G. (1984) *Drama as Education.* Harlow, Essex: Longman.

Boomer, G. (1992) *Negotiating the Curriculum: Education for the 21st Century.* Sydney: Ashton Scholastic.

Bruner, J. (1996) *The Culture of Education.* Cambridge, MA: Harvard University Press.

Davis, D. and Lawrence, C. (eds) (1986) *Gavin Bolton: Selected Writings.* London: Longman.

Freire, P. (1972) *Pedagogy of the Oppressed.* London: Penguin.

Gardner, H. (1993) *The Arts and Human Development.* New York: Basic Books.

Habermas, J. (1972) *Knowledge and Human Interests* (J. Schapiro, trans.). London: Heinemann.

Heathcote, D. (1988) *Drama and Social Change: Dorothy Heathcote 1984 New Zealand Lectures.* Auckland: Kohia Teachers Centre.

Lane, J. (1998) Unpublished drama journal for MTeach, University of Sydney.

Lovat, T. and Smith, D. (1995) *Curriculum: Action on Reflection Revisited*, 3rd edn. Wentworth Falls, Sydney: Social Science Press.

Medway, P. (1980) *Finding a Language: Autonomy and Learning in School.* London: Chameleon.

Morgan, N. (1998) Positioning drama in the arts. *Adem*, **4**, 8–11.

Northcott, F. (1998) Unpublished drama journal for MTeach, University of Sydney.

Patterson, K. (1991) Living in a peaceful world. *The Horn Book Magazine*, January, pp. 32–38.

Titchen, A. M. (2000) *Professional Craft Knowledge in Patient-centred Nursing and the Facilitation of its Development.* University of Oxford D. Phil Thesis. Oxford: Ashdale Press.

Wagner, B. J. (1995) A theoretical framework for improvisational drama. *National Association for Drama in Education*, **19**(2), 61–70.

# 25

# Research supervision: mystery and mastery

**Margot Pearson**

## Introduction

Research supervision as a subject attracts constant reference from both students and supervisors to traditions harking back to medieval Europe, and stories of trials, ordeals and obstacles to overcome. The use of colourful terminology, such as reference to 'death and glory' topics with uncertain outcomes, indicates the potential for excitement, passion, even glamour, and for failure, depression and hurt. The air of mystery is part of the attraction for some because there is no formula, and every case or student is different; as is every outcome where the goal is to make an original contribution to knowledge. Some metaphors in use perpetuate the air of mystery with references to 'rites of passage' and initiation. Other metaphors such as 'apprentice' for students and 'parenting' for supervisors (Cullen et al., 1994; Clegg and Gall, 1998) position students as younger and subordinate. This position might seem to be one of anachronistic paternalism in graduate education as we enter the twenty-first century where the mean age of candidates in Australia, as in the USA, is in the mid-30s (LaPidus, 1997; Pearson and Ford, 1997). It can also appear contrary to a strong expectation that 'good' students will be independent. Thus the metaphors mask unexamined attitudes and values, which can be part of a less attractive syndrome of what Schön (1987) calls strategies of 'mystery and mastery' in which students and supervisors can get caught in a behavioural world that inhibits reflection and learning, where difficult matters are kept private and unable to be discussed.

At the same time there are greater external pressures for quality in graduate education and for institutional accountability from students, governments and employers (Pearson and Ford, 1997). In particular there is growing interest in preparing postgraduates for employability in the workplace, since academia is no longer the main employment destination. These pressures are leading to a move from the traditional to a more instrumental approach to research education. As at the undergraduate level, there is pressure to replace personal and informal processes of socialization and acculturation with explicit intellectual formation and skills development (Scott, 1995, p. 2). This move accompanies a growing consensus that the goal of PhD candidature is not some earth-shaking original finding or theory in one's field, but a period of supervised study and research at the end of which a candidate has demonstrated the capacity to undertake independent research and has produced a thesis which contains: original data, or use of data analysis; coherence of argument and presentation; and competence in technical, conceptual and contextual analysis (Cullen et al., 1994, p. 55). In other words, research supervision is becoming more clearly a form of professional education (Pearson, 1996). This general situation obviously applies to the preparation of PhD students in the health care professions, whether they are registered within their own health science faculty or within another faculty within the university.

The move to effecting change in research education and supervision is, however, constrained by a lack of pedagogic theory and understanding. Research supervision is not always recognized as a form of teaching. The term more frequently used is 'training'. Professional development for supervisors too is referred to as 'supervisor training'. So the educative processes for both research students and research supervisors are potentially limited by a reduced view of what could be involved. For the idea of training can conjure up a narrow practical focus on 'how to' as technique, and can reinforce the prejudice that 'learning by doing' is sufficient on its own, or with little formal structure. We are caught in the contradiction of the unexamined nature of research education and supervision, which relies on experiential learning but does not recognize it as a legitimate form of education and learning with its own dynamic.

This situation is not surprising when we consider that academic teaching has long been dominated in all professions, including those in health care, by the teaching of propositional knowledge (knowing-that) rather than knowing-how. Barnett (1994, pp. 47–49) describes the move underway in our epistemic framework in higher education to legitimize various forms of knowing-how, but this change is more evident in some professional faculties, for example, nursing and occupational therapy. Calls for change, particularly to broaden the PhD degree, are often met with curriculum responses such as coursework, short courses and workshops for skills of an essentially generalist and generic nature; these can perpetuate the approaches that the academic community is comfortable with for teaching propositional knowledge.

An alternative response is to look more closely at what students and supervisors are doing and how they might learn the expertise they will need to be independent professional researchers, scholars and effective supervisors. In doing this we will at the same time take research education and supervision out of the realm of mystery and metaphor, and seek to give it visible and public form, a form which might constitute a framework to structure supervisory interaction and supervisory development for various research and professional fields, including health care research education and supervision.

## Developing expertise in research and scholarship

### The content of expertise in research and scholarship

In a study of supervision (Cullen et al., 1994), we asked a group of students to document their activity on a weekly basis. Unsurprisingly, student logs described much day-to-day activity where the practicalities included specific tasks from the mundane to the challenging, such as setting up experiments, organizing a field trip, photocopying, analysing results, reading, writing and attending seminars; they included personal and financial concerns, such as getting sick, working part-time, applying for scholarship extensions, exercising and going on holiday.

Our studies confirmed that research students are learning in addition to the knowledge they are producing:

- **professional and technical competence** – to design and conduct investigations, choose appropriate methodologies, learn and use various techniques for analysis, new equipment, statistics packages, and so on;
- the **management of self and others** – the logistics of research, e.g. putting together equipment, technicians, documents and other materials; self-management, particularly for juggling responsibilities and time; management of others, whether technicians, supervisors or other academics;
- ways to **engage with the research community** – strategies for accessing a peer network of other students/researchers; experience in mixing with other academics in relevant fields, and becoming part of a culture as a colleague;
- as an additional task, **learning to write appropriately**.

In contrast to much of their previous formal study, research students are being asked to learn non-propositional knowledge, the knowledge of how to function as a professional researcher and scholar, and they are learning it through the practical experience of producing knowledge and social interaction. This knowledge, which Higgs and Titchen (1995) call professional craft knowledge (PCK), encompasses the more obvious knowledge of how to conduct a research project – what Phillips and Pugh (1994) call the 'craft of research'. It also embraces the more invisible 'tacit knowledge', which includes the capacity to generate original ideas, reframe problems, and have confidence as autonomous professionals in their judgment, and the capacity to evaluate the work of others and oneself, which is necessary for professional growth (Phillips and Pugh, 1994, pp. 19–20). In addition to 'know-how', PCK encompasses 'know-who', the facility to access current knowledge, which often is not to be found in written publications, but through formal and informal communication and interaction in communities of practitioners, researchers and academics (Marceau,

1997, p. 4.3). In professional fields such as health care, both know-how and know-who will be of significance in negotiating the complexities of researching professional practice in the workplace. This is an especially sensitive matter where the workplace is the researcher's place of employment (Brennan, 1995).

## Approaches to acquiring PCK

Recognition of PCK and its nature leads to considering how best to develop it in the context of research education. In doing this I propose to look at approaches which focus on the doing of the research and the imparting of PCK as a form of situated learning. Well known is the approach developed by Schön for educating professionals to learn what he calls the 'art of their practice', where they deal with situations of uncertainty, instability and uniqueness. Across professions Schön sees a pattern of 'reflective conversation with the situation' (Schön, 1983, p. 268). In his later work, Schön draws on the work of Dewey to elaborate what this might mean for educating professionals, stating that since students cannot be taught what they need to know they can be coached. This involves getting students to see for themselves the relationships between the means and methods employed and the results achieved. In coaching, according to Schön, the teacher and student engage in a dialogue which facilitates reciprocal reflection-in-action (Schön, 1987).

### *Coaching*

The term 'coach', like 'apprenticeship', is often used loosely in discussions of research supervision, functioning more as a metaphor than an educational strategy. It is therefore useful to look at an approach to developing expertise where coaching is one of a set of methods drawn from studies of traditional apprenticeship, and studies of successful, apprentice-style approaches to teaching the practice of reading, writing and mathematics in school settings. This approach is called 'cognitive apprenticeship' because it refers to the learning of cognitive and metacognitive skills, the 'externalisation of processes that are usually carried out internally' (Collins et al., 1989, p. 457). The model for cognitive apprenticeship includes three groups of pedagogical methods (Collins et al., 1989, pp. 481–483). The core methods, designed to help students acquire an integrated set of cognitive and metacognitive skills are:

- **Modelling**, where an expert carries out a task so students can observe and build a conceptual model of the process required to complete the task. In cognitive domains experts can externalize the process by verbalizing their thought processes.
- **Coaching**, which consists of observing students carry out a task and offering hints, feedback, reminders and new tasks aimed to bring their performance closer to expert performance.
- **Scaffolding**, which refers to providing supports such as cue cards or intermediate-level tasks to help students perform the task, with the removal of such support termed **fading**.

Additional methods are designed to help students gain conscious access to and control of their problem-solving strategies:

- **articulation**, where students articulate their knowledge, reasoning or problem-solving processes in a domain;
- **reflection**, facilitating student comparison of their problem-solving processes with those of an expert, and the development of an 'internal cognitive model of expertise'.

A final method, promoting student autonomy both in solving problems and in formulating problems to be solved, is:

- **exploration**, where students are pushed to frame and solve questions and problems that are interesting to them, while the expert 'fades out' direction.

Overall, the approach fosters students becoming metacognitive participants in their learning, and an 'overt function of the role of teacher [is] to help students develop this awareness' (Ryan and Quin, 1994, p. 19), a similar outcome to Schön's reflection-in-action.

If we look at reports of research supervisors of their practice through the lens of cognitive apprenticeship as an educational strategy, it gives more distinct form to supervision as a teaching process. In interviews (Cullen et al., 1994; Pearson and Ford, 1997), experienced supervisors described various strategies which are similar to those cited as coaching with scaffolding, modelling, articulation and exploration, for example:

It's important to start the students *[whose background is not strong]* with something fairly structured and concrete . . . It's good if you can find a little problem . . . A problem that is accessible and they ought to be able to do in a couple of months when they've got some mastery of the topic. *[It]* may or may not form part of their actual thesis . . . You've got to get them to the point where they feel some confidence in being able to take something on and not be put off by the open-ended nature of the problem, or even by the fact that it's really up to them to define the problem . . .

(Cullen et al., 1994, p. 52)

. . . the first thing that happens is I would give the students several papers and say the thing I am trying to do right now is this . . . So read this, read this, read this and then come and have a chat. So we have a chat and then I say, well now would you like to try to prove this theorem, would you like to try a simulation, would you like to try a trial design using the package bound by the conjecture. So you give them some small task . . . so that the person isn't overwhelmed . . .

(Cullen et al., 1994, p. 53)

Moreover, reflection and critique are a feature of learning in various disciplines. In science fields, regular laboratory sessions are held where research project progress and results are discussed. In some disciplines student groups, with or without a supervisor, hold regular sessions where relevant current literature is read and discussed. An example of how modelling, articulation and reflection can occur in a group setting comes from the report of the practice of a supervisor from the social sciences by Pearson and Ford (1997). This supervisor held a series of seminars with her PhD students focusing on theory and practice. One student appreciated the opportunity to present her own research design and data collection to the group for feedback, and explained:

The most recent seminar was presented by a woman who is writing up her data, presenting the results of her interviews and surveys. For me, currently in the data collection phase, this was a valuable discussion. It was exciting to see what is around the corner, the shortcuts, the mistakes, the different choices to be made.

(Pearson and Ford, 1997, p. 48)

Another approach to modelling effective professional practice and legitimizing divergent approaches to problem-solving is given within the context of co-supervision in the following example:

In recent years, I've supervised two PhD students who have been located in a lab where the principal of that lab and I have done collaborative work. We've basically been interested in the same problem. We don't plan experiments together, and, in fact, he's adopted one approach to the problem, and I've adopted another, but we have a common interest in comparing the results that we're getting with the different approaches.

With regard to co-supervision, the way that we've operated is that his lab has regular meetings every couple of weeks where everyone in his lab talks about their work, and I've gone to those meetings. And I hold meetings for people in my lab once a week, and students . . . that I'm co-supervising participate at my meetings.

(Pearson and Ford, 1997, pp. 55–56)

### *Reflective conversation on practice*

The importance of dialogue and reflective conversation on practice cannot be underestimated. Recognition of this is significant in research education where it is usual for students to initiate much of their contact with supervisors and other experts (Pearson, 1996). Indeed Phillips and Pugh (1994, pp. 52–53) assume the need for such initiative, and they suggest as a strategy for students in learning their craft, a student-initiated version of modelling. They advise students to observe established good researchers in the appropriate discipline, noting the practices, skills and techniques they are using, and to practise the use of techniques such as questionnaires or maintaining lab equipment in a non-thesis exercise.

However, in following their own arrangements students may limit the opportunity for dialogue and reflection about the detail and 'artistry' of professional research technique and expertise. It is in dialogue with a student about actual problems that this expertise is shared through feedback which is highly situated (Schön, 1983; Collins et al., 1989). Moreover, an expert has developed the ability to reframe problems and to identify possible strategies from an extensive repertoire built up over time. From this repertoire the expert tests out in practice new hypotheses in a form of exploration which

Schön sees as similar to Lewin's notion of action research, where the practitioner's reflection on knowing-in-action gives rise to actionable theory (Schön, 1995, p. 31). It is through such conversation with supervisors and other experts that students can extend their repertoire and learn to evaluate their own work and that of others. In this process they are extending the curriculum beyond the competence needed to complete their research project, towards developing their expertise as a future professional.

An account of the way in which a supervisor can encourage the development of expertise and the student's professional repertoire in an area often left to student initiative comes from Bruce (1996). Bruce has developed a reflective model for building expertise in reviewing the literature, based on the recognition that many students do not bring sufficient competence to the task. She advises supervisors to encourage students to keep a journal for the literature review and other parts of their work, and suggests strategies for supervisory sessions, similar to the methods of cognitive apprenticeship, such as:

- talking with students about reflective practice and discussing the relevance to reviewing literature;
- modelling the reflective approach by sharing how they plan, write and evaluate literature reviews;
- helping students to move through parts of the reflective cycle (for literature reviews) during supervisory sessions (coaching, articulation);
- encouraging cooperative learning by asking students to share their plans and implementations with each other, and to help each other reflect on the outcomes and make new plans (Bruce, 1996, p. 249).

### *Mentoring*

Clarifying the activity of coaching the research apprentice can help to establish the province of mentoring, which is a term often used interchangeably with coaching. Coaching is a strategy for developing research expertise. Mentoring concerns supporting students in managing their candidature in the context of their evolving personal development and career goals. Many students have, with varying degrees of intensity, early feelings of loss of control and confusion as they confront the challenge of not knowing. It is this challenge which underlies much of the documented emotional experience of the 'rite of passage' (Cullen et al., 1994). Many students find themselves managing complex arrangements across sites to get their research completed. Increasingly, students are also concerned with their future in an uncertain graduate employment market. In this context, mentoring is a leadership role which requires sustained dialogue, but is not necessarily part of 'hands on' supervision (Pearson and Ford, 1997, p. 112). Depending on circumstances, mentoring can be provided productively by the principal supervisor, shared by co-supervisors, or come from someone who is outside the immediate context of the student's lab or department.

## Implications for supervisor development

### *Coaching supervisors*

At one level there is an obvious parallelism in how supervisor development might proceed. Opportunity for experiential learning, reflection and coaching might be made available for supervisors by pairing new supervisors with experienced ones, with some structure for feedback and reflection. Another approach would be to set up a form of clinical supervision whereby new supervisors discuss their relationships and critical incidents with an experienced supervisor in a developmental programme. (Critical companionship, as described in Chapter 10, offers one such approach.) Group sessions discussing supervision can lead to professional conversation about practice and issues. Some of these might involve students giving feedback on their experience. Workshops for supervisors can provide opportunities to rehearse strategies and discuss them with others. Moreover, an advantage of distinguishing more clearly the processes of coaching and mentoring could be to enable co-supervisors to negotiate their distinct responsibilities more effectively.

### *Developing a professional conversation on research education*

However, there is another level at which supervisors must consider their task in educating professionals. There is a need for supervisors to reflect on and critique research education. If we accept that doing a research degree is both part of producing knowledge and a form of higher education rather than training, then we can follow Barnett's (1990) argument to establish whether we have achieved a quality outcome that is more than technique, for both the education of the students and the professional development of the supervisors. Barnett's criteria for appropriate knowledge-oriented activity for higher education are social interaction, personal commitment, the development of the mind, consideration of values, and openness to critical scrutiny. The last means scrutiny at all levels: specific findings, concepts, theories, frameworks of assumptions, practices, truth criteria, fundamental perspectives and orientation, and even 'the entire apparatus of the discipline as a whole' (Barnett, 1990, p. 44). These elements allow for a conversation in which the parties try to sustain and advance mutual understanding, and which is open-ended.

Another part of that conversation should concern the nature of appropriate knowledge and ways of knowing for academics and professionals in different contexts. For research students will find themselves caught in this debate, whether they are located in health care organizations or seek to work there, or whether they become academic researchers. General talk of differing cultures and values is insufficient. Learning how to negotiate the differences is another component of the professional expertise of a researcher and scholar, as the balance of research carried out in universities, health care organizations and other agencies changes (Pearson and Ford, 1997, pp. 50, 109–111). Students who have developed and articulated their cognitive and metacognitive skills in their research domain will be more sensitive to context and better able to be adaptive.

## Conclusions

If we accept the argument that research education is a form of professional education then we can begin to articulate what is being learned in addition to completing a research project. In this chapter I have given an example of how an approach described as cognitive apprenticeship might be used to give a structure to strategies such as coaching, and a language for reflection on such a strategy. It is important, however, to appreciate that this example is given for its heuristic value; it is not a recipe nor intended to be. It is a structure that could be embedded in a series of ongoing conversations grounded in the practice of research and scholarship. Context and purpose are important in the learning of skills, whether at the meta-level of reflection on professional practice or when reflecting on specific tasks. It is for this reason that professional craft knowledge must be learnt by supervisors and students who are working together, sharing expertise and experience. In this respect research education is as highly individualistic as supervisors always claim. What can be developed at the generic level are forms, structures, frameworks and language for articulation and reflection, so that the conversations are open and public.

## Acknowledgements

Some of the data and the quotations from interviews used in this chapter come from two studies (Cullen et al., 1994; Pearson and Ford, 1997) on graduate education funded under the Evaluations and Investigations Program, Department of Employment Training and Youth Affairs, Canberra, Australia.

## References

Barnett, R. (1990) *The Idea of Higher Education*. Buckingham: SRHE/Open University.

Barnett, R. (1994) *The Limits of Competence*. Buckingham: SRHE/Open University.

Brennan, M. (1995) Education doctorates: Reconstructing professional partnerships around research? *The Australian Universities Review*, **38**(2), 20–22.

Bruce, C. (1996) From neophyte to expert: Counting on reflection to facilitate complex conceptions of the literature review. In *Frameworks for Postgraduate Education* (O. Zuber-Skerrit, ed.), pp. 239–253. Lismore, Australia: Southern Cross University.

Clegg, S. and Gall, I. (1998) The discourse of research degrees supervision: A case study of supervisor training. *Higher Education Research and Development*, **17**(3), 323–332.

Collins, A., Brown, J. S. and Newman, S. E. (1989) Cognitive apprenticeship: Teaching the crafts of reading, writing and mathematics. In *Knowing, Learning and Instruction* (L. B. Resnik, ed.), pp. 453–494. Hillsdale, NJ: Erlbaum.

Cullen, D. J., Pearson, M., Saha, L. J. and Spear, R. H. (1994) *Establishing Effective PhD Supervision*. Canberra: Australian Government Publishing Service.

Higgs, J. and Titchen, A. (1995) Propositional, professional, and personal knowledge in clinical reasoning. In *Clinical Reasoning in the Health Professions* (J. Higgs and M. Jones, eds), pp. 129–146. Oxford: Butterworth-Heinemann.

LaPidus, J. B. (1997) Issues and themes in postgraduate education in the United States. In *Beyond the First Degree* (R. G. Burgess, ed.), pp. 21–39. Buckingham: Open University/SRHE.

Marceau, J. (1997) *The High Road or the Low Road? Alternatives for Australia's Future. A Report on Australia's Industrial Structure.* North Sydney: Australian Business Foundation.

Pearson, M. (1996) Professionalising PhD education to enhance the quality of the student experience. *Higher Education*, **32**, 303–320.

Pearson, M. and Ford, L. 1997, *Open and Flexible PhD Study and Research*, DEETYA, Australian Government Publishing Service, Canberra.

Phillips, E. M. and Pugh, D. S. (1994) *How to Get a PhD.* Milton Keynes: Open University Press.

Ryan, G. L. and Quin, C. N. (1994) Cognitive apprenticeship and problem based learning. In *Reflections on Problem Based Learning* (S. E. Chen, R. Cowdroy, A. Kingsland and M. Ostwald, eds), pp. 15–33. Sydney: Australian Problem Based Learning Network.

Schön, D. (1983) *The Reflective Practitioner.* New York: Basic Books.

Schön, D. (1987) *Educating the Reflective Practitioner.* San Francisco: Jossey-Bass.

Schön, D. (1995) Knowing-in-action: The new scholarship requires a new epistemology. *Change*, November/December, pp. 27–34.

Scott, P. (1995) *The Meanings of Higher Education.* Buckingham: Open University/SRHE.

# 26

# Research and professional craft knowledge

**Anne Parry**

The central focus of this chapter concerns the relationship between professional craft knowledge and research: the need for each health care profession to assume responsibility for presenting and legitimizing its unique core of knowledge of everyday practice; and how substantial, credible and socially valuable intelligence-in-action may be revealed and articulated to the benefit of the professions themselves, their practitioners, students, and clients or patients, and the development of health care provision.

For convenience, 'health care professions' is used to cover the professions whose scope was defined by medicine for most of the twentieth century: nursing; the orthodox therapy professions of occupational therapy, physiotherapy, and speech and language therapy; radiography; and chiropody/podiatry. An important element of their emancipation and development of identities separate to that of medicine has been construction of separate knowledge bases. They are, however, beset by an abiding problem: explication of their professional craft knowledge (Brown and McIntyre, 1993) – the largely hidden or tacit, cognitive but not psychomotor, intuitive procedural and practical knowledge that guides everyday clinical activities.

## Characterization of professional knowledge

The nature of professional knowledge has exercised many philosophers (see Eraut, 1994, p. 15), and lately educators and educationalists in the health care professions have themselves begun to articulate the distinction between knowledge that underpins practice and enables action and professional **know-how** that is inherent in action. Knowledge is understood to consist of 'scientific' or empirically derived and theoretical knowledge and 'pre-scientific' knowledge or knowledge of everyday practices (Frolov, 1984).

Fifty years ago, Ryle (1949) distinguished between 'knowing that' and 'knowing how'. **Knowing that** is propositional knowledge derived through research and scholarship, that is publicly available for teaching and learning, public scrutiny and information, for improving clinical practice in textbooks, for journal articles, research and audit reports, course handouts and so on. **Knowing how** is non-propositional knowledge acquired by practitioners through practice and experience. It corresponds to prescientific knowledge, underlies daily practice and is largely hidden. Ryle viewed it as 'intelligence-in-action' that constantly evolves through experiential learning but does not require the knower to articulate underlying personal theories. According to Parry and Stone (1991a), it is a combination of logic and heuristics, tricks of the trade, rules of thumb, the ability to reason from partial knowledge and to make reasonable guesses – the stuff that is the mark of professional thinking but is not amenable to capture and being written down and codified. Polyani (1967) coined the term 'tacit knowledge' to describe that which we know but cannot tell. Parry and Stone's work with physiotherapists (Parry and Stone, 1991b) substantiates Eraut's assertion that findings from a relatively new area of research, knowledge elicitation, show that people do not know what it is they know (Eraut, 1994, p. 15).

The clinical reasoning process of experienced practitioners is largely unconscious, and key aspects of knowing are embedded in action and transmitted by practical example. Consequently, students are required to spend a significant amount of time learning their craft through demonstration, practice and feedback, but that knowledge is not cast in a publicly available form. The public may, however, share with a profession recognition of outstanding practitioners, people who, as Schön described, are not distinguished by more professional knowledge per se but more 'wisdom', 'talent', 'intuition' or 'artistry' (Schön, 1987).

From their extensive studies of medical problem-solving, Elstein et al. (1979) suggest that almost spontaneous **intuitive** solutions to diagnostic problems are reclaimed from individuals' schemata, their personal concepts and theories, stored in long-term memory. However, as shown by the investigation by Vernon et al. (1998) of podiatrists' and chiropodists' interpretations of shoe wear marks, assumptions about the dependability of intuitive knowledge may be dangerous; experience may cause practitioners to develop individual and different schemata, which is another reason for codifying professional craft knowledge and building theory.

Although Elstein and co-authors concluded that medical judgment is more an art than a science, they were focusing on diagnosis and, consequently, ignored the reasoning of post-diagnostic treatment. Based on his observations of professionals in action, Schön refers to both 'artistry in situations of uniqueness and uncertainty' (Schön, 1983, p. 165) and the artfulness of reflection (Schön, 1991). As Wood (1996, p. 626) claims for occupational therapy, it appears that most advanced knowledge for the role of practitioners of health care professions has become manifest through the practices of 'many extraordinarily skilled (and a few genius) practitioners'. Jean Ayres and Berti Bobath, for example, have had important clinical reverberations within their own professional areas, respectively occupational therapy and physiotherapy. Bobath was undoubtedly an artist; through working with her, many physiotherapists and occupational therapists have benefited, primarily intraprofessionally, from her direct tutelage and her reputation. Pat Davies, an early pupil of Bobath, is a prime example of how experiential learning and reflection-on-action can facilitate both evolution of intelligence-in-action and transformation of intuition and artistry to propositional knowledge (Davies, 1985, 1990).

## The need to legitimize the core knowledge of practice

Most occupations commonly recognized as professions control access to information valuable to the public (Goodlad, 1984). However, in the case of the health professions, while, as Eraut claims (1994, p. 6), each profession appears to keep 'occupational knowledge within the guild', important knowledge is hidden even to the profession itself. Although Eraut (1994, p. 15) asserts that there is 'increasing acceptance that important aspects of professional competence and expertise cannot be represented in propositional form and embedded in a publicly accessible knowledge base', the challenge is to identify what might be revealed and the possible strategies for doing so. It is important for a number of reasons. For example, the work of professions is constantly changing and the direction of change is the product of powerful competing interests which vary from country to country. The smaller health care professions can identify with Meerabeau's (1998, p. 398) complaint that 'nursing often seems to be trying to find a small voice in a discourse created by other, far louder, voices'. The exhortation of Harrison and co-authors about the comprehensibility of economic analyses to health service clinicians and managers is equally appropriate to professional craft knowledge: 'If information is not accessible, it cannot be used in the decision making process within the operational health care field. If relevant research evidence cannot be understood, it will not impact upon clinical practice and thus will have little practical value' (Harrison et al., 1998, p. 340).

The move to universities and other higher education institutions from professional colleges outside the mainstream higher education system is another reason to legitimize the core knowledge of practice. Although this move conferred academic respect on the professions, they are still considered to be academically unstable because they are seen to be dependent for their academic credibility on discipline-based courses in the biomedical or social sciences taught by academics of those disciplines. Furthermore, making the training and education of practitioners more academic solidified a consequence of qualifying examinations. Increasing areas of professional knowledge became codified and publicly available in books, journal articles, handouts, workbooks and other texts needed to prepare students for traditional examinations of propositional knowledge, in particular the discipline-based theories and concepts derived from bodies of coherent, systematic knowledge (e.g. the role of psychological or sociological theories in physiotherapy and nursing) and generalizations and practical principles in the applied field of professional action (see Eraut, 1994, p. 43).

In terms of Broudy's model (Broudy et al., 1964, cited by Eraut, 1994), replication and application of knowledge are the technical and vocational modes of use of propositional knowledge. Interpretation and association, or the intuitive capacity to digest, distil and select from previous experience, are the professional modes. Discussing 'professional craft knowledge', Higgs and Titchen (1995) referred to 'theories-in-use' and likened health practitioners' ability to interpret incomplete and ambiguous data and to identify implications which are not directly deducible from explicit data to Benner's concept of 'intuitive knowledge', which is based on experience and imagination (Benner, 1984).

**Theories-in-use** arise from action science, a body of work developed in recent decades, in particular by Argyris and Schön (1974). Central to action science is identification of the theories that practitioners use to guide their behaviour. The key distinction is between the **espoused theories** that an individual claims to follow and the theories-in-use that can be inferred from action. They may be the same or they may be different, and the practitioner may be unaware of any inconsistency. Argyris and Schön claim that it is possible to identify theories-in-use by reflection on action and, importantly, to use these theories to predict the consequences of their implementation.

A third reason to legitimize the core knowledge of practice is the 'crisis in confidence in professional knowledge', the so-called 'theory–practice gap' (Schön, 1987). According to Schön (1987, p. 10), by the mid-1980s there was growing concern about the increasing gap between research-based propositional knowledge taught to students in the professions and the practical knowledge and 'actual competencies required of practitioners in the field'. Ten years later, Hunt et al. (1998) found that physiotherapy graduates perceived important gaps between knowledge and skills gained in their university education and those required in the workplace, and highlighted the need for change in educational preparation.

Some explanation for the crisis may be offered by the multilayered concept of postmodernity that alerts us to a variety of contemporary social and cultural changes taking place within many 'advanced' societies (Lyon, 1994). Most of us have encountered the cultural dimension of postmodern debate in discussion of the apparent fragmentation of art and architecture, film and music. Lyon emphasizes the social dimension of postmodernity: i.e. if modernity refers to the social order that emerged following the Enlightenment, postmodernity refers to a new type of society structured around consumers and consumption rather than workers and production. Rapid change in delivery of health care, shifting political concerns and reduction of purpose and goals to performance criteria are examples of the postmodern condition that induces **apocalyptic unease**.

As research and publication have increased many-fold in the last decade, it is difficult to know the extent to which practitioners' reported feelings of exhaustion and depersonalization (Scutter and Goold, 1995) and stress (Donohue et al., 1993) are themselves new phenomena. However, if graduates are to be enabled to develop the knowledge and skills necessary to cope in the changing professional workplace, we cannot continue to hide behind the simple notion that the knowledge of a profession is specialized and distinct from that of any other profession or occupation but not amenable to explication. Rather, in order to advance professional practice, we need to empower ourselves to speak with authority about our professional practice by legitimizing professional craft knowledge and assimilating it into the model of propositional knowledge.

This task is related to the current worldwide drive towards research-based practice but is essentially different from it. That is, the concept of **evidence-based medicine** is being promoted on the same linear model of 'technical rationality' castigated by Schön (1983): identify problem, search literature, analyse results using techniques like meta-analysis, synthesize guidelines for practice. The randomized controlled trial (RCT) is the gold standard, the controlled study without randomization the silver standard, and less rigorous group comparison designs the bronze standard (Basmajian and Banerjee, 1996, pp. 1–4), because they are amenable to systematic review (Chalmers and Altman, 1995). While Rolfe (1988) sees nursing in thrall to the social sciences and still subject to the tyranny of the RCT, Roberts (1994) has referred to the 'hegemony of medicine' and Higgs and Titchen (1998) to the 'hegemony of scientific knowledge', both of which have conspired in equal measure to convince physical therapists in the USA and physiotherapists in the

UK, Australia, Canada and Scandinavia to adopt the orthodox **scientific/positivist** or **logical empiricist** world view and its research methods. This is the dominant paradigm, and Robertson's (1995) analysis of 272 articles published in *Physical Therapy* revealed the increasing use of group comparison designs even though many questions from physiotherapy practice are not amenable to them.[1]

Modernity has achieved a great deal in science, technology and democratic politics but has been a mixed blessing. From one perspective, as the product of the Enlightenment, the logical empiricist paradigm represents a liberating step for human society, releasing itself from the bonds of superstition. From another perspective, however, it is a movement to narrow our view of the world, even to monopolize knowing in the hands of an elite few. On the one hand it has taught us the value of critical public testing of knowledge, but on the other it has separated the researcher from the subject of his or her research, striving for objective knowledge. Matthews (1998) claims that the scientific community is so squeamish about subjectivity that it does not question the plausibility of statistically significant findings from RCTs. More importantly for practitioners, Eraut (1994, p. 17) contends that findings which are expressed in terms of probabilities can offer only 'limited guidance to professionals making decisions about individual cases' unless there is further evidence about their typicality. In such circumstances, great weight is attached to professional judgment, to 'wise judgment', another example of the use of professional craft knowledge that it should be possible to reveal.

## From theory-based practice to practice-based theory

According to Rolfe (1988, p. 1), not only is 'the application of generalizable, research-based knowledge to unique, person-centred practice, the so-called "research-based practice" advocated by the Department of Health, one of the main causes of the theory–practice gap' in nursing, but there is a growing mistrust among nurses that 'academic knowledge can offer anything of relevance to practice situations'. Other authors have criticized the notion of nursing theory on the grounds that nursing is practice-based and, therefore, should be understood rather than explained (Allmark, 1995), and have even suggested that the move towards academic status of nurse-teachers is misplaced (Mallik, 1993).

While there is a tension between developing knowledge which has academic currency and knowledge which has relevance to practice, several authors have offered alternative views. Dale (1994) suggests that the problem is not a gap between theory and practice but a gap between the ways in which nurse-teachers and practitioners use theory. Dale identifies three types of knowledge – propositional, practice and experiential – and, in keeping with Brown and McIntyre's (1993) metaphor of 'professional craft knowledge', suggests that development of the second two types of knowledge is the key to dealing with the relationship between theory and practice. Ashworth and Longmate (1993) assert that nurses are continually theorizing and, therefore, that theory is an essential element of the way in which expert nurses practise. They argue that there is a rich interconnection between reflection and practical action. This is one of the main themes of a recent article on the intertwinement of theory in practice in physiotherapy: that scientific principles and clinical practices are mutually dependent and that more detailed insight is required into the way that scientific principles are translated and transformed in application (Lettinga et al., 1999).

## Revealing professional craft knowledge

Ryle (1949, p. 30) proposed that 'effective practice precedes the theory of it', and Schön (1987) advocated exploring the 'swampy lowlands' of actual practice. Clearly, before interventions can be evaluated we need to find a vocabulary and language to describe our professional craft knowledge so that it is open to public scrutiny, we can facilitate the learning of students, and then design research that evaluates clinical effectiveness. Consequently, the 'million dollar question' is: what research strategies are suited to research that focuses on unearthing the knowledge that practitioners use and making it public and consensual? Of necessity, these strategies must be exploratory in nature in an area that has had little or no previous research. In order to change the status of professional craft knowledge, it is necessary to develop theoretical ideas which will either complement existing ideas or represent new ways of thinking. At the same time, we must seek to close the gap between the practicalities, uncertainties and general messiness of both the clinical process and the research process and the more formal and patterned world of theory.

The methods that can be employed fit Denzin and Lincoln's (1994) description of qualitative research. They cite the description by Nelson et al. (1992, p. 2) of the methodology of research in cultural studies as being 'a bricolage', which may be likened to a quilt in which material is pieced together to create a pattern or a montage in which different images are superimposed to create a picture. The choice of practice is 'pragmatic, strategic and self-reflective' and a construction fitting the specifics of a complex situation emerges. Indeed, while biomedical scientists appear focused within a single paradigm, researchers in the professions can employ whatever strategies, methods or empirical materials are to hand. The choice depends on the research question that is asked, which, in turn, depends on the context in which it is asked. From an analysis of 346 articles in 68 Swedish doctoral dissertations in physiotherapy, Ekdahl and Nilstun (1998) found that design and data analysis overwhelmingly reflected the nomothetic, or generalizing, approach of the logical positivist paradigm, but that many also asked questions related to the meaning of experience. They concluded that physiotherapists are eclectic in their approach and combine elements from different paradigms.

In comparison with the pre-active design and deductive reasoning of logical empiricist researchers, qualitative researchers use inductive analysis: categories, themes and patterns are not imposed prior to data collection but arise from the data. Unlike the objective and impersonal standpoint adopted towards subjects in theory-testing scientific research, approximating the way physical scientists treat atoms and particles, qualitative theory-building approaches take a much more involved and close-up viewpoint of the participants. The interpretivist paradigm of many researchers reflects an attempt to obtain in-depth understanding and interpretation of the situation or other phenomena rather than an attempt to capture 'objective' reality; the goal is to connect the parts to the whole by emphasizing meaningful relationships that operate in the social world that is studied, rather than to establish a cause and effect relationship.

Health care practitioners are not in a unique position. Their situation is very similar to that of teachers. Cochran-Smith and Lytle (1993) have argued that they, as practitioners, should have greater control of the research agenda and should be encouraged to have greater confidence in their professional knowledge. Furthermore, Altricher et al. (1993) have argued that it is essential to make teachers' knowledge public. Revelation of the professional craft knowledge of all practitioners, therefore, requires a research culture in which researchers can collaborate in and facilitate practitioner research.

Action research has evolved from the work of Lewin (1946), whose cycle of planning, action and fact-gathering was the forerunner of Elliott's (1980) action research spiral. Feminist researchers have stressed that action research should be about change (see Bannister et al., 1994), and Cohen and Manion (1980, cited by Bannister et al., 1994) state that action research is appropriate when 'specific knowledge is required for a specific problem in a specific situation, or when a new approach is to be grafted on to an existing system'. Widely used in education to empower teachers and to affirm their professional judgment, action research is probably the most widely practised participative research approach. Winter (1998, p. 59) claims that it 'uses criteria for good practice quite directly to guide the process of inquiry, because action research can be thought of as an idealized version of professional practice itself'. It lends itself to exposing professional craft knowledge because the research question arises out of the problems of practitioners and the analysis of the situation is in situ.

Bond and Walton (1998), for example, drew on an action research project with mothers of children who had been sexually abused and colleagues in a social work team to explore the scope offered by practitioner research to extend learning on the part of social workers, their managers, service users and educators, and to generate self-help and organization change. It illustrates research-mindedness in practice and shows what can be achieved when dissemination of findings is taken seriously.

Winter (1998) also focuses on the form of the participatory relationship required to give voice to others, particularly minority groups within the wider community. He cites Bishop's example of management of social care to illustrate participation. Bishop (1995) arranged a series of brainstorming sessions to collect social workers' perceptions of the task, organized their ideas, circulated them for comment and then drew up a guidelines document.

Titchen and Binnie (1994) have described an action research strategy for generating and testing theory in a way that is subordinate to and conditioned by improving practice. It requires a prior observational study to generate a set of tentative principles which are tested, refined and retested through the action research spiral. This can be likened to Lewin's (1946) 'reconnaissance' and the need to ensure that the basic conceptual framework is adequate for understanding what the problem is. They also aver that action research partnerships of practitioners and researchers permit the coexistence and compatibility of 'practice thinking' and 'research thinking'.

Schön (1983, p. 165) sees practice as 'a kind of research . . . Inquiry is a transaction with the situation in which knowing and doing are inseparable'. His rationale stresses **reflection-on-action** as well as reflection-in-action. Justifying actions will encourage the analytical process and can be used to facilitate articulation of 'theories-in-use'. Morse (1991) utilized the techniques of grounded theory (Strauss and Corbin, 1994) to analyse interview data and develop a model for describing the various types of relationship that are negotiated between nurses and patients. The model was presented to the participants for verification and was modified according to their comments, suggestions or questions. The grounded theory approach strongly underlines the human dimension of society, emphasizing the way in which individuals play a part in constructing their social environment. Thematic content analysis (Burnard, 1991), a more distanced stance, was used by Innes (1998) to identify the coping strategies used by radiographers to manage the stress of coping with postgraduate education and full-time work.

Case-based or idiographic meanings are an important element of qualitative research, and research has shown how **story-telling** or narratives are characteristic of the way various health care practitioners reason out issues they meet in their practice; for example, Hunter (1991) about doctors, Mattingly and Fleming (1994) about occupational therapists, and Benner (1984) about nurses. Hunter (1991) argues that because the case is the basic unit of thought in medicine, however scientific clinical knowledge may be, it is narratively organized and communicated. Discourse analysis is now a well-established method in psychology, and experienced researchers may be able to produce sets of meanings that operate independently of the intentions of practitioners, patients and clients. Story-telling may facilitate practitioners' understanding of their experiences and be a conduit towards theorizing about their practice.

## Publication

According to Winter (1998, p. 53), 'one of the central themes in thinking about action research is the relationship between knowledge and cultural authority'. This is true about all explication of professional craft knowledge, and it may underlie identification of a theory–practice gap in nursing. As education of practitioners moved from hospital-based professional schools to the universities and other higher education institutions, the locus of knowledge creation shifted. It shifted so far that some nurses perceived a unidirectional hierarchical relationship between themselves and researchers who had lost touch with clinical reality but who built theory that was disseminated as clinical guidelines (Rolfe, 1988; Mallik, 1993). Without the comment and feedback stage of the action research spiral, this process does not foster research-mindedness in practitioners but sows seeds of doubt about the fundamental issue of ownership of the knowledge of a profession. Professional craft knowledge is possessed by the practitioners. The role of researchers is to give greater voice to practitioners by revealing it. The role of journals is to allow those voices to be heard.

Researchers have an obligation to disseminate their findings and to expose their methods to scrutiny, but attitudes can have a profound effect not only on what is published and how it is published but even on the methodologies employed. Ekdahl and Nilstun (1998) suggest that one reason why so few of the physiotherapy research articles that they analysed eschewed quantitative data to focus on description and understanding was fear of not getting the article published because the research would not conform to the medical model. This is compounded by pressure to publish in highly rated research journals because some potential research funding agencies use journal hierarchies to rate the 'track record' of applicants. Bond and Walton (1998, p. 124) have commented on the gatekeeping practices of academic journals that 'reinforce rather than bridge the separation between readerships of and contributors to' them and to 'trade magazines'. Salvage (1998, p. 22) has complained of 'the snobbery of nurse academics who refuse not only to publish in popular journals but also dissuade students from reading what they sniffily refer to as "the comics"'.

It is too simplistic to suggest that the choice is between writing for an identified audience or for 'brownie points', but disconfirming statements about the status of professional journals may not only dissuade authors from submitting to them but also cause practitioners to doubt themselves, their understanding of their own practice and, indeed, to doubt whether they have any right to ownership of professional knowledge. Rather, journal editors need to try to create an atmosphere which values the needs and goals of all sections of their professions and provides an outlet for knowledge and ideas which enable researchers and practitioners to connect.

Salvage (1998) says that nurse researchers 'have the luxury of being able to . . . simultaneously publish the full account [of their research] in *NT Research* and a more condensed version in *Nursing Times*'; the latter is bought by more than 80 000 nurses, midwives and health visitors every week. The researchers of most professions could present their research in different ways for different purposes in research journals and magazines, since many national professional associations produce both a journal and a magazine, such as *Physiotherapy* and *Physiotherapy Frontline,* in their subscription services. The *British Medical Journal* and the *New England Journal of Medicine* show, however, that there is room in highly rated journals for a wide variety of articles to meet the diverse needs of readers. As O'Connor (1978, p. 14) writes, journals are a kind of multi-authored book and 'editors must define or re-define the aims and scope of their journals and choose articles and other features congruent with those aims'. If, in hope of raising the status of their journals, editors, referees and their committees expect authors to meet specific, ritualized criteria, the gap between researchers and professionals will widen. Alternatively, imaginative use of sections of journals can give them broad relevance and appeal.

Huth (1990, p. 5), editor of *Annals of Internal Medicine*, writes that 'a powerful test of audience is "who cares", a close relative of "so what"'. Practitioners who care are at both ends of explication of professional craft knowledge; they possess the craft knowledge, and publication of revelations about it must enable them to identify with it, contest any guidelines that are reputed to be based on it, develop research-mindedness, and most importantly, own it. The question 'so what?' returns us to the beginning of this chapter and the reasons for doing research in professional craft knowledge.

## Note

1 But for the publications of Shepard, Jenson and associates this might beg a question about the difference between physiotherapy and physical therapy (see, e.g., Shepard, 1987; Jensen, 1989; Shepard et al., 1993).

## References


Allmark, P. (1995) A classical view of the theory-practice gap in nursing. *Journal of Advanced Nursing*, **22**, 18–22.

Altricher, H., Posch, P. and Somekh, B. (1993) *Teachers Investigate Their Work.* London: Routledge.

Argyris, C. and Schön, D. A. (1974) *Theory in Practice: Increasing Professional Effectiveness.* San Francisco: Jossey-Bass.

Ashworth, P. and Longmate, M. A. (1993) Theory and practice: Beyond the dichotomy. *Nurse Education Today*, **13**, 321–327.

Bannister, P., Burman, E., Parker, I., Taylor, M. and Tindall, C. (1994) *Qualitative Methods in Psychology: A Research Guide.* Buckingham: Open University Press.

Basmajian, J. V. and Banerjee, S. N. (eds) (1996) *Clinical Decision Making in Rehabilitation: Efficacy and Outcomes.* New York: Churchill Livingstone.

Benner, P. (1984) *From Novice to Expert: Excellence and Power in Clinical Nursing Practice.* London: Addison Wesley.

Bishop, L. (1995) An approach to managing changing professional roles through exploring 'What is inspection?' MSc dissertation, Anglia Polytechnic University.

Bond, M. and Walton, P. (1998) Knowing mothers: From practitioner research to self-help and organisational change. *Educational Action Research*, **6**(1), 111–127.

Broudy, H. S., Smith, B. O. and Burnett, J. (1964) *Democracy and Excellence in American Secondary Education.* Chicago: Rand McNally.

Brown, S. and McIntyre, D. (1993) *Making Sense of Teaching.* Milton Keynes: Open University Press.

Burnard, P. (1991) A method of analysing interview transcripts in qualitative research. *Nurse Education Today*, **11**, 461–466.

Chalmers, I. and Altman, D. (1995) *Systematic Reviews.* London: BMJ Publishing Group.

Cochran-Smith, M. and Lytle, S. (1993) *Inside/Outside: Teacher Research and Knowledge.* New York: Teachers College Press.

Cohen, L. and Manion, L. (1980) *Research Methods in Education.* London: Croom Helm.

Dale, A. E. (1994) The theory-practice gap: The challenge for nurse teachers. *Journal of Advanced Nursing*, **20**, 521–524.

Davies, P. M. (1985) *Steps to Follow: A Guide to the Treatment of Adult Hemiplegia.* Berlin/New York: Springer Verlag.

Davies, P. M. (1990) *Right in the Middle: Selective Trunk Activity in the Treatment of Adult Hemiplegia.* Berlin/New York: Springer Verlag.

Denzin, N. and Lincoln, Y. (1994) Introduction: Entering the field of qualitative research. In *Handbook of Qualitative Research* (N. Denzin and Y. Lincoln, eds), pp. 1–17. Thousand Oaks, CA: Sage.

Donohue, E., Nawawl, A., Wilker, A., Schindler, T. and Jette, D. (1993) Factors associated with burnout in Massachusetts rehabilitation hospitals. *Physical Therapy*, **73**, 750–761.

Ekdahl, C. and Nilstun, T. (1998) Paradigms in physiotherapy research: An analysis of 68 Swedish doctoral dissertations. *Physiotherapy Theory and Practice*, **14**(4), 159–169.

Elliott, J. (1980) Action research in schools: Some guidelines. In *The Theory and Practice of Education* (J. Elliott and D. Whitehead, eds). Cambridge: Cambridge Institute of Education.

Elstein, A. S., Shulman, L. S. and Sprafka, S. A. (1979) *Medical Problem Solving: An Analysis of Clinical Reasoning*. London: Harvard University Press.

Eraut, M. (1994) *Developing Professional Knowledge and Competence*. London: The Falmer Press.

Frolov, I. (ed.) (1984) *Dictionary of Philosophy*. Moscow: Progress Publishers.

Goodlad, S. (1984) Introduction. In *Education for the Professions: Qius Custodiat?* (S. Goodlad, ed.), pp. 4–16. Guildford, Surrey: NFER-Nelson/Society for Research into Higher Education.

Harrison, K., Gray, K. and Barlow, J. (1998) Evaluation of clinical interventions: Effectiveness, efficiency and equity. *British Journal of Therapy and Rehabilitation*, **5**(8), 396–401.

Higgs, J. and Titchen, A. (1995) The nature, generation and verification of knowledge. *Physiotherapy*, **81**(9), 521–530.

Higgs, J. and Titchen, A. (1998) Research and knowledge. *Physiotherapy*, **84**(2), 72–80.

Hunt, A., Adamson, B. and Harris, L. (1998) Physiotherapists' perceptions of the gap between education and practice. *Physiotherapy Theory and Practice*, **14**(4), 125–138.

Hunter, K. M. (1991) *Doctors' Stories: The Narrative Structure of Medical Knowledge*. Princeton, NJ: Princeton University Press.

Huth, E. J. (1990) *How to Write and Publish Papers in the Medical Sciences*. Baltimore: Williams & Wilkins.

Jensen, G. M. (1989) Qualitative methods in physical therapy research: A form of disciplined enquiry. *Physical Therapy*, **69**(6), 492–500.

Innes, J. (1998) A qualitative insight into the experiences of post graduate radiography students: Causes of stress and methods of coping. *Radiography*, **4**, 89–100.

Lettinga, A., Siemonsma, P. C. and van Veen, M. (1999) The intertwinement of theory and practice in physiotherapy: A comparative analysis of NDT and MRP as an example. *Physiotherapy*, **85**(9), 476–490.

Lewin, K. (1946) Action research and minority problems. *Journal of Social Issues*, **2**, 34–46.

Lyon, D. (1994) *Postmodernity*. Buckingham: Open University Press.

Mallik, M. (1993) Theory-to-practice links. *Senior Nurse*, **13**(4), 41–46.

Matthews, R. (1998) *Facts Versus Factions: The Use and Abuse of Subjectivity in Scientific Research*. Cambridge: European Science and Environment Forum.

Mattingly, C. and Fleming, M. (1994) *Clinical Reasoning: Forms of Inquiry in Therapeutic Practice*. Philadelphia: F. A. Davis.

Meerabeau, E. (1998) Immigrants to the New World: Nursing as an academic discipline. *NT Research*, **3**(5), 388–392.

Morse, J. M. (1991) Negotiating commitment and involvement in the nurse-patient relationship. *Journal of Advanced Nursing*, **16**, 455–468.

Nelson, C., Treichler, P. A. and Grossberg, L. (1992) Cultural studies. In *Cultural Studies* (L. Grossberg, C. Nelson and P. A. Treichler, eds), pp. 1–16. New York: Routledge.

O'Connor, M. (1978) *Editing Science Books and Journals*. London: Pitman Medical.

Parry, A. and Stone, S. (1991a) Capturing the basics: The development of an expert system for physiotherapists. *Physiotherapy*, **77**(3), 222–226.

Parry, A. and Stone, S. (1991b) Redeeming expert knowledge. In *Proceedings of XI International Conference of the World Confederation for Physical Therapy*, book II, pp. 603–605. London: WCPT/Chartered Society of Physiotherapy.

Polyani, M. (1967) *The Tacit Dimension*. London: Routledge.

Roberts, P. (1994) Theoretical models of physiotherapy. *Physiotherapy*, **80**(6), 361–366.

Robertson, V. J. (1995) A quantitative analysis of research in *Physical Therapy*. *Physical Therapy*, **75**(4), 313–322.

Rolfe, G. (1988) The theory-practice gap in nursing: From research-based practice to practitioner-based research. *Journal of Advanced Nursing*, **28**(3), 672–679.

Ryle, G. (1949) *The Concept of Mind*. London: Hutchinson.

Salvage, J. (1998) Editorial. *Nursing Times*, **94**(28), 22.

Schön, D. A. (1983) *The Reflective Practitioner*. London: Temple Smith.

Schön, D. A. (1987) *Educating the Reflective Practitioner*. San Francisco: Jossey-Bass.

Schön, D. A. (1991) *The Reflective Practitioner: How Professionals Think in Action*. London: Temple Smith.

Scutter, S. and Goold, M. (1995) Burnout in recently qualified physiotherapists in South Australia. *Australian Journal of Physiotherapy*, **41**, 115–118.

Shepard, K. F. (1987) Qualitative and quantitative research in clinical practice. *Physical Therapy*, **67**(12), 1891–1894.

Shepard, K. F., Jensen, G. M., Schmoll, B. J., Hack, L. M. and Gwyer, J. (1993) Alternative approaches to research in physical therapy: Positivism and phenomenology. *Physical Therapy*, **73**(2), 88–101.

Strauss, A. and Corbin, J. (1994) Grounded theory methodology: An overview. In *Handbook of Qualitative Research* (N. Denzin and Y. Lincoln, eds), pp. 273–285. Thousand Oaks, CA: Sage.

Titchen, A. and Binnie, A. (1994) Action research: A strategy for theory generation and testing. *International Journal of Nursing Studies*, **31**(1), 1–12.

Vernon, W., Parry, A. and Potter, M. (1998) Preliminary findings in a Delphi study of shoe wear marks. *Journal of Forensic Identification*, **48**(1), 22–35.

Winter, R. (1998) Finding a voice – thinking with others: A conception of action research. *Educational Action Research*, **6**(1), 53–67.

Wood, W. (1996) Legitimizing occupational therapy's knowledge. *American Journal of Occupational Therapy*, **50**(8), 626–634.

# 27

# Professional craft knowledge and power relationships

**Annette Street**

Power relationships and forms of knowledge are entirely different things and yet are inexorably linked. The task of this chapter is to delineate the ways these interrelationships work as a basis for ways to rethink, re-act and resist the exercise of propositional power that marginalizes professional craft knowledge. To begin this task it is important to explore the way we write and speak and act with regard to power.

### Power is not a commodity

Everyday discussions and most texts treat power as a commodity, something that one person or group has to the detriment of others. Thus we speak of people who have the **power to** achieve something, have **power over** someone, can **empower** another, are **powerful** or are **powerless**. Each of these terms carries a meaning that suggests that power is an object we either have or don't have. Comprehending how language shapes our understanding of the world is important here. If we think in terms of dichotomies of the 'haves' and the 'have nots' then we create a picture that is static and polarized. The point I want to make in this chapter is that power is not an object which can be 'had' but a force which circulates (Foucault, 1977). It can be likened more to a process than a product. Power can be used but not held. This is an important and liberating point. It provides us with a picture of our world where opportunities to exercise power are available for anyone, although social and personal circumstances mean some people have many more opportunities afforded to them than others. An understanding of how power is used to privilege certain kinds of knowledge over other kinds can open up possibilities to subvert the status quo. It may facilitate different ways of thinking, which lead to changed action or the knowledge of when and how to refrain from action (Street, 1995).

The argument has been made in this book that propositional power is afforded more status than professional craft knowledge, and thus those who are aligned with these forms of knowledge are accordingly afforded more status. This point is particularly obvious when we think about doctors, nurses and patients. Equating medical, nursing and patients' knowledges with a hierarchical ordering of propositional, professional craft and lay knowledges is both artificial and misleading. It reduces the complexities of these knowledges and their interrelationships. It sharpens and demarcates hierarchical boundaries between doctors, nurses and patients that are blurred and often fluid. It also disguises the effects of power relationships at work.

## Medical knowledge and power relationships

### Medical use of professional craft knowledge

Doctors are highly educated in terms of propositional knowledge. They are taught to adhere to the gold standard of the randomized control trial as the method by which the most reliable and rigorous knowledge can be obtained. Scientific propositional knowledge is rewarded by social and professional status. Medicine has strongly aligned its knowledge base with science and has been afforded the status that scientists enjoy, while being financially remunerated for medical craft skills in a way that scientists are not. This financial reward has brought with it the other trappings of social success – opportunities to move in those social circles where decision-making occurs and sinecures are available. In the past this social status along with political alliances has enabled doctors to create a monopoly of referral processes and prescribing rights (Willis, 1983).

Very few doctors actually ever use this scientific method to obtain knowledge themselves; rather, they are consumers of propositional knowledge which informs their professional craft knowledge. Frequently, doctors sit in a consulting room and face a person who reports a jumble of seemingly unrelated symptoms. The doctor asks some probing questions, narrows down possibilities, discards some symptoms as not part of the presenting problem and finally comes up with a tentative diagnosis, which is often confirmed by laboratory tests. Effective doctors work with the person to make sense of their illness in the context of their lives. They may provide advice and education that is health promoting and related to ongoing management of the condition. Thus they use their professional craft knowledge to determine the person's health problem and the appropriate treatment regime to assist. Yet invariably whenever doctors speak of their knowledge they emphasize the scientific base (Turner, 1987). They so tightly align their use of scientific knowledge with their practice that their usage of medical craft knowledge is rarely described in any more detail than 'clinical practice'. They contend that what they do in their consulting rooms is scientific, rather than being craft knowledge based on scientific knowledge or created in order to use propositional knowledge in the particular case (see Chapter 2). They claim the right of experts to define 'what constitutes a sick or insane client, but they also determine the limits of possibilities for the study, treatment and management of the objectified client' (Cheek and Rudge, 1993, p. 276).

Similarly, much of surgery is physical work. The capacity to cut, bend, break, reattach and suture are all parts of the surgeon's repertoire of surgical craft knowledge. Surgery requires scientific knowledge, but much experimental surgery precedes scientific trials; it is an outgrowth of craft knowledge that may then become the basis of a controlled scientific trial to test efficacy. Yet again, surgical knowledge is underpinned by the scientific propositional knowledge of anatomy and physiology.

The value of professional craft knowledge is emerging as a counterbalance to the dominance of propositional knowledge. In 1998 I attended the American Psychiatric Association's annual meeting. As a feminist sociologist who is interested in what counts as knowledge, I asked myself, 'whose knowledge was afforded the most status?', 'who was chosen to speak at the main public lectures?' and 'what were the key topics?' It was interesting to note that those who were chosen to speak to thousands at the huge public lectures were either psychiatrists interested in the latest directions in polypharmacy, neurologists or neuropsychiatrists. Again, propositional knowledge was the dominant public discourse of this event. However, competing discourses became apparent throughout the course of the proceedings. Concerns were aired that supporting such a strong partnership with pharmacologists and neuroscientists denied the therapeutic craft knowledge of 'talk therapy' that has been the basis of psychoanalysis. These debates were not resolved. Such debates form an ongoing undercurrent in medicine and represent its joint heritage from science and the craft of medical practice; the reason that medicine is sometimes discerningly described as an art and a science.

## Knowledge and power relationships in nursing

Historically, nurses have had a less secure basis from which to describe their practice. Debates in the nursing literature of the 1970s and 1980s raged as nurses tried to decide whether nursing was an art or a science; or if doctors cured and nurses cared. These dichotomous debates occurred because of the need for nurses to articulate their practice in ways that enabled them to gain professional credence and overthrow their image as doctors' handmaidens. Some nurses opted to develop nursing science and to emulate the scientific alliances made by their medical colleagues. Others chose to emphasize the caring and holistic elements of nursing. More recently, the practice has been to merge the two directions to describe the nurse as a holistic, reflective and technologically capable practitioner able to utilize evidence-based knowledge, to coordinate, plan and provide care. This role requires the exercise of both propositional and professional craft knowledge but, in the eyes of the public, nursing is not afforded the status of other disciplines that also use these combinations of knowledge forms. There are distinctive differences in the roles of doctors and nurses. These distinctions are becoming more evident with the advent of telemedicine and computerized patient monitoring systems. Such systems enable medical staff to remain in their hospital office away from patient care and to monitor information about the patient on computer screens. Unless operating, doctors are able to undertake most of the diagnosis from the scientific data available and stay remote from the messiness of patient care. It is nurses who wipe up vomit and faeces, collect sputum, and deal with fungating wounds. Nurses provide the kind of comfort and technological care that requires them to stay close to the person and the technology. It is nurses who hear the family stories or notice that something is wrong that is not being monitored on the screens. Nurses organize for other health professionals to become involved or coordinate discharge care. Yet these activities are essentially based on nurses' craft knowledge, which inevitably has its base in the propositional nature of the physical sciences, philosophy, sociology, psychology or education, but which is interpreted in nursing action that is polished through mentoring, experience and practice.

Nursing is a generic label for a multitude of nursing specialties that require different forms of propositional knowledge and different opportunities to exercise power. Intensive care nurses are often revered for their technological skill that demonstrates their propositional knowledge in ways that appear more sophisticated than that of their peers working in mental health or medical nursing. Links with high technology and close working relationships with medical staff are a necessary part of practice in intensive care environments. Yet each specialty depends on sophisticated scientific knowledge. The use of propositional knowledge may be invisible to the person who watches a nurse giving a dying man a bed bath or teaching an asthmatic child how to use a peak flow meter. Too often these activities are related to the tasks of family life and, as such, carry the low status of private sphere activities when compared with those that belong in the public domain. The subjective and relational aspects of private domain knowledge are undervalued in comparison to objective, scientific and technical public domain knowledge.

## The exercise of nursing power

Although nursing professional craft knowledge does not provide nurses with the same social status, fiscal rewards or opportunities to control health care directions as their medical colleagues enjoy, they nevertheless have opportunities to exercise power in multiple ways. The personal and sometimes intimate contact with patients and their families enables many nurses to exercise power as information-givers, as patient advocates, as coordinators of care, and to receive the benefits of the interpersonal relationships in the healing or dying process (Street, 1992). This exercise of professional craft power may be in the best interests of patients, their families, allied health staff and medical staff, or it may not. In a recent study (Aranda and Street, 1999), nurses demonstrated how the alliances they formed with dying patients through close nurse–patient relationships enabled them to respond in sophisticated ways to these patients' needs. The position that each nurse took up at any given time was negotiated with the patient or was developed through a preparedness to transgress professional discourses on distancing practices in order to assist patients to take as much control as they desired. In this way, power circulated through the structuring of intersubjective nurse–patient relationships in which the subjective view of experience of each party is taken into account. The nurse as healer empowered the patient through knowledgeable and sensitive practice; likewise patients empowered themselves to become their own healers with nursing support. This notion of nurses as healers is described further by Titchen in Chapter 9. In addition, McCormack and Titchen delineate in Chapter 12 ways in which patients can be helped to make decisions about their care that are authentic in the context of who they are and of their lives.

However, not all power is exercised wisely in nursing practice. Nurses may use power through their actions, their projections or their assumptions. Much that passes under the rubric of the 'best interests of the patient' can be found to be in the best interest of the nurses, catering staff, medical staff or hospital administration (Street, 1995). Nurses can withhold information, ignore patients, project their needs and beliefs onto the patients, be Anglo-centric in their practice, compete with allied health and medical staff and engage in horizontal violence, taking out their frustrations on their peers. They may be obstructive with medical and administrative staff and exercise power inappropriately over staff of lesser status such as cleaners, ward clerks or patient care attendants. These misuses of power contravene the provision and continuity of effective patient care, disrupt nurse–patient and staff relationships, and deny the healing potential of quality nursing care (May, 1993).

## The patient experience

The capacity for nurses to use and abuse power is mirrored in the patient's experience. When ill people become 'patients' they find themselves subject to intimate intrusions into their physical and mental well-being by a range of health professionals. They discover that they are required to discuss sensitive topics about their bodies and malfunctions with a constant stream of strangers. They learn that there are processes and routines which are nurse-controlled and to which they are expected to conform (May, 1992). They become the object of the medical gaze and subject to the scrutiny and actions of multiple health professionals (Foucault, 1977). Their actions and responses are under constant surveillance, and the interpretation of this information is made behind closed doors. Their story has to be endlessly repeated in a myriad of contexts. Their socioeconomic situation is elicited and documented whilst their social and familial relationships have to be acted out in public and become part of the domain of knowledge that is evaluated in relation to their 'case'. Many people claim access to knowledge of their health problems and offer competing and confounding advice. Patients and their relatives are often afraid to complain about difficulties relating to their treatment or care because they fear a lack of attention or mistreatment in the future (May, 1992). Helpless families can resort to bribes such as chocolates and flowers for the nurses to ensure good care for their loved one.

The exercise of power occurs not only in what is **known** about the patient's physical body, social situation and social relationships. Power is also exercised in numerous physical ways through the daily routine of hospital or community care. In hospitals, patients are expected to dress in night attire during the day, eat at designated times, in bed, and from a limited choice of menu. They are expected to allow themselves to be washed or showered routinely each day and to conform to the image of what nurses consider is a tidy bed area with a clean, tidy patient (Street, 1995). They learn to tolerate intrusive questions about bowels and bladders in public and discover the need to adapt to the specified expectations of a 'good patient'. They learn to accept being exercised and pummelled by physiotherapists or provided with medications and other treatments by nurses for their 'own good'. They learn that they need to satisfy social workers that they can pay their bills and cope at home with family issues, whilst also explaining to occupational therapists how they will manage to function with diminished activity levels. Part of the illness experience concerns coming to terms with the opportunities for health professionals to exercise their propositional and professional craft knowledge in relation to the patient.

Health professionals also exercise power in the way that they reframe and reformulate patients' lay knowledge of their symptoms and conditions to represent it in medicalized forms (Wellard, 1996). This activity silences or marginalizes the patient voice. The language of propositional knowledge or professional craft knowledge prevails. Benign breast lumps are named and the woman finds she has a **disease** – fibrocystic breast disease – and an associated care regime.

Yet when health professionals deconstruct their own practices they may exercise power in the best interests of the patient (Drevdahl, 1995). This may occur through practices of interpreting the illness experience in ways that help patient and family to exercise power through informed and participatory decision-making processes. Patient- and family-centred care has been part of the professional literature for some time, but there are too few instances of consistent practice where it is evident that processes are in place to ensure its continuity. The work of Titchen (Chapter 9) sets out the processes and practical strategies of skilled companionship that offers a new way of working **with** patients and their families. (See also Chapter 16.)

### The exercise of patient power

Patients are able to exercise power in a variety of ways that assist or disrupt the healing process. Patients who have serious or chronic conditions often become experts in understanding the complexity of their condition and its management in everyday life. Patient advocacy and self-help groups often provide access to propositional knowledge about the condition and professional craft knowledge concerning its management. Engagement with these groups may provide the patient and family with the confidence and knowledge to recognize their rights, to challenge disempowering structures, to question treatment regimes, to participate in decision-making and to act as advocates for others. Patients learn that they can refuse treatment, be 'non-compliant' with drug regimes, use a range of other practices and therapies without disclosure to the physician, and exercise their right to require second, third and fourth opinions.

However, the exercise of power by patients does not always achieve better health care or effective therapeutic relationships with health professionals. Patients and carers can become aggressive in the demands they place on health care professionals' time and expertise. They can deliberately demand extra service by constantly ringing their bells or calling out, be unsympathetic to the care needs of other patients, and have unreal expectations of the unit resources or the availability of the community service. Manipulative patients are not always aggressive. For example, some 'dear old ladies' can exercise power through the tyranny of niceness (Street, 1995). Attention-getting behaviours are part of some patients' repertoires that assist them to take more control. Thanking the very busy nurse for a service provided and then sweetly asking for just one more little task to be done is a pattern that may be repeated constantly.

## Moving on: reformulating power relations

Although it is evident that the status associated with propositional power means that doctors are able to exercise power more readily and more effectively than either other health professionals or patients, the seeming hierarchy of power relations is not fixed. It is inherently unstable. This situation has important ramifications. An understanding that power relations are constantly exercised in a capillary action that can be re-formed, reframed and reconstituted means that change is always possible. Change can occur at macro policy and health system levels; it can also occur at the micro level of daily interactions (see, e.g., Binnie and Titchen, 1999). Comprehension of the inherent fragility of these strategies and their attendant social relationships is also liberating. Situations are not set in concrete. Strategies, traditions and routines can always be resisted, restructured or reclaimed.

Nurses have a profound and intimate ongoing engagement with the subjective bodies of ill or injured people (Lawler, 1991). They may engage in objectifying practices but their professional craft knowledge is bound up in the intersubjectivity of the nurse–patient relationship and its effects in care for the whole person (Aranda and Street, 1999). The development of partnerships in body care between nurses and patients can be healing and life-enhancing, even in the face of terminal illness (van der Riet, 1998).

Patients too have deep and specific knowledge of their particular body, with, in some instances, a more generalized knowledge of the illness experiences of others with similar health conditions (Lawler, 1997). They can readily learn to objectify their subjective experience and speak about the affected part of the body as if it was separate to themselves. Sometimes this is a survival strategy, as evident in the account by Gallagher, a severely disabled woman, who describes herself as 'just a head' (Fassett and Gallagher, 1998). The work of Fassett, a skilled nurse, allowed Gallagher to reconstruct her health care experience in a way that was more enabling and healing for her as a person. Gallagher reconfigured her views of herself in ways that were meaningful for her and affirmed her intellect.

In my work with colleagues we have engaged in various participatory processes to examine and reconstruct practice in ways that are more empowering. We use action research and feminist participatory processes to affirm professional craft knowledge and chart the ways that power can be shared in partnerships with patients. These processes enable us to deconstruct the power relations at work and to reconstruct our actions in ways that deliberately attempt to circulate power amongst us. In this way no one group is able to exercise power without contestation. Our initial work was with nurses (Street, 1995; Street and Walsh, 1998; Blackford and Street, 1999); then we included doctors and other health professionals (Punyahortra and Street, 1998); and finally, we are involving all those whose situation will be affected by the actions – patients/clients and other stakeholders (Street, 1998). These strategies enable us to work **with** others to contest the status quo and to construct ways of using professional craft knowledge to facilitate healing, in ways that take account of the differences of race, gender, class and ability. They allow us to journey with sick people on their own terms.

## References

Aranda, S. and Street, A. (1999) Being authentic and being a chameleon: Nurse–patient interaction revisited. *Nursing Inquiry*, **5**(2), 75–82.

Blackford, J. and Street, A. (1999) The potential of 'peer' clinical supervision to improve nursing practice. *Clinical Effectiveness in Nursing*, **2**(4), 205–212.

Binnie, A. and Titchen, A. (1999) *Freedom to Practise: The Development of Patient-Centred Nursing*. Oxford: Butterworth-Heinemann.

Cheek, J. and Rudge, T. (1993) The power of normalisation: Foucauldian perspectives on contemporary Australian health care practices. *Australian Journal of Social Issues*, **28**(4), 271–284.

Drevdahl, D. (1995) Coming to voice: The power of emancipatory community interventions. *Advances in Nursing Science*, **18**(2), 13–24.

Fassett, D. and Gallagher, M. R. (1998) *Just a Head.* St Leonards, NSW: Allen & Unwin.

Foucault, M. (1977) *Discipline and Punish: The Birth of the Prison.* New York: Pantheon.

Lawler, J. (1991) *Behind the Screens: Nursing Somology and the Problem of the Body.* Melbourne: Churchill Livingstone.

Lawler, J. (ed.) (1997) *The Body in Nursing.* Melbourne: Churchill Livingstone.

May, C. (1992) Nursing work, nurses' knowledge, and the subjectification of the patient. *Sociology of Health and Illness*, **14**(4), 472–487.

May, C. (1993) Subjectivity and culpability in the constitution of nurse–patient relationships. *International Journal of Nursing Studies*, **30**(2), 181–192.

Punyahortra, S. and Street, A. (1998) Exploring the discursive construction of menopause for Thai women. *Nursing Inquiry*, **5**(2), 96–103.

Street, A. (1992) *Inside Nursing.* New York: SUNY Press.

Street, A. (1995) *Nursing Replay.* Melbourne: Churchill Livingstone.

Street, A. (1998) From soulmates to stakeholders: Issues in creating quality postmodern participatory research relationships. *Social Sciences in Health*, **4**(2), 119–129.

Street, A. and Walsh, C. (1998) Nursing assessments in New Zealand. *Journal of Advanced Nursing*, **27**, 553–559.

Turner, B. (1987) *Medical Power and Social Knowledge.* London: Tavistock.

van der Riet, P. (1998) The sexual embodiment of the cancer patient. *Nursing Inquiry*, **5**(4), 248–257.

Wellard, S. (1996) Family connections? Exploring nursing roles with families in home-based care. *Nursing Inquiry*, **3**(1), 57–58.

Willis, E. (1983) *Medical Dominance: The Division of Labour in Australian Health Care.* Sydney: George Allen and Unwin, Australia.

# Section Four

---

# Reflections

# 28

# A dynamic framework for the enhancement of health professional practice in an uncertain world: the practice–knowledge interface

**Angie Titchen and Joy Higgs**

In this book we have explored practice knowledge from two main perspectives: from the frame of reference of the (health) professions, whose practice knowledge is the focus of this book, and from the point of view of the individual professional, whose practice knowledge is in a constant state of critique and redevelopment. In Chapter 1 we examined different images for the nature of practice knowledge (an anemone, a kaleidoscope, a labyrinth and a river), presenting practice knowledge as a phenomenon which is multifaceted, living, changeable, evolving and constructed. Our key message at that point was that expert health professionals seamlessly integrate three forms of practice knowledge in action, i.e. propositional knowledge, professional craft knowledge and personal knowledge. Given that academia and the professions themselves have previously valued propositional knowledge above the other forms of knowledge and have placed more emphasis on the application of theory to practice than on the integration of the three forms of knowledge, this book has attempted to redress this imbalance. We have focused on the nature of professional craft knowledge and its relationships and integration with propositional and personal knowledge.

In Chapter 2, Higgs and Andresen created the metaphor of weaving to portray the development of a profession's knowledge base (within the broader context of the evolution of the knowledge of the ages reflected in the weaving of a never-ending tapestry) and the development of an individual professional's knowledge base (reflected in the weaving of personal carpets). The theme of practice knowledge generation was examined in a number of chapters in the book. A more sophisticated view of how research evidence can be used in patient care has been offered, in which it is recognized that practitioners cannot merely take research findings and/or theories 'off the shelf' and apply them to a particular episode of patient care; they have to do work, either to judge whether the findings and/or theories are useful in this specific case, or to create new professional craft knowledge in order to particularize the research and/or theories and make them relevant to the given context. As a whole, this book has examined ways in which this knowledge creation and its validation can be undertaken by practitioners, practitioner-researchers and researchers, and how these processes can be facilitated in students and less experienced practitioners. It has been proposed that such practices are based on the notion of constructivism and that metacognition, deliberative reflection and professional artistry play key roles in the use, acquisition and creation of professional practice knowledge.

This final chapter integrates the many threads woven throughout this book to focus on a third key dimension of practice knowledge. That, beyond the nature and development of practice knowledge, is the incorporation into practice of the individual's and the profession's evolving practice knowledge base which stands in a reciprocal, mutually-enhancing relationship with practice-generated knowledge. We examine the practice–knowledge interface with reference to a number of themes developed in this book, and introduce a framework for the enhancement of health professional practice for the uncertain world of health care. This framework has three parts: the practice–knowledge dialectic, practice development and the facilitation of professional agency.

## The practice–knowledge dialectic

There is an essential unity between knowledge and practice which could be considered a dialectic relationship (Higgs, 1999). A dialectic may be defined as 'the philosophic process of reconciling the contradictions of experience in a higher synthesis' (Hayward and Sparkes, 1982, p. 309). This merger, through the confrontation of the differences between the two phenomena (knowledge and practice) 'results in a higher order process that transcends and encompasses them both' (Kolb, 1984, p. 29). We can think of this as a dialectic: doing–knowing.

The value of dialectics in discussing the nature of professional practice in postindustrial (postmodern) society lies in the reality that much of the role and success of professionals is entwined in their capacity to deal effectively with the contradictions they face. In the world of professional practice, where we are dealing with the multiple variables of human life and the inexactness of professional knowledge and practice, success and excellence lie in harnessing the relevant strengths of the contradictory choices and options facing us, and producing a higher synthesis of these choices. Herein lies the essence of the practice–knowledge dialectic.

In Fig. 28.1 we depict three important dimensions of this relationship and its success.

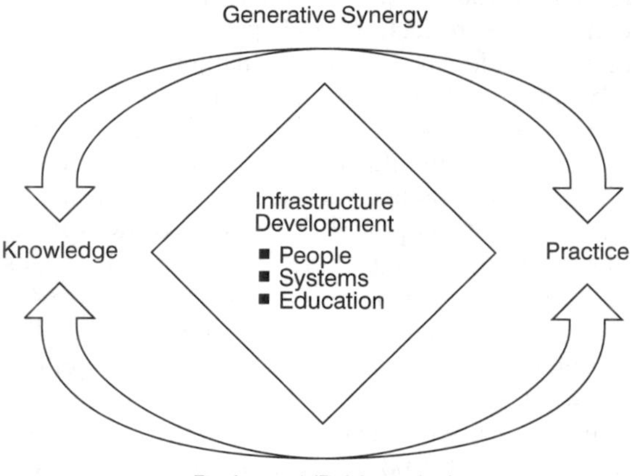


**Figure 28.1** The knowledge–practice dialectic

The first is the synergy of generation of knowledge and the evolution of practice, the development of each acting as a catalyst to the enhancement of the other. The second dimension is reciprocal appraisal (and reappraisal), in that a central responsibility of professionals is to continually appraise/evaluate their knowledge and practice as part of assuring quality in their practice roles. These two dimensions are explored in part two of the professional practice framework: practice development. The third dimension is the infrastructure development which is essential for the promotion of professional agency. This discussion is developed in part three of the framework: facilitating professional agency.

## Practice development

To examine this factor we revisit the metaphor of a river of knowledge (introduced in Chapter 1 and developed in Chapter 7), focusing on a particular part of the evolution of knowledge, reflective evaluation. We use the image of a pool within a river system to illustrate this process, this review of knowledge. In the quiet time of watching reflections in the pool we envisage the concentric ripples[1] which form when something (some new idea or disturbance) is tossed by the turbulence of the main stream of the river into the centre of the still pool, disrupting its smooth surface (see Plate 4, at the front of Section 3, p. 119).

Each ripple represents a theme relating to practice knowledge and its impact on professional practice, which has emerged in the book. These themes show where we have arrived in our understanding of practice epistemology, its development and its connection with the development of expertise, and reveal some of the obstacles facing the health care professions as they develop their epistemologies in a postmodern era.

### *Practice*

At the heart of our dreaming pool lies practice: we are committed to the notion that professional practice not only must be theory-based, but also needs to be founded on practice-based theory. (See Fig. 28.2, also Chapters 7 and 26.) Such theory, generated by practitioners themselves, sometimes with the support of outside researchers, replaces the modernist idea that grand theory and certainty can be sought by the health professions.

The current context of uncertainty and rapid change has resulted from a number of trends over

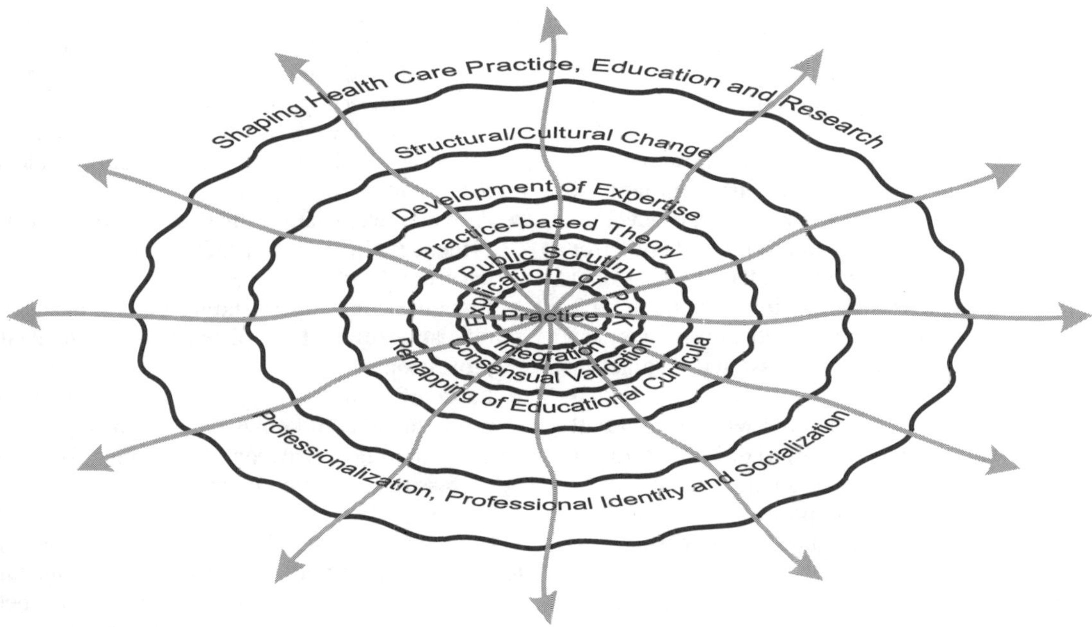


**Figure 28.2** Practice development

the past 20 or so years which have significantly impacted on professional practice, including postmodernism and globalization. Postmodernism (see Andresen, 1998) can be considered to be a broad, varied and diffuse intellectual and artistic period which has provided a critical standpoint or historical phase of transition, an attitude of radical scepticism towards things, particularly towards history, towards values, towards grand theories and certainty. Postmodernism has brought a time of critical reflection and judgments about where we have been and where we are going. It has prompted a pendulum swing back from the dizzy extreme of scientific-empirical confidence and certainty that had been the hallmark of modernism during the first half of the twentieth century. The 'postmodern dis-position' is characterized by moments which manifest fundamental dimensions of individuals and reflect personally held values (Higgs, 1998). As postmodernism wanes in the early twenty-first century, we can reflect that one of its most salient qualities, in the hands of a large army of vocal proponents, has been that whilst it stands as the 'ultimate critic' of every other intellectual position, it fails dismally in being self-critical (L. Andresen, personal communication).

'*Globalization* refers to the increasing unification and interconnectedness of the world and its nations. It is manifested in global economic restructuring (particularly in terms of multinational companies, foreign loans/debts and interdependence of national economies), increased global communication (with overwhelming immediacy and magnitude of information and news), ever-growing international involvement and influence on the political, military and human dimensions of life, rapid dissemination of technological advances and new dimensions in travel speed and scope' (Higgs et al., 1999, p. 33). Within this context health professionals seek to practise and generate knowledge in confusing circumstances, at local and global levels, in addition to having to cope with the uncertainty of dealing with people in what Schön (1983) describes as the messiness of professional practice.

### *Developmental strategies*

Rippling out from the heart of the pool is the developmental strategy for making professional craft knowledge more explicit. As this knowledge is disclosed, it is **integrated** with propositional and personal knowledge. The next ripple or theme of activity in the developmental strategy is the **public scrutiny** and **consensual validation** of this new knowledge. In the next, **practice-based theory** is further developed and tested using qualitative and quantitative empirical research and evaluation. Professional educators **remap educational curricula** to include emerging professional craft knowledge and the more fully developed practice-based theories.

Underneath all these ripples (and now forming one of its own) has run the **development of expertise**. This ripple has rested on the development and testing of facilitation strategies for helping practitioners to explicate their professional craft and personal knowledge, integrate them with propositional knowledge and critically review and test the resulting professional practice knowledge.

The next ripple represents the wider **structural and cultural changes** and **reconfiguration** of professionalization, professional identity and socialization that will support the evolution of knowledge and the development of expertise and vice versa. These changes are brought about through practice development approaches located in critical social science where there is an intent to transform practice, at the same time as generating new knowledge about how to carry out the change effectively.

Finally, we reach the edge of the pool, which is constantly eroded and re-formed by the lapping ripples. Over time and with intent, the ripples transform the social and political landscape in health care. In the new landscape, changed power relationships allow patients and families to be genuinely involved in decisions about their care, enabling their voices, along with those of health care practitioners, to be heard and acted upon by policy and funding decision-makers. Thus, the voices of patients, families and practitioners become as loud as those of politicians and traditionally influential lobbyists, helping to shape health care practice, education and research.

To some readers, this dreaming may seem just that: unobtainable as a reality or merely wishful thinking, given the obstacles that have to be overcome. Taking each ripple or theme in turn, we set out these obstacles and crystallize the authors' and our own key ideas on ways forward, born of practice wisdom (for further reading see Scott, 1990), professional artistry, rigorous research and visionary thinking.

## Explication and integration of professional practice knowledge forms

Right at the heart of our framework there are significant obstacles to be overcome, including:

- Predominant valuing of propositional knowledge in some of the health professions (e.g. medicine and physiotherapy) and in parts of others (e.g. occupational therapy and nursing).
- A narrow view of evidence-based practice in which research evidence is the only evidence that counts.
- A naive expectation that acting on research evidence alone will produce certainty in an uncertain world.
- Ignorance, misunderstanding or not seeing the relevance of practice epistemology in the health professions.
- Lack of understanding about the nature of professional craft knowledge and the integration and interplay between the three forms of professional practice knowledge.

Convincing reasons for all forms of knowledge to be equally valued by practitioners, educators, researchers and research funders have been advanced in this book. First, research into expertise has shown that practice in uncertain, messy situations requires professional practice knowledge based on a mixture of propositional knowledge, professional craft knowledge and personal knowledge. (See Chapters 8 and 14; see also Kennedy, 1987.) Second, research-based evidence must be particularized by the practitioner in order to provide effective, personalized care. Nevertheless, Maxwell's Chapter 13 alerts us, as advocates of professional craft knowledge in the health professions, to the danger of going too far in countering the dominance of propositional knowledge and reproducing situations similar to that in performing arts. There, professional craft knowledge is valued above propositional knowledge. Maxwell argues that the latter is disregarded by many actors and their educators at the expense of critical reflection.

The book has helped to elucidate the nature of professional craft knowledge and to demonstrate the complexity of this form of knowledge and its relationships with propositional and personal knowledge. These complexities have been largely ignored in professional education and lifelong learning. And examination of the ways in which professional craft knowledge is acquired, used and created through practice has been neglected by researchers. Many authors in this book have argued that professional craft knowledge, whether it relates to education, practice or research, cannot be acquired independently of the education, practice or research experience. (See Chapters 15, 17, 19,

20, 22 and 23.) In addition, it has been found that the acquisition, use and creation of professional craft knowledge are inseparable and that professional craft knowledge can be used both consciously and unconsciously by practitioners.

The relevance of health professional researchers knowing about epistemology could be challenged. For example, Robertson (1996, p. 535) argues that 'a claim that knowing about theories of the nature of knowledge is necessary to generate or validate knowledge is mistaken'. She states that 'scientists have not needed to know about theories of knowledge to contribute to their fields over the decades and centuries'. In a paper replying to these arguments (Higgs and Titchen, 1998), we agreed that researchers **can** generate knowledge through research without understanding the nature of knowledge. However, we argued that this method-focused approach is inadequate. Rather, it is highly desirable, if not essential, that researchers make informed decisions about the goals and methodologies they develop to answer their research questions and understand the knowledge they are seeking to generate.

In this book we extend this debate and propose that practitioners and researchers need to be aware of, and value equally, the three forms of professional practice knowledge because the focus of attention needs to be broadened if professional craft and personal knowledge are to be explicated for public scrutiny. All practitioners are accountable for their practice and thus have a responsibility to review critically their professional knowledge base and make it publicly available. Practitioners, therefore, need to know the nature of this dynamic knowledge base, so that they can explore its complexity and particularity, contribute to developing the practice epistemology of the profession and participate in the never-ending process of critical appraisal, extension and review of the profession's knowledge base. (See Chapters 7 and 26.) If practitioners know how they generate professional craft knowledge and how they use it (and personal knowledge) to particularize propositional knowledge, then they will be better able to facilitate the metacognitive and deliberative reflective processes that this requires in less experienced practitioners. (See Chapter 8.)

These processes are illuminated in chapters by Walker on the sociocultural theory of participation in cultural practice/activities (Chapter 3), Titchen on critical companionship (Chapter 10), Dewing on supported reflection in clinical supervision (Chapter 16), and Best and Edwards on clinical practicums or placements (Chapter 21). These authors show how practitioners and students can be helped to develop an understanding of their practice epistemology through development of their metacognitive ability. Introducing students and practitioners to epistemology and its relevance to professional practice and research and helping them to challenge unquestioned assumptions about evidence-based care could also be considered by educators and facilitators of experiential learning.

Whilst it is recognized that the more tacit, less accessible aspects of professional craft and personal knowledge may never be fully expressible in words, they can be expressed through the use of creative arts media. Simons and Ewing (Chapter 24) show how the arts can be used by educators and facilitators of experiential learning. In addition, we demonstrate in this book how word imagery (anemone, kaleidoscope, labyrinth) and metaphor (river) can be used to express the more subtle complexities and nuances of creating a practice epistemology in a postmodern era.

### Practice-based theory and the remapping of educational curricula

In addition to the obstacles above, further difficulties need to be addressed in seeking to develop practice-based theory using qualitative research approaches, and remapping curricula to include this theory and all forms of professional practice knowledge. These obstacles include the following:

- Health professions have a preference for predictive theories deductively derived (often modifying and testing theories developed by other disciplines), rather than interpretive, explanatory theories inductively derived from studying health professionals' own perspectives on their practice. This is reflective of the medical model/scientific approach to knowledge generation, historically supported in the professionalization of the health professions.
- There is a lack of explicit recognition that personal development is a key part of becoming and developing as a professional. Health sciences education emphasizes professional development and has traditionally accentuated health professionals' 'clinical' role rather than their personal input to health care.
- Disproportionate weighting of propositional knowledge occurs in explicit curricula and in assessments of clinical knowledge, leading to

students perceiving professional craft and personal knowledge development as less important and less valid than the acquisition of scientific facts and theories.

- Within implicit clinical education curricula, clinical educators may model professional craft and personal knowledge that is outmoded or no longer considered appropriate (e.g. practical strategies for realizing paternalism, depersonalization and objectification of patients).

Currently, our practice epistemologies are unbalanced, as Richardson (see Chapter 6) suggests, by the masculinization of knowledge. More balance could be achieved by increasing our valuing of women's ways of knowing. (See Belenky et al., 1986; Pinkola Estes, 1994.) Thus, work will have to be done to legitimize a new core knowledge of practice and to give it academic credibility. (See Chapters 7 and 26.) Perhaps this work is more likely to come about as more people understand practice epistemology and the nature of expertise and professional artistry. They might begin to see the value of qualitative research approaches for developing more balanced practice epistemologies. Then the need to develop the professional craft knowledge of doing such research will become clear; research supervisors and their students could use cognitive apprenticeship as suggested by Pearson (see Chapter 25) to develop this knowledge. Guided by Parry (see Chapter 26), members of the professions could also give clear messages to journal editors about the kind of work that should be published in order to develop balanced practice epistemologies.

If curriculum planners begin to value equally all three kinds of professional practice knowledge and propositional knowledge that is inductively derived from practice, then the remapping of curriculum content and process would probably eventuate. The curriculum would include these kinds of knowledge and the professional practice knowledge of agency in an uncertain world, and would recognize the important role that personal frames of reference play in professional practice. Planners would design new educational and assessment strategies, such as scaffolding or support by more able learners, or using creative arts to help students acquire and integrate the three forms of professional practice knowledge. Educators are likely to need support in developing genuinely integrated curricula and in using new strategies to help their students mature intellectually, emotionally and psychologically. This support could be offered through debate, critique and curriculum development support.

Educators are probably already aware of the significant role that the clinical practicum, or placement, plays in facilitating learning. However, they may not be so aware that the practicum is the best context for facilitating the multifaceted learning process of acquiring professional craft knowledge, developing awareness of how personal frames of reference influence us as professionals, and how both these kinds of knowledge are integrated with propositional knowledge. Gaining knowledge of the nature and changeability of practice culture can also be effectively facilitated in the practicum. Thus these contexts can prepare students for changing participation in changing communities of practice (see Chapters 3 and 21) and for developing a personal research process. The effectiveness of the context is dependent, of course, on the quality of clinical educators, supervisors, mentors or critical companions in terms of their clinical and facilitation expertise and ability to articulate their knowledge bases. The quality of clinical education can be improved through outside support and through the shared learning experiences, for both educator and student, that the practicum context makes possible.

It must be recognized that cultural practices imbue the implicit values of role models and that these values will influence the substance of the professional craft knowledge acquired and the extent of personal maturation that can occur in beginning and less experienced practitioners. Many authors here have offered prescriptions about the need for clinical role models who are able to explicate practical strategies for giving patient-centred, effective, up-to-date care. As we read this literature we become aware that practitioners may need help to explore implicit values which may result in care that is no longer consistent with the emerging emphasis on health care values of person-centredness, holism and caring. Conroy, for example (see Chapter 23), points out the negative effects on students' moral development of role models who implicitly value scientific reductionism rather than holistic and caring ethical approaches. The reductionist approach frequently presents professional craft knowledge as a limited, 'unscientific' commodity, reflecting uncritical thinking, outdated ideas and values. The emphasis of this book, quite to the contrary, presents professional craft knowledge as complementary to propositional knowledge and as a valuable and essential tool in health sciences education and health care.

### The development of expertise

In addition to the above obstacles, the development of expertise faces the following hindrances:

- Health care organizations often do not understand the nature of professional expertise and, therefore, do not provide appropriate structures (such as clinical career ladders and performance outcomes) and cultures for the development or use of professional expertise.
- Expert practitioners are often unable to articulate their practice epistemology and/or have poorly developed facilitation skills for helping less experienced professionals to develop expertise.
- If a learning culture does not genuinely exist, practitioners may resist developmental programmes, even when support in the form of mentorship, supervision or critical companionship is beginning to be provided by the organization. Without confidence in the system, practitioners can see these strategies as a management surveillance tool designed to disempower them and take away their clinical autonomy and responsibility (Tirchen *et al.*, 1999).
- There is a general belief that practice research is carried out by outsider researchers from academic institutions and not by practitioners themselves.
- Expert practitioners may be unfamiliar with practitioner-research approaches to generating knowledge about their practice and creating the conditions (structural/cultural) in which the development of expertise will flourish.
- If practitioners wish to engage in practice research, there may be a lack of understanding and support from academic institutions.

A number of aspects of professional expertise have been examined in several chapters in this book. (See Chapters 8–14.) From this exploration the notion of professional artistry has emerged as a hallmark of expertise. Chapter 1 (see Table 1.1) presented professional artistry as an advanced level of clinical competence characterized by a unique, highly skilled approach to clinical practice built up through extensive introspective and critical reflection upon, and review of, clinical practice. This artistry is essential in professional agency in a world of practice where ends are uncertain and risks have to be taken. It is dependent on all three forms of professional practice knowledge, their interplay and integration and subsequent use in professional judgment. This knowledge moves beyond a focus on technical expertise towards caring conceptualized as an ethical stance (see Chapter 18) which is person-centred, authentic (see Chapter 12) and an interpersonal process (see Chapter 9). Mediation between the three kinds of knowledge and the creation of new professional practice knowledge can be viewed as the evolution of knowledge from a constructivist view. This evolution and the use of this knowledge in everyday practice require metacognition and deliberative reflection.

## The facilitation of professional agency

Agency refers to the capacity to act independently, responsibly and capably. In a professional context we could reasonably expect the health professional (agent) to demonstrate technical competence, the ability to interact effectively with people, and the capacity to adapt to and influence changing contexts. Agency is reflected in a new model for health practitioners proposed by Higgs and Hunt (1999). (See also Chapter 8.) This model, called the 'interactional professional', is particularly suited to the rapidly changing global context of health care. The interactional professional demonstrates the following characteristics:

- technical competence;
- interpersonal competence;
- the ability to interact with and change the context of practice;
- the capacity to demonstrate professional responsibility in serving and enhancing society;
- social responsibility;
- system interactivity;
- situational leadership.

Drawing on these ideas and the ripples or themes developed in part 2 of our framework, i.e. practice development, we propose that professional agency (in the health professions) can be epitomized in three factors: professional artistry, practice wisdom and professional expertise (see Fig. 28.2).

These characteristics involve the professional heart, mind, body and spirit, and will. The task of helping practitioners to develop their expertise and agency is likely also to involve infrastructure development (people, systems and education). In particular, agency requires effective systems (e.g. supportive cultures), staff development and education at pre-entry, in-service and postgraduate levels, all occurring within learning, empowerment cultures.

The development of professional agency can be facilitated by self-directed learning, peer learning, staff and systems development. Titchen (2000) investigated the role of experienced professionals in facilitating the expertise/agency of other professionals. She characterized this task as an experiential learning journey in which an expert practitioner journeyed together with a less experienced practitioner on physical, emotional, psychological, social and metaphysical levels. She and other authors in this book have stressed that expert practitioners need help to become effective facilitators of such enablement and learning. First, they need to explicate their professional practice knowledge; second, they need to understand their practice epistemology, so that they can facilitate others' construction, testing and verification of professional practice knowledge; third, they need to develop skills to facilitate others' metacognition, deliberative reflection, critique and critical dialogue and review of their own practice.

A variety of facilitation strategies have been offered in this book:

- **action research** – where practitioners simultaneously transform and investigate their own practice; e.g. exploring how to effectively help beginning practitioners to become more aware of their values and personal frames of reference and how these influence their work with patients;
- **practitioner research** – where practitioners explore an aspect of their practice without an attempt to change it; for instance, uncovering their professional craft knowledge of working with people with dementia;
- **scaffolding or support by more able learners** – e.g. clinical supervisors, critical companions/friends helping less experienced practitioners to dialogue critically with themselves and their practice, enhance self-regulation and self-reflection and thus metacognitive skills and processes;
- using **creative arts media** to acquire and integrate professional practice knowledge – e.g. learning about self and others, professional artistry and working collaboratively with patients, families and colleagues both intra- and inter-professionally.

## System and culture development

Beyond the development of individuals, the promotion of professional agency requires system development, for example developments in pro-

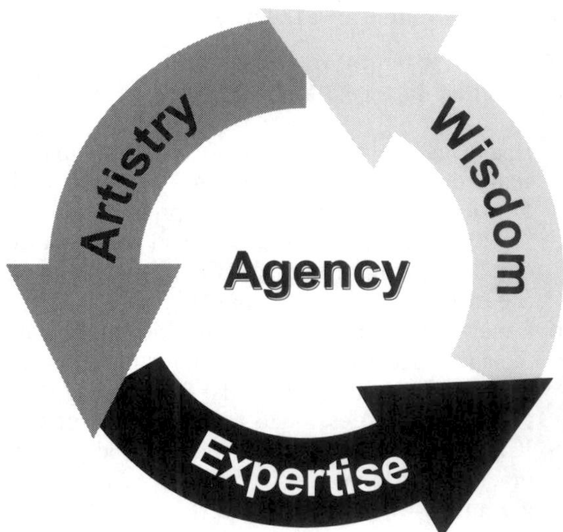


**Figure 28.3** Professional agency

fessions, practice, education and research. This relates to the two outer ripples in our practice development model (Fig. 28.2).

System change requires structural and cultural developments, changes in professionalization, professional identity and professional socialization, and developments in practice, education and research that both provide the framework for health care and represent the products of system development.

Professions are responding to postmodern demands by reconfiguring professionalism with a greater patient-centred focus. This book supports this trend and advocates professions viewing their knowledge bases as resources for patients and their families. This goal requires professionals to understand and be able to articulate their professional craft knowledge. Professional socialization into a differentiated community of practice also requires the explication of clear professional identities as well as a recognition of the value of creating professional cultures which share patient-centred values.

Professional socialization is a topic about which much has been written (e.g. Cant and Higgs, 1999). This book has contributed to this discussion by illustrating ways in which professional identity can be facilitated and shaped by enhancing the teaching of professional craft knowledge in on-campus learning and clinical practicums, staff development and practice development. In addition, collaborative research approaches could reveal how expert practitioners offer their professional practice knowledge in ways that patients and families can understand and use in informed decision-making about their care. Explicated professional craft knowledge could also be used to establish the key professional practice knowledge that distinguishes professions, and to promote understanding of knowledge that professions have in common. Being clearer about each other's knowledge bases, the professions can work together more effectively for the benefit of patients. This, in turn, is likely to lead to greater valuing of what each profession has to offer. Through our journey of exploration of practice knowledge in writing this book we have reached the conclusion that professional craft knowledge is a key in the reconfiguration of professionalization, professional identities and socialization.

Postmodern society requires new approaches and widespread changes to health care and the structures and cultures of its organizations. Changes in roles and relationships within educational systems will be necessary in both academic and clinical settings. For example, expert practitioners who see themselves as authorities in their field and who use didactic clinical teaching strategies may need help to see themselves as learning resources working alongside less experienced practitioners within collegiate relationships. In traditional relationships between health care and academic/educational communities, academics are the ones who have tended to research practice and set up programmes for **practitioners** to address the deficits in their practice. Postmodern relationships are rather more reciprocal, in that academics value practitioners' professional practice knowledge, seeking to learn from it and to use it in curriculum development. Thus, collaborative education and research programmes are established in which academics learn and work **with practitioners**. Collaborative inservice educational programmes and courses are designed to focus on each others' strengths rather than deficits. Thus, academics can access professional artistry and practitioners can benefit from the expert facilitation of educators in terms of explicating their knowledge and learning how to help others to learn. (See Titchen and Higgs, 1995.) For such collaboration to occur, it is likely that health care organizations and educational institutions will need to establish learning cultures that value professional artistry and see learning as part of a professional's everyday work. Unfortunately, in many organizations and institutions the culture is rather the antithesis, and learning and the development of expertise are largely unsupported and undervalued (Binnie and Titchen, 1999). Collaborative systems require participants to overcome unconducive cultures. Titchen et al. (1999) report that practitioners experience a variety of oppressive environments, such as hierarchical blame cultures.

Practice development is a strategy to address the goal of promoting culture and system change. We support a practice development approach located within a critical social science tradition. Critical social science is a way of studying and generating knowledge which views the world critically and seeks to redress power imbalances. Use of a critical social science philosophy, in this context, enables a rigorous approach to practice development that attempts to improve the development of expertise, the evolution of professional practice knowledge and the involvement of practitioners and patients in policy decision-making. Improvement is brought about by transforming the structures, roles, power relationships or cultures that currently prevent the new practices being implemented. There is also an attempt to gain theoretical and practical insights and understandings, through research, debate and critique, not only about the socio-historical, cultural and political factors that shape current practice, thinking and values and hinder change, but also about how to address those factors to bring about the desired changes. From our experience of practice development approaches working in a critical social science tradition, we propose that academic and health care organizations, working in collaborative partnerships, could successfully create learning and empowerment cultures. These partnerships could take the form of critical companionships, where the academic organization acts as a critical companion for the health care organization (Titchen et al., in press). For further information on how to bring about structural and cultural change, see Ward et al. (1998), Cutcliffe et al. (1999), Jackson et al. (1999a, b) and McCormack et al. (1999).

For health professionals and their patients to shape health care practice, education and research by influencing policy and funding, it will be necessary to change power relationships between practitioners and their patients, between doctors and other health care professionals, and between practitioners/patients and policy/funding decision-makers both locally and nationally. Overcoming obstacles to system development (such as entrenched, traditional relationships and difficulties in the articulation of professional craft knowledge to policy or funding decision-makers) requires practice development using a critical social science perspective. (See Chapter 27.) In particular, power differentials between doctors and other health professions are likely to reduce as the unique contribution of each health profession to patient care becomes clarified. Changed power relationships between practitioners and their patients would be helped by practitioners being able to articulate particularized propositional knowledge to their patients in ways that are not jargonistic and alienating. Thus, professional practice knowledge becomes a negotiable resource for patients and their families, rather than a source of power and control. This resource offers a greater role for patients and families in decision-making not only about their own care, but also about the delivery of existing and new services.

Much attention is currently being given by governments to enabling people who use and deliver health services to have a say in shaping these services and influencing local health providers. Research has been commissioned to find out how such empowerment and participation can be facilitated. The time is right, therefore, for helping patients and practitioners to empower themselves to speak with authority about their health care experiences and practices, respectively.

## Conclusions

In drawing together the various topics and themes presented in this book we have created a three-part framework which explores the practice–knowledge interface. The three parts of the framework are: the practice–knowledge dialectic, practice development and the facilitation of professional agency. We contend that the generation of knowledge from practice and the enhancement of practice through knowledge requires that we value and continue to expand our understanding of the higher order phenomenon, **the practice–knowledge dialectic**. It also requires working individually and collectively to expand our practice knowledges and knowledge-led practices like ripples in the pool of understanding, and using this knowledge, experience and practice skills to facilitate individual and group professional agency.

The six themes, or ripples, contained within our dreaming pool carry important messages for new millennium practitioners, educators and researchers. These messages relate to individual practitioners, health care and educational organizations and their cultures, professional identity, empowerment and the evolution of knowledge within a constructivist view. These factors link with the patient's world and with the deliberative reflection and metacognition of the practitioner. Yet the reflective 'time out' is but part of the overall knowledge–practice (river) system. This dynamic system of professional practice combines action and knowledge which are explicit and structured with underlying living images and mystery. It is time for the new streams of thinking presented in this book to be exposed and buffeted by mainstream thinking and culture and by competing vested interests, flowing alongside the mainstream and, in time, becoming confluent with it. Ancient wisdom tells us, 'do not push against the river'. So we will join its flow strengthened by our analysis, shape its course and transform the landscape through which it travels to the restless sea.

## Notes

1 In Chapter 7, Titchen and Ersser propose a developmental strategy for making professional craft knowledge more explicit. They suggest that consensual validation of new and existing professional craft knowledge could come about in ever-widening circles like the ripples in the pool, from the local group of professional colleagues, through regional and national forums, to publication and the Internet.

## References


Andresen, L. (1998) The *assets* of academia: Thoughts regarding our intellectual and moral value-capital. *HERDSA News*, **20**(3), 16–17.

Belenky, M. F., Clinchy, B. M., Goldberger, N. R. and Tarule, J. M. (1986) *Women's Ways of Knowing: The Development of Self, Voice and Mind*. New York: Basic Books.

Binnie, A. and Titchen, A. (1999) *Freedom to Practise: The Development of Patient-Centred Nursing*. Oxford: Butterworth-Heinemann.

Cant, R. and Higgs, J. (1999) Professional socialisation. In *Educating Beginning Practitioners: Challenges for Health Professional Education* (J. Higgs and H. Edwards, eds), pp. 46–51. Oxford: Butterworth-Heinemann.

Cutcliffe, J., Jackson, A., Ward, M., Cannon, B. and Titchen, A. (1999) Practice development in mental health nursing: Part 1. *Mental Health Practice*, **2**, 27–31.

Hayward, A. L., and Sparkes, J. J. (1982) *The Concise English Dictionary*. Ware: Omega Books.

Higgs, C., Neubauer, D. and Higgs, J. (1999) The changing health care context: Globalization and social ecology. In *Educating Beginning Practitioners: Challenges for Health Professional Education* (J. Higgs and H. Edwards, eds), pp. 30–37. Oxford: Butterworth-Heinemann.

Higgs, J. (1999) Doing, knowing, being and becoming in professional practice. In *Proceedings of the MTeach Post-Internship Conference 27–28 Sept 1999*. University of Sydney, http://alex.edfac.usyd.edu.au/conference 99/Keynotes/higgs.htm.

Higgs, J. and Hunt, A. (1999) Redefining the beginning practitioner. *Focus on Health Professional Education: A Multi-Disciplinary Journal*, **1**(1), 34–48.

Higgs, J. and Titchen, A. (1998) Research and knowledge. *Physiotherapy*, **84**, 72–80.

Higgs, P. (1998 ) Philosophy of education in South Africa: A revision. *Studies in Philosophy and Education*, **17**(1), 1–16.

Jackson, A., Ward, M., Cutcliffe, J., Titchen, A. and Cannon, B. (1999a) Practice development in mental health nursing: Part 2. *Mental Health Practice*, **2**(5), 20–25.

Jackson, A., Cutcliffe, J., Ward, M., Titchen, A. and Cannon, B. (1999b) Practice development in mental health nursing: Part 3. *Mental Health Practice*, **2**(7), 24–30.

Kennedy, M. (1987) Inexact sciences: Professional education and the development of expertise. *Review of Research in Education*, **14**, 133–168.

Kolb, D. A. (1984) *Experiential Learning – Experience as the Source of Learning and Development*. Englewood Cliffs, NJ: Prentice-Hall.

McCormack, B., Kitson, A., Manley, K., Titchen, A. and Harvey, G. (1999) Towards practice development – a vision in reality or a reality without vision? *Journal of Nursing Management*, **7**, 255–264.

Pinkola Estes, C. (1994) *Women Who Run With Wolves: Contacting the Power of the Wild Woman*. London: Rider Books.

Robertson, V. J. (1996) Epistemology, private knowledge, and the *real* problems in physiotherapy. *Physiotherapy*, **82**, 534–539.

Schön, D. (1983) *The Reflective Practitioner: How Professionals Think in Action*. New York: Basic Books.

Scott, D. (1990) Practice wisdom: The neglected source of practice research. *Social Work*, **35**(6), 564–568.

Titchen, A. (2000) *Professional Craft Knowledge in Patient-Centred Nursing and the Facilitation of Its Development.* DPhil thesis, University of Oxford; Oxford: Ashdale Press.

Titchen, A., Dewing, J., McCormack, B. and Manley, K. (1999) *Realising Clinical Effectiveness and Clinical Governance Through Clinical Supervision*. Royal College of Nursing Institute Open Learning Pack. Abingdon, Oxon: Radcliffe Medical Press.

Titchen, A., Butler, J. and Kay, R. Transforming practice. In *Professional Practice in Health, Education and the Creative Arts* (J. Higgs and A. Titchen, eds). Oxford: Blackwell Science (in press).

Ward, M. F., Titchen, A., Morrell, C., McCormack, B. and Kitson, A. (1998) Using a supervisory framework to support and evaluate a multiproject practice development programme. *Journal of Clinical Nursing*, **7**, 29–36.

# Index